Emergency Medicine

Editors

FRED WU
MICHAEL WINTERS

PHYSICIAN ASSISTANT CLINICS

www.physicianassistant.theclinics.com

Consulting Editor
JAMES A. VAN RHEE

July 2017 • Volume 2 • Number 3

ELSEVIER

1600 John F. Kennedy Boulevard • Suite 1800 • Philadelphia, Pennsylvania, 19103-2899

http://www.theclinics.com

PHYSICIAN ASSISTANT CLINICS Volume 2, Number 3
July 2017 ISSN 2405-7991, ISBN-13: 978-0-323-53146-7

Editor: Jessica McCool
Developmental Editor: Casey Potter

Physician Assistant Clinics (ISSN: 2405–7991) is published quarterly by Elsevier Inc., 360 Park Avenue South, New York, NY 10010-1710. Months of issue are January, April, July, and October. Periodicals postage paid at New York, NY and additional mailing offices. Subscription prices are $150.00 per year (US individuals), $205.00 (US institutions), $100.00 (US students), $210.00 (Canadian individuals), $257.00 (Canadian institutions), $100.00 (Canadian students), $150.00 (international individuals), $257.00 (international institutions), and $100.00 (international students). Foreign air speed delivery is included in all *Clinics* subscription prices. All prices are subject to change without notice. POSTMASTER: Send address changes to *Physician Assistant Clinics*, Elsevier Periodicals Customer Service, 11830 Westline Industrial Drive, St. Louis, MO 63146. Customer Service Health Sciences Division, Subscription Customer Service, 3251 Riverport Lane, Maryland Heights, MO 63043. **Customer Service: 1-800-654-2452 (U.S. and Canada); 314-447-8871 (outside U.S. and Canada). Fax: 314-447-8029. E-mail:** journalscustomerservice-usa@elsevier.com **(for print support);** journalsonlinesupport-usa@elsevier.com **(for online support).**

Reprints. For copies of 100 or more, of articles in this publication, please contact the Commercial Reprints Department, Elsevier Inc., 360 Park Avenue South, New York, NY 10010-1710. Tel. 212-633-3874; Fax: 212-633-3820; E-mail: reprints@elsevier.com.

Physician Assistant Clinics is covered in *MEDLINE/PubMed (Index Medicus)* and *EMBASE/Excerpta Medica, Current Contents/Clinical Medicine, and ISI/BIOMED.*

PROGRAM OBJECTIVE
The goal of the Physician Assistant Clinics is to keep practicing physician assistants up to date with current clinical practice by providing timely articles reviewing the state of the art in patient care.

TARGET AUDIENCE
Physician Assistants and other healthcare professionals.

LEARNING OBJECTIVES
Upon completion of this activity, participants will be able to:
1. Review topics in pediatric emergency medicine.
2. Discuss developing topics in drug and antibiotic stewardship in emergency medicine.
3. Recognize best practice in integumentary, orthopedic, and respiratory emergencies, among others.

ACCREDITATION
The Elsevier Office of Continuing Medical Education (EOCME) is accredited by the Accreditation Council for Continuing Medical Education (ACCME) to provide continuing medical education for physicians.

The EOCME designates this enduring material for a maximum of 15 *AMA PRA Category 1 Credit*(s)™. Physicians should claim only the credit commensurate with the extent of their participation in the activity.

All other healthcare professionals requesting continuing education credit for this enduring material will be issued a certificate of participation.

DISCLOSURE OF CONFLICTS OF INTEREST
The EOCME assesses conflict of interest with its instructors, faculty, planners, and other individuals who are in a position to control the content of CME activities. All relevant conflicts of interest that are identified are thoroughly vetted by EOCME for fair balance, scientific objectivity, and patient care recommendations. EOCME is committed to providing its learners with CME activities that promote improvements or quality in healthcare and not a specific proprietary business or a commercial interest.

The planning committee, staff, authors and editors listed below have identified no financial relationships or relationships to products or devices they or their spouse/life partner have with commercial interest related to the content of this CME activity:
Krysta Jade Arnold, BS, MSPAS, PA-C; Karimeh Borghei, MSN, FNP-C, PA-C; Kevin Burns, PA-C; Jeffrey Callard, PA-C, BS; Bartholomew Cambria, PA-C; Bryce Campbell, MPH, PA-C; Amanda P. Coté, MHS, PA-C; Aaron Cronin, DSc, PA-C; Joseph Daniel; Jon Femling, MD, PhD; Anjali Fortna; Jordan Gleason, PA-C; Jed Grant, MPAS, PA-C; Carson R. Harris, MD, FACEP, FAAEM, DABAM; Jamie L. Hodes, MSPAS, PA-C; Casey Jackson; Clint Kalan, MMSc, PA-C; James Kilmark, PA-C, MS; Joshua F. Knox, MA, PA-C; Jessica McCool; Hoodo Mohamed, PA-C, MS; Jonathan D. Monti, DSc, PA-C; Karen A. Newell, MMSc, PA-C, DFAAPA; Lynn Scherer, MS, PA-C; Tanya Schrobilgen, MS, PA-C; Michelle Lynn Seithel, BS, MSPAS, PA-C; Cary J. Stratford, PA-C, DFAAPA; Dennis Tankersley, MS, PA-C; James Van Rhee, MS, PA-C; Ann R. Verhoeven, MMSc, PA-C; Ryan Voccia, MMS, PA-C; Lara West, PA-C; Katie Widmeier; Mary Jo P. Wiemiller, MS, PA-C; Katie Williams; Michael Winters, MD, FACEP, FAAEM; Fred Wu, PA-C, MHS; Kayla Zappolo, MS, PA-C.

UNAPPROVED/OFF-LABEL USE DISCLOSURE
The EOCME requires CME faculty to disclose to the participants:
1. When products or procedures being discussed are off-label, unlabelled, experimental, and/or investigational (not US Food and Drug Administration [FDA] approved); and
2. Any limitations on the information presented, such as data that are preliminary or that represent ongoing research, interim analyses, and/or unsupported opinions. Faculty may discuss information about pharmaceutical agents that is outside of FDA-approved labelling. This information is intended solely for CME and is not intended to promote off-label use of these medications. If you have any questions, contact the medical affairs department of the manufacturer for the most recent prescribing information.

TO ENROLL
The CME program is available to all Physician Assistant Clinics subscribers at no additional fee. To subscribe to the Physician Assistant Clinics, call customer service at 1-800-654-2452 or sign up online at www.physicianassistant.theclinics.com.

METHOD OF PARTICIPATION

In order to claim credit, participants must complete the following:

1. Complete enrolment as indicated above.
2. Read the activity.
3. Complete the CME Test and Evaluation. Participants must achieve a score of 70% on the test. All CME Tests and Evaluations must be completed online.

CME INQUIRIES/SPECIAL NEEDS

For all CME inquiries or special needs, please contact elsevierCME@elsevier.com.

Contributors

CONSULTING EDITOR

JAMES A. VAN RHEE, MS, PA-C
Associate Professor, Program Director, Yale School of Medicine, Yale Physician Assistant
Online Program, New Haven, Connecticut

EDITORS

FRED WU, PA-C, MHS
Program Director, Emergency Medicine PA Residency, University of California San
Francisco-Fresno, Fresno, California

MICHAEL WINTERS, MD, FACEP, FAAEM
Associate Professor of Emergency Medicine and Medicine, University of Maryland School
of Medicine, Program Director, Combined EM/IM Program, Co-Director, Combined
EM/IM/Critical Care Program, University of Maryland Medical Center, Baltimore, Maryland

AUTHORS

KRYSTA JADE ARNOLD, BS, MSPAS, PA-C
Physician Assistant, Emergency Department, University of Missouri Hospitals and Clinics,
Columbia, Missouri

KARIMEH BORGHEI, MSN, FNP-C, PA-C
UC Davis CTSC Clinical Research Center, Sacramento, California

KEVIN BURNS, PA-C
Co-Director, Emergency Medicine PA Residency, Department of Emergency Medicine,
Yale Emergency Medicine, Yale New Haven Hospital, New Haven, Connecticut

JEFFREY CALLARD, PA-C, BS
Lead Administrative PA, Emergency Physicians Medical Group, Director PA/NP Post
Graduate Emergency Medicine Fellowship, Department of Emergency Medicine,
St Joseph Mercy Hospital, Ann Arbor, Michigan

BARTHOLOMEW CAMBRIA, PA-C
Administrative Director, Six Sigma Black Belt, Lead PA, Department of Emergency
Medicine, Northwell Health, Staten Island University Hospital, Staten Island, New York

BRYCE CAMPBELL, MPH, PA-C
PA Resident, Department of Emergency Medicine, Yale Emergency Medicine, Yale New
Haven Hospital, New Haven, Connecticut

AMANDA P. COTÉ, MHS, PA-C
Physician Assistant, Emergency Medicine, Albany Medical Center, Albany, New York

AARON CRONIN, DSc, PA-C
Director of Research, Assistant Professor, US Army/Baylor EMPA Residency Program, Department of Emergency Medicine, Madigan Army Medical Center, Joint Base Lewis McChord, Tacoma, Washington

JON FEMLING, MD, PhD
Department of Emergency Medicine, University of New Mexico School of Medicine, Albuquerque, New Mexico

JORDAN GLEASON, PA-C
PA Resident, Department of Emergency Medicine, Yale Emergency Medicine, Yale New Haven Hospital, New Haven, Connecticut

JED GRANT, MPAS, PA-C
Assistant Professor, PA Program, University of the Pacific, Sacramento, California

CARSON R. HARRIS, MD, FACEP, FAAEM, DABAM
Professor, Department of Emergency Medicine, Consultant, Minnesota Poison Control System, Medical Director, Valhalla Place Addiction and Mental Health Services, University of Minnesota Medical School, Eagan, Minnesota

JAMIE L. HODES, MSPAS, PA-C
Physician Assistant, Emergency Medicine, Albany Medical Center, Albany, New York

CLINT KALAN, MMSc, PA-C
Department of Emergency Medicine, University of New Mexico School of Medicine, Albuquerque, New Mexico

JAMES KILMARK, PA-C, MS
Lead Clinical PA, Emergency Physicians Medical Group, Lead PA, PA/NP Collaborative Team, Department of Emergency Medicine, St Joseph Mercy Hospital, Ann Arbor, Michigan

JOSHUA F. KNOX, MA, PA-C
Clinical Associate Professor, Physician Assistant Studies, Marquette University, Milwaukee, Wisconsin

HOODO MOHAMED, PA-C, MS
Department of Emergency Medicine, St Joseph Mercy Hospital, Ann Arbor, Michigan; Director, St Joseph Mercy Saline Urgent Care, Saline, Michigan

JONATHAN D. MONTI, DSc, PA-C
Director, Assistant Professor, US Army/Baylor EMPA Residency Program, Department of Emergency Medicine, Madigan Army Medical Center, Joint Base Lewis McChord, Tacoma, Washington

KAREN A. NEWELL, MMSc, PA-C, DFAAPA
Assistant Professor, Director of Didactic Education, PA Program, Emory University School of Medicine, Atlanta, Georgia

LYNN SCHERER, MS, PA-C
Associate Director of APC Services; Program Director EMPA Residency, Department of Emergency Medicine, Albert Einstein Healthcare Network, Philadelphia, Pennsylvania

TANYA SCHROBILGEN, MS, PA-C
Associate Program Director, EMPA Fellowship, Arrowhead Regional Medical Center, Colton, California

MICHELLE LYNN SEITHEL, BS, MSPAS, PA-C
Physician Assistant, Emergency Department, University of Missouri Hospitals and Clinics, Columbia, Missouri

CARY J. STRATFORD, PA-C, DFAAPA
Emergency Services of New England Inc, Springfield, Vermont

DENNIS TANKERSLEY, MS, PA-C
Program Director, EMPA Fellowship, Lead PA, Department of Emergency Medicine, Arrowhead Regional Medical Center, Colton, California

ANN R. VERHOEVEN, MMSc, PA-C
Director, Emergency Medicine Physician Assistant Residency Program, Emergency Medicine Department, Regions Hospital, Saint Paul, Minnesota

RYAN VOCCIA, MMS, PA-C
Physician Assistant, Emergency Medicine, Albany Medical Center, Albany, New York

LARA WEST, PA-C
Director of Postgraduate PA Education, Department of Emergency Medicine, Northwell Health, Staten Island University Hospital, Staten Island, New York

MARY JO P. WIEMILLER, MS, PA-C
Clinical Associate Professor, Physician Assistant Studies, Marquette University, Milwaukee, Wisconsin

KAYLA ZAPPOLO, MS, PA-C
Physician Assistant, Department of Emergency Medicine, Albert Einstein Healthcare Network, Philadelphia, Pennsylvania

Contents

> Anaphylaxis is a serious, rapidly developing allergic reaction that, if untreated, may result in death. Signs and symptoms may affect multiple body systems; mortality most frequently results from compromise of the airway and the respiratory system or from hemodynamic collapse. Epinephrine is the primary treatment of anaphylaxis, and should be used early in the management of any patient with concern for a life-threatening allergic reaction. Supportive therapy also may be provided. Patients discharged after treatment of anaphylaxis should receive education on the condition and should be discharged with an epinephrine auto-injector to treat future anaphylactic reactions.

> Back pain is ubiquitous and a common presenting symptom to the emergency department that is often triaged as a low-acuity complaint. Most back pain is mechanical and self-limited. However, back pain can be the sole or major complaint of serious underlying etiologies. A careful history and physical examination is critical in assessing for a potential emergency. Aortic dissection, aortic aneurysm, spinal and paraspinal infections, and cauda equina syndrome require a high index of suspicion. Key features from the history and physical examination should guide appropriate workup using proper imaging and laboratory studies.

> This article discusses 4 potentially lethal rashes and their management: staphylococcal toxic shock syndrome (TSS), meningococcemia, erythema multiforme (EM), and toxic epidermal necrolysis. A staphylococcal TSS rash may be confused with sunburn or flush associated with the fever; desquamation occurs in late stages. Meningococcemia is caused by an aerobic gram-negative diplococcus. The rash is present on the mucosa, palms, and soles. EM is an inflammatory skin eruption characterized by target lesions. Mucosa may or may not be involved. Toxic epidermal necrolysis is caused by antiepileptics and antibiotics. Diagnosis is usually made clinically with the presence of Nikolsky sign.

Abdominal pain, pelvic pain, and vaginal bleeding are common symptoms in emergency departments. It is essential in the care of these patients to assume that everyone is pregnant until proved otherwise. The general approach to patients with abdominal/pelvic pain and/or vaginal bleeding should be similar regardless of pregnancy status, first addressing the patient's airway, breathing, and circulation before proceeding with a more in-depth evaluation. It is important in the evaluation of all pregnant patients to rule out life-threatening diagnoses first, and stay cognizant that pregnant patients may have symptoms that are secondary to a non–pregnancy-related diagnosis.

A careful history and physical examination should be completed on all patients presenting with fever. Children who have fever without a source or concerning physical examination findings should undergo diagnostic evaluation. Clinical decision tools can be used to further risk stratify febrile children. Children over 28 days who appear well and meet low risk criteria can be discharged home with close outpatient follow-up. Admission and appropriate antibiotic therapy should be initiated for any child who is under 28 day old or who appears ill, is unable to maintain hydration, or does not have appropriate follow-up.

Skin and soft tissue infections are an incredibly common and sometimes life-threatening presentation to the emergency department. These can be classified as either purulent or nonpurulent infections, each with their own etiologies. Appropriate antimicrobials for nonpurulent infections and prompt incision and drainage of purulent infections are the mainstays of treatment. Necrotizing skin and soft tissue infections are an incredibly dangerous form of purulent and nonpurulent infections that necessitate early surgical intervention.

Whether treating traumatic lacerations or burns, understanding the factors that affect patient healing is key to providing good patient care. Type, location, and tissue type involvement are only a portion of what physician assistants must consider in managing wounds. Patient comorbidities, socioeconomic factors, and access to care must also be kept in mind. Taking all of the elements discussed in this article into account when determining the best methods for wound care/repair and specialist involvement is the only way to ensure the best chances of success for the patients.

Poisoning is currently the leading cause of injury-related death in the United States. Drugs, both pharmaceutical and illicit, cause most poisoning deaths. The top 5 substance categories causing fatalities are sedative/hypnotics/antipsychotics, cardiovascular drugs, opioids/acetaminophen in combination, stimulants and street drugs, and alcohols. There were an estimated 1.1 million emergency department visits for drug poisoning annually between 2008 and 2011. This article reviews the critical management principles of acute toxic drug ingestions for emergency medicine physician assistants, focusing on the importance of toxidrome recognition. Included is a list of substances that can cause death in toddlers with a single dose.

Although there are clear guidelines for the treatment of patients with end-organ damage (hypertensive crisis), there is little evidence to guide the evaluation of asymptomatic patients with elevated blood pressure in the ED. A reasonable approach is to attempt to ascertain the baseline blood pressure, determine if there is a high probability of occult end-organ damage, avoid nonbeneficial diagnostic studies, reduce further risk to patients by initiating conservative treatment in the ED, and allow the primary care provider to bring patients to the goal blood pressure. Generally acute treatment is not indicated and may possibly be harmful.

Orthopedic-related injuries and illnesses, a leading cause of emergency department (ED) malpractice claims and dollars paid, are commonplace in the ED. Prompt and accurate recognition of conditions requiring specialty intervention remains a vital emergency clinician skill. This article provides emergency clinicians a cognitive framework of how to best approach the evaluation of potential orthopedic emergencie and briefly reviews several critical orthopedic emergencies encountered in the ED.

Emergency department providers routinely prescribe antibiotics to treat common and life-threatening infections. Whenever antibiotics are used, biologic pressure is placed on bacteria, promoting resistance. Excessive antibiotic use facilitates the emergence, persistence, and transmission of antibiotic-resistant bacteria and increases health care costs. Contemporary research demonstrates that antibiotics are frequently overprescribed in ambulatory settings, including the emergency department. Responsible antibiotic use, known as antimicrobial stewardship, includes the appropriate use of antimicrobials to improve patient outcomes, reduce microbial resistance, and decrease the spread of multidrug-resistant infections.

Treatment guidelines for appropriate use of antibiotics in the emergency setting are described in this review.

Karen A. Newell

Headache is an extremely common complaint in the acute care setting. Given that the cause of headache is very broad, it is vital that the clinician be able to recognize and initiate emergent management of the life-threatening causes. The history and presenting signs and symptoms are key elements in the identification of life-threatening causes for adult headache. This article reviews the risk factors associated, clinical presentation, diagnostic work-up, and initial management of subarachnoid hemorrhage, cerebral venous sinus thrombosis/cerebral venous thrombosis, giant cell arteritis/temporal arteritis, and meningitis/encephalitis.

Jeffrey Callard, James Kilmark, and Hoodo Mohamed

Eye complaints account for approximately 2% of emergency department (ED) visits in the United States annually. The history and physical examination are essential portions of the evaluation of these complaints. There are several tools to assist the emergency provider in the diagnosis and evaluation of eye problems, including the slit lamp, ophthalmoscope, tonometry, and ocular ultrasound. In this article, the authors cover the common ED presentations for ocular emergencies. Specifically, the article focuses on the historical and physical examination findings that will help readers to recognize the red flags in eye and vision complaints.

Amanda P. Coté, Jamie L. Hodes, and Ryan Voccia

Chest pain is a common chief complaint in the emergency department and is associated with several serious diagnoses. Because of its potential morbidity and mortality, many patients have admissions and work-ups that are not necessary. Determining which patients are at low risk for major adverse cardiac events could benefit both patients and the health care system. The History, Electrocardiogram, Age, Risk Factors, Troponin (HEART) pathway is a recently developed scoring system that has shown promise in determining which patients may be safely discharged with outpatient follow-up.

PHYSICIAN ASSISTANT CLINICS

RELATED INTEREST

Medical Clinics of North America
May 2017 (Vol. 101, Issue 3)
Emergencies in the Outpatient Setting
Joseph F. Szot, *Editor*

THE CLINICS ARE AVAILABLE ONLINE!
Access your subscription at:
www.theclinics.com

PHYSICIAN ASSISTANT CLINICS

FORTHCOMING ISSUES

October 2017
Cardiology
Daniel Thibodeau, Editor

January 2018
Urology
Todd J. Doran, Editor

April 2018
Ocean Audiology
Laura A. Kirk, Editor

RECENT ISSUES

April 2017
Infectious Disease
Robert A. Paxton, Editor

January 2017
Endocrinology
Ellen D. Mandel (D.B.), Editor

October 2016
Pediatrics
Kristyn Lowery, Brian Wingrove, and
Genevieve A.N. DelRosario, Editors

RELATED INTEREST

Medical Clinics of North America
May 2017 (Vol. 101, Issue 3)
Emergencies in the Outpatient Setting
Joseph H. Stahl, Editor

THE CLINICS ARE AVAILABLE ONLINE!
Access your subscription at:
www.theclinics.com

Foreword

Emergency Medicine

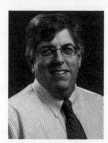

James A. Van Rhee, MS, PA-C
Consulting Editor

I was all ready to submit my foreword for this issue when I heard the sad news that one of the first PAs I worked with, the one who mentored me in my first hospitalist job, had passed away. I am sure only a few of you knew him. He was never a leader in PA education, never on faculty, nor served as a program director. He never held national or state office. I didn't think there are any articles in any journal with his name attached. He never was outspoken about an issue troubling PAs. He is what I would call the everyperson PA, a PA who day in and day out provided care to patient after patient, never looking for glory, just wanting to provide relief for people suffering.

He graduated in the early 1970s and often told the story of going to office after office to find his first job; back then there were not three to five jobs for every PA. He spent most of his interviews explaining what a PA was. When I met him for the first time, he had been a PA for years, and he mentored me in my job as a hospitalist PA and in oncology. He taught me the hospital system, clinical procedures, how to work with a wide variety of attending physicians, but most importantly, he taught me the things they never teach you in PA school. The little things. The things that make a difference in a patient's care.

We all have a person like this early in our career, or at least I hope everyone does. The person who helps us grow. He allowed me become a preceptor of PA students in the hospital we worked. This was my first foray into education, and I caught the education bug. I have gone on to educate hundreds of students, and I hope that I have been able to pass on to the students a few of the things he passed on to me.

So I say farewell and goodbye to my friend and colleague, Drew Robinson, PA-C. Drew, you will be missed. I hope that every newly graduating physician assistant gets a chance to work and learn from someone like you.

In this issue we are focusing on emergency medicine. Fred Wu and Dr Michael Winters have put together another excellent issue. All of the topics are pertinent not only to those in emergency medicine but also to those in all other areas of medicine as well. If

Physician Assist Clin 2 (2017) xv–xvi
http://dx.doi.org/10.1016/j.cpha.2017.04.002
2405-7991/17/© 2017 Elsevier Inc. All rights reserved.

you are in orthopedics, Stratford provides an excellent review of Back Pain Emergencies, and Monti and Cronin cover Orthopedics Pearls and Pitfalls. Burns, Campbell, and Gleason cover Anaphylaxis, Cambria and West look at Lethal Rashes, an article you don't want to miss- Kalan and Femling review Skin and Soft Tissue Infections, and to finish the area of dermatology, Tankersley and Schrobilgen look at the Pitfalls of Wound Management. Looking for a review of Deadly Drug Ingestions? Then the article by Verhoeven and Harris has you covered. Headache Mistakes You Don't Want to Make: Easily Missed Diagnoses by Newell and Ocular Emergencies by Callard, Kilmark, and Mohomad are excellent reviews of these two important areas. Scherer and Zappolo cover Pregnancy Disasters in the First Trimester. And, there is more; as you can see, this issue has something for everyone.

I hope you enjoy the seventh issue of *Physician Assistant Clinics*. Our next issue will provide you with a review of the latest in cardiology.

James A. Van Rhee, MS, PA-C
Program Director, Yale School of Medicine
Yale Physician Assistant Program
100 Church Street South, Suite A250
New Haven, CT 06519, USA

E-mail address:
james.vanrhee@yale.edu

Website:
http://www.paonline.yale.edu

Preface

High-Risk Emergency Medicine

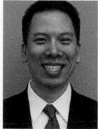 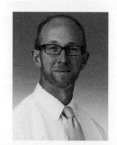

Fred Wu, PA-C, MHS   Michael Winters, MD, FACEP, FAAEM
Editors

In 1960, four Navy corpsmen returned from their military service and enrolled in the first physician assistant (PA) training program at Duke University. Since the time of these initial graduates, PAs have become an integral component to the health care system. In fact, there are currently more than 108,000 certified PAs, a 35% increase from just 5 years ago. Most certainly, this number will continue to increase, as PA graduates expand their roles in numerous areas of medicine. Emergency medicine is the third most popular specialty for PAs, with more than 11,000 PAs practicing in academic and community emergency departments, freestanding emergency departments, and urgent care centers. Within the emergency department, PAs can manage acute care patients, fast-track patients, and patients placed under observation in collaboration with their physician colleagues.

The evaluation and management of the emergency department patient can be complex and challenging. Patients often present during the critical early hours of illness, when signs and symptoms of serious disease can be subtle and easily overlooked. It is during these times when lives can be saved, or lost. It is during these times when the stakes are high for both the patient and the provider. In this issue of *Physician Assistant Clinics*, we have focused on high-risk complaints that are seen daily in emergency departments across the country. These high-risk complaints include headache, pediatric fever, skin and soft tissue infections, chest pain, back pain, first-trimester bleeding, and anaphylaxis. For the topics contained in this issue, we provide a current, evidence-based review with attention to conditions that are high risk for poor patient outcome and high medicolegal risk for PAs. With this information, we feel strongly that the practicing PA can provide efficient, high-quality care to the emergency department patient.

Authors were selected for this issue based on their expertise and reputation as outstanding PA educators. These authors represent a diverse group of emergency medicine PAs from both community and academic acute care settings. The pearls

Physician Assist Clin 2 (2017) xvii–xviii
http://dx.doi.org/10.1016/j.cpha.2017.04.001
2405-7991/17/© 2017 Elsevier Inc. All rights reserved.

and pitfalls discussed by these authors are truly invaluable, and we sincerely thank them for their contributions. Undoubtedly, this text will save lives!

Importantly, we would like to thank the PAs who we have the privilege of working alongside at our respective institutions. You are inspirational and provide us with the motivation to improve our own clinical practice. Finally, we would also like to thank our families for providing us with the opportunity to work on such an important contribution to the emergency medicine PA literature. Your love and support mean the world to us.

Fred Wu, PA-C, MHS
Emergency Medicine PA Residency
University of California San Francisco – Fresno
155 North Fresno Street
Fresno, CA 93701, USA

Michael Winters, MD, FACEP, FAAEM
University of Maryland School of Medicine
University of Maryland Medical Center
110 South Paca Street
6th Floor, Suite 200
Baltimore, MD 21201, USA

E-mail addresses:
fwu@fresno.ucsf.edu (F. Wu)
mwinters@em.umaryland.edu (M. Winters)

Anaphylaxis

Kevin Burns, PA-C[a],*, Bryce Campbell, MPH, PA-C[b],
Jordan Gleason, PA-C[b]

KEYWORDS

- Anaphylaxis • Epinephrine • Steroid • Allergy

KEY POINTS

- Anaphylaxis is a serious, rapidly developing allergic reaction that may result in death if untreated.
- Anaphylaxis may affect a variety of organ systems, with mortality most associated with compromise of the airway, breathing, or circulatory status.
- The mainstay of treatment for anaphylaxis is epinephrine. Any patient with clinical signs of anaphylaxis should receive intramuscular epinephrine, with consideration for intravenous epinephrine in cases of hemodynamic collapse.
- Adjunctive therapies to epinephrine in the treatment of anaphylaxis include steroids, antihistamines, inhaled bronchodilators, and intravenous fluids. Although beneficial, they do not supplant epinephrine as definitive management.
- Patients who are stable for discharge from the emergency department should receive education about their condition, and should be discharged with an epinephrine autoinjector for use in future anaphylactic reactions.

INTRODUCTION

The term "anaphylaxis" was first introduced into the medical lexicon in 1902 by the French physiologist Charles Richet.[1] Richet, along with colleague Paul Portier, presented the term during a lecture to the Societé de Biologie in Paris regarding their discovery of what is now known as anaphylaxis.[2] Richet and Portier exposed dogs to a small dose of sea anemone toxin in an attempt to allow the dog to develop an immunity to the substance. The initial exposure caused little significant reaction; however, after a second exposure of the same dosage several days later, the animals developed wheezing, bloody vomitus, and died within 25 minutes. The term "anaphylaxis" was

Disclosure Statement: The authors have nothing to disclose.
[a] Emergency Medicine PA Residency, Department of Emergency Medicine, Yale Emergency Medicine, Yale New Haven Hospital, 464 Congress Avenue, Suite 260, New Haven, CT 06519, USA; [b] Department of Emergency Medicine, Yale Emergency Medicine, Yale New Haven Hospital, 464 Congress Avenue, Suite 260, New Haven, CT 06519, USA
* Corresponding author.
E-mail address: Kevin.burns@yale.edu

Physician Assist Clin 2 (2017) 345–356
http://dx.doi.org/10.1016/j.cpha.2017.02.002
physicianassistant.theclinics.com

coined, meaning "lack of protection."[2] For his work on the topic of anaphylaxis, Charles Richet was awarded the 1913 Nobel Prize in Physiology or Medicine.

Anaphylaxis has been defined as a serious allergic reaction that is rapid in onset and may cause death.[3] The World Allergy Organization (WAO) has established more formal clinical criteria for the diagnosis of anaphylaxis (Boxes 1 and 2) that describe anaphylaxis as being likely if a patient meets at least one of a combination of several different clinical complaints.[4] Although comprehensive, the WAO criteria involve multiple components that may be challenging to recall at the bedside. Some emergency medicine providers have proposed more straightforward criteria: any allergic reaction that may compromise the airway, breathing, or circulation should be treated as an anaphylactic reaction.[5]

Anaphylaxis is typically the result of an immunologic response to a foreign substance. Most commonly this is the result of an immunoglobulin E (IgE)-dependent response, but depending on the triggering agent, may be caused by a host of other mechanisms (Fig. 1). Initial exposure to the offending agent results in the binding of IgE to receptors on the mast cells and basophils. After a second exposure, antigen binds with the IgE to activate mast cells and basophils, causing the release of a variety of chemical mediators throughout the body. Mediators such as histamine, tryptase, leukotrienes, prostaglandins, cytokines, and platelet-activating factor flood the systemic circulation.[6] These chemicals induce bronchoconstriction, vasodilation, and

---

Box 1
World Allergy Organization clinical criteria for diagnosis of anaphylaxis

Anaphylaxis is highly likely when any 1 of the following 3 criteria is fulfilled:

1. Acute onset of an illness (minutes to several hours) with involvement of the skin, mucosal tissue, or both (eg, generalized urticaria, itching or flushing, swollen lips-tongue-uvula)
   AND AT LEAST 1 OF THE FOLLOWING:
   a. Respiratory compromise (eg, dyspnea, wheeze-bronchospasm, stridor, reduced peak expiratory flow [PEF], hypoxemia)
   b. Reduced blood pressure or associated symptoms of end-organ dysfunction (eg, hypotonia [collapse], syncope, incontinence)
   OR

2. Two or more of the following that occur rapidly after exposure to a likely allergen for that patient (minutes to several hours)
   a. Involvement of the skin-mucosal tissue (eg, generalized urticaria, itch-flush, swollen lips-tongue-uvula)
   b. Respiratory compromise (eg, dyspnea, wheeze-bronchospasm, stridor, reduced PEF, hypoxemia)
   c. Reduced blood pressure or associated symptoms (eg, hypotonia [collapse], syncope, incontinence)
   d. Persistent gastrointestinal symptoms (eg, crampy abdominal pain, vomiting)
   OR

3. Reduced blood pressure after exposure to known allergen for that patient (minutes to several hours)
   a. Infants and children: low systolic blood pressure (age-specific) or greater than 30% decrease in systolic blood pressure
   b. Adults: systolic blood pressure of less than 90 mm Hg or greater than 30% decrease from that person's baseline

Data from Simons FE, Ardusso LR, Dimov V, et al. World allergy organization anaphylaxis guidelines for the assessment and management of anaphylaxis. J Allergy Clin Immunol 2011;127(2):593.e3.

Box 2
Key treatments

- Rapid administration of intramuscular (IM) epinephrine for hypotension, dyspnea, or significant edema of the airway.

- Administer epinephrine with slow intravenous (IV) push if there is imminent airway loss, profound hypotension, or worsening symptoms despite IM epinephrine.

- In addition to IV epinephrine, consider treating supraglottic and laryngeal edema with aerosolized epinephrine while preparing to establish a definitive airway.

- Hypotension should be treated with aggressive fluid resuscitation using a crystalloid solution.

- Corticosteroids and antihistamines (H_1 and H_2) should be used as a supplementary therapy in addition to epinephrine and fluids.

---

increase vascular permeability, resulting in the life-threatening clinical sequelae of an anaphylactic reaction. On rare occasions, anaphylaxis can also be triggered by non-IgE mechanisms, such as IgG, the complement system, and nonimmunologic causes that result in direct activation of the mast cells and basophils.

The true prevalence of anaphylaxis in the general population is unknown. Wood and colleagues[7] reported a prevalence in the United States of at least 1.6% to 7.7% across the population surveyed. A review of a European population estimated that 0.3% of the those in Europe experience an episode of anaphylaxis over the course of their lives.[8] There also appears to be a relationship between age and risk of anaphylaxis. Children age 4 years and younger have been found to have rates of anaphylaxis almost 3 times higher than that of other age groups.[9]

Clinical Features

The symptoms and clinical features of anaphylaxis are multisystemic and **Tables 1** and **2** list the frequency of symptoms. Anaphylaxis may occur within seconds, or be delayed more than an hour after an exposure. More rapid reactions are associated with a higher mortality.[10] Anaphylaxis is primarily a clinical diagnosis. History may confirm exposure to a possible allergen, such as a new drug, food, or sting. However, there is no gold standard diagnostic test, and the diagnosis of anaphylaxis should be considered in any rapidly progressing multisystem illness.[11] Early clinical features of anaphylaxis include pruritus of the palms and soles, tingling of the mouth and tongue, generalized warmth, tightness in the chest, and a lump in the throat. Up to 90% of patients have urticaria or angioedema. Urticaria, defined as edema of the upper dermis, appears as raised erythematous wheals in evanescent pruritic patches. Angioedema, which involves the deep dermis, is often described as puffy, nonpitting areas of skin or mucous membrane. Angioedema is generally painless and nonpruritic.[12]

Edema of the larynx can result in upper airway obstruction and is the most common cause of death from anaphylaxis. The onset can be sudden and mimic that of foreign body obstruction or sudden cardiac death. Angioedema of the oropharynx, lips, and tongue is less likely to cause airway obstruction, but should be treated promptly and aggressively, as it may progress to laryngeal edema. Bronchospasm is a common symptom in anaphylaxis, but tends to be less severe unless the patient has a preexisting history of asthma.[12] Other common mucous membrane manifestations seen in anaphylaxis include rhinitis, nasal obstruction, chemosis, and conjunctivitis.[12]

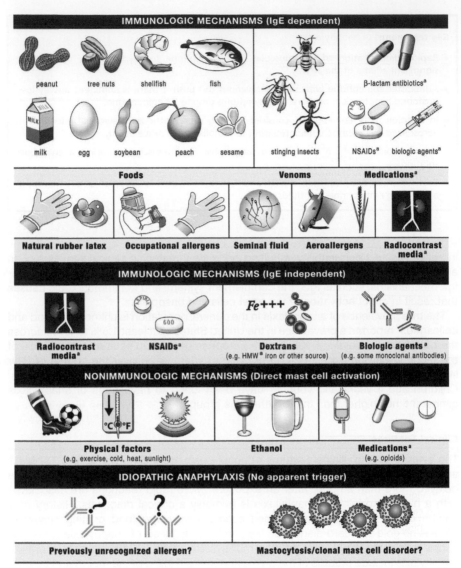

Fig. 1. Causes of anaphylaxis. HMW, high molecular weight; NSAIDs, non-steroidal anti-inflammatory drugs.[a] Trigger anaphylaxis by more than one mechanism. (*Data from* Simons FE, Ardusso LR, Bilò MB, et al. World Allergy Organization anaphylaxis guidelines: summary. J Allergy Clin Immunol 2011;127(2):589; with permission.)

The second most common cause of death after laryngeal edema is refractory hypotension. Defined as a symptomatic drop in systolic blood pressure of 20 to 30 mm Hg, this is typical of anaphylaxis when a patient is initially presenting with dizziness, syncope, or sudden death.[13]

Abdominal pain and cramping are often overlooked symptoms of anaphylaxis. These symptoms are most commonly seen in food-mediated reactions. Angioedema of the gut lining results in nausea, vomiting, diarrhea, and rarely hematochezia.

Table 1
Clinical features of anaphylaxis

Organ System	Signs and Symptoms
Cardiovascular	Hypotension, tachycardia, dizziness, lightheadedness, syncope, confusion, weak pulse, decreased urine output
Dermatologic	Hives, swelling, itching, warmth, redness; angioedema, swelling of the deep dermal layer: lips, eyes, hands, nonpruritic tingling
Gastrointestinal	Abdominal pain, cramping, diarrhea, vomiting
Gynecologic/ Obstetric	Uterine cramping, mucosal edema and erythema, vulvovaginal itching, preterm labor
Neurologic	Irritability, anxiety, somnolence, lethargy, feeling of "impending doom," headache, seizure
Respiratory	Coughing, wheezing, shortness of breath, stridor, chest pain, intercostal/ accessory muscle use, hoarseness, dysphagia, throat tightness (globus), deep dermal swelling of the lips, uvula, tongue, airway obstruction, sudden death
Ocular/Ear nose throat	Lid edema, redness, chemosis, tearing, itching, mucosal swelling, nasal congestion/rhinorrhea, itching

Symptoms of acute coronary syndrome, Takotsubo cardiomyopathy, ventricular tachycardia, and nonspecific ST-T wave changes are reported in anaphylaxis. These symptoms are attributed to decreased perfusion secondary to hypotension, hypoxemia, and iatrogenic epinephrine therapy. It is believed that histamine and cytokines also may induce coronary vasospasm and cardiac dysrhythmias.[14]

A biphasic mediator release can occur in up to 20% of cases, causing recurrence of symptoms hours to days after the initial exposure.[15] This concern for recurrence of

Table 2
Frequency of anaphylaxis signs and symptoms

Signs and Symptoms	Frequency in Anaphylaxis, %
Cutaneous	
Urticaria and angioedema	62–90
Flushing	45–55
Pruritus without rash	2–5
Respiratory	
Dyspnea, wheeze	45–50
Upper airway angioedema	50–60
Rhinitis	15–20
Hypotension, dizziness, syncope, diaphoresis	30–35
Abdominal	
Nausea, vomiting, diarrhea, abdominal pain	25–30
Miscellaneous	
Headache	5–8
Substernal pain	4–5
Seizure	1–2

Data from Lieberman P, Nicklas RA, Oppenheimer J. The diagnosis and management of anaphylaxis practice parameter: 2010 update. J Allergy Clin Immunol 2010;126(3):480.e35; with permission.

symptoms may affect decisions regarding disposition of these patients (see the section "Disposition," later in this article).

MANAGEMENT
Epinephrine

The treatment of anaphylaxis is similar to that of all critically ill patients in the emergency department. There must be a rapid assessment of the patient's overall condition by first evaluating the patient's airway, breathing, and circulation. When the clinical criteria defining anaphylaxis are met, the patient should receive epinephrine immediately.[3] However, the provider's gestalt should never be overlooked, as many patients will present without clearly meeting all the parameters of the WAO definition and should still be treated with epinephrine. Examples include a patient with a history of near-death anaphylaxis to peanuts who ingested peanuts and presents within minutes experiencing urticaria and generalized flushing.[3]

All published guidelines clearly identify epinephrine as the first-line medication for the treatment of anaphylaxis.[16] Epinephrine has potent life-saving alpha-1 adrenergic vasoconstriction effects on the small arterioles in most body organ systems. This vasoconstriction decreases mucosal edema, preventing and reducing upper airway obstruction, and increases blood pressure, preventing and reducing shock. The beta-1 adrenergic effects lead to increased rate and force of cardiac contractions. The beta-2 effects lead to bronchodilation and decreased release of histamine, tryptase, and other mediators of inflammation from mast cells and basophils.[17] The initial dose of epinephrine for anaphylaxis is 0.3 to 0.5 mL (1:1000 dilution) administered as an intramuscular (IM) injection. Children should receive 0.01 mg/kg up to a maximum of 0.3 mL.[18] Epinephrine is best absorbed in large muscle groups, and ideally the vastus lateralis (lateral thigh) should be the primary site used for IM injections.[19] The dose of epinephrine can be repeated every 5 to 15 minutes based on clinical effect.[3]

Hypotension generally responds to IM epinephrine and intravenous fluid resuscitation. However, if hypotension persists, intravenous (IV) epinephrine may be given. The most common error in the treatment of anaphylaxis is too much epinephrine given too quickly, precipitating cardiac dysrhythmias and chest pain.[12] A push dose preparation of epinephrine can be achieved by using 1 mL of 1:10,000 epinephrine diluted in 5 to 10 mL of normal saline and given as a slow IV push over 3 to 5 minutes. If life-threatening symptoms continue, the dose may be repeated. Alternatively, an epinephrine drip can be started by using 1 mL of 1:1000 dilution of epinephrine in 250 mL of 5% dextrose in water, infused at 1 to 10 μg/min (0.014–0.14 μg/kg per minute).[18] It is believed that a continuous infusion of epinephrine may be preferred over intermittent push doses, which have been linked to adverse outcomes. If cardiac arrest ensues during the treatment of anaphylaxis, the aforementioned treatment regimen should be discontinued and advanced cardiac life support algorithms should be followed.[12] Although caution should be exercised with the administration of epinephrine to elderly patients and those with established coronary artery disease, epinephrine should never be withheld from a patient with true anaphylaxis.

Aerosolized epinephrine may be considered in the setting of severe angioedema. Racemic epinephrine 2.25% solution, 0.5 mL in 3.5 mL saline, or epinephrine 1:1000, 5 mL can be administered via nebulizer. This may decrease supraglottic and laryngeal edema while preparations are made for a definitive airway.[12]

Patients with severe allergies or prior anaphylaxis will frequently carry an epinephrine autoinjector (EAI). The development of commercial autoinjectors has allowed patients and families to be able to self-administer the correct dose of IM epinephrine without the medical training needed to draw up and administer a drug using a standard vial and syringe. Autoinjectors are generally available in both pediatric (0.15 mg) and adult (0.3 mg) formulations. In the United States, commonly prescribed brand name EAI's include EpiPen/EpiPen Jr. (Mylan Inc., Canonsburg, PA) and Adrenaclick (Amedra Pharmaceuticals, Horsham, PA). Although primarily used in the community, some have advocated for the use of EAIs within the hospital to limit medication errors. Kanwar and colleagues[20] presented a case series of iatrogenic epinephrine overdoses within their institution. One solution that was proposed was to stock crash carts with EAIs clearly labeled "use only for anaphylaxis" to avoid the inadvertent administration of cardiac arrest dosage epinephrine. Recent research has shown that EAIs are underused in the emergency treatment of anaphylaxis in the community; noninvasive sublingual epinephrine administration is being proposed as an alternative treatment. Studies have shown sublingual administration of epinephrine 40 mg from tablet formulation achieves an epinephrine plasma concentration similar to those obtained after epinephrine 0.3 mg IM.[21] Fast-disintegrating sublingual epinephrine may be a feasible alternative to IM epinephrine that warrants further development.[22]

Often, patients will have received epinephrine in the prehospital setting before initial emergency department evaluation. During the initial emergency department assessment, it is imperative to fully assess the patient for alternative causes of his or her complaints, as well as any adverse reactions to the previously given epinephrine, before the administration of additional anaphylaxis treatments.[12]

Second-Line Medications

Aside from the use of epinephrine in the anaphylactic patient, there are other treatments currently used in the emergency department for management of anaphylaxis. It is important to note that there is limited evidence to support improvement in survivability, morbidity, and mortality with the use of second-line medications. Depending on the patient's symptoms, treatment modalities include antihistamines, β (beta)-2 agonists, supplemental oxygen, and glucocorticoids. None of these treatments should ever be considered curative or sufficient in the treatment of the anaphylactic patient without concomitant use of epinephrine.

Patients in early anaphylaxis may present with cutaneous symptoms of flushing, urticaria, pruritus, or nonspecific rashes. In these patients, an H_1 antihistamine medication, such as diphenhydramine at a dose 50 mg (1–2 mg/kg for pediatric patients), may be given as a slow IV push. If IV or intraosseous access is not readily available, IM or oral medications (of identical doses) may be given as well, with an expected slower onset of effect.[23] Lin and colleagues[24] demonstrated that the addition of an H_2 antihistamine, such as ranitidine or cimetidine, will improve the urticaria and heart rate at 2 hours post administration when compared with diphenhydramine alone. This study specifically used ranitidine 50 mg IV in the test group, but by theory of extrapolation and class-effect, other H_2 antihistamine may provide similar results. There was no significant difference between the test and control groups in comparing angioedema, erythema, blood pressures, and other varied symptoms.[25]

Patients who are experiencing wheezing or bronchospasm that are refractory to the initial IM epinephrine dose, or are continuing to have difficulty with oxygenation, may benefit from a more selective β-2 adrenergic medication,[23] such as albuterol, levalbuterol, or terbutaline. Nebulized albuterol at 2.5 mg is a reasonable initial dosage. Persistent bronchospasm may require additional doses, including the potential use of continuous nebulized albuterol at 15 to 20 mg/h.

Glucocorticoid medications, such as hydrocortisone, methylprednisolone, and dexamethasone, have not been proven to be effective in the acute phase of anaphylaxis due to their delayed onset of action. This class of medications may play a role in the "protracted" or "biphasic" immune response that sometimes occurs in anaphylactic patients. There is no current literature to support the efficacy of a short-term "burst" (3–5 days) of glucocorticoids in comparison with a single dose. Therefore, it is currently recommended to give only 1 dose at the onset of symptoms.[16,25,26] There have been no studies to date looking at the efficacy of hydrocortisone compared with dexamethasone or any other combination of glucocorticoids in anaphylaxis.[26]

Intravenous Fluids

Anaphylaxis, if untreated, may progress to anaphylactic shock (a subset of distributive shock). In these instances, treatments must be aggressive and specific to the patient's clinical condition. Unless otherwise contraindicated, patients with anaphylaxis should be given crystalloid boluses. This is especially important for patients with hypotension (Table 3). Normal saline is typically the intravenous fluid of choice and tends to remain in the intravascular space longer than dextrose-containing fluids. If the patient is fluid responsive, then he or she may benefit from continued administration of crystalloids, as long there is no contraindication to such (eg, depressed ejection fraction, end-stage renal disease).[23]

Vasopressors

For the patients who are not fluid responsive, or who may need some restriction in volume-expansion treatments, other vasoactive medications may be implemented in addition to epinephrine. Dopamine, norepinephrine, and vasopressin all may be considered as adjunctive therapies for the hypotensive patient. Methylene blue limits vasodilation through the inhibition of nitric oxide cyclic guanosine monophosphate, and also may be considered as an alternative for the patient with refractory hypotension.[27]

In the subset of patients who are prescribed β-adrenergic antagonists, there have been multiple case studies reporting increased bronchospasm and refractoriness to initial doses of epinephrine. These patients may require multiple IM doses of epinephrine, as well as an epinephrine IV infusion. Although being on a β-blocker does not increase one's risk of developing anaphylaxis, it is important to recognize if the patient is taking these medications, as glucagon at a dose of 1 to 5 mg may need to be administered IM. If it is not, the epinephrine may work only at the α receptors, causing a reflexive vagal response, ultimately worsening the hypotension.[23,28–35]

Patients who have failed all standard interventions and who are approaching complete vascular collapse also may be considered as candidates for extracorporeal

Table 3 Hypotension definitions in anaphylaxis	
Age	Systolic Blood Pressure, mm Hg
Term neonates, 0–28 d	<60
Infants, 1–12 mo	<70
Children, >1–10 y	<70 + (2 × age in y)
Beyond 10 y	<90

Data from Lieberman P, Nicklas RA, Oppenheimer J. The diagnosis and management of anaphylaxis practice parameter: 2010 update. J Allergy Clin Immunol 2010;126(3):480.e35; with permission.

membrane oxygenation, where available, to serve as a bridge until they are able to recover from the initial episode.[27]

DISPOSITION

Discharging a patient who presented with anaphylaxis can occur after an observation period and after the patient's symptoms have resolved. During this period, the patient should be observed for a protracted or biphasic reaction.[15,36] Although these reactions are seemingly rare, occurring less than 0.25% of the time, they have the potential to be fatal.[37] Unfortunately, the time frame for this reaction to occur has been documented to be anywhere from 5 minutes up to 4 days after the initial response.[38] Because observation of all patients with anaphylaxis for up to 4 days is clinically impractical, current practice guidelines suggest time frames of 4 to 8 hours, depending on the patient's history.[36] Grunau and colleagues[37] demonstrated a 0.18% rate of clinically important biphasic reactions, 2 of which were patients who failed to meet criteria for anaphylaxis on their initial emergency department visits. Given the relative rarity and unpredictable time frame of the biphasic reaction, and the capacity for the patient to self-medicate at home with EAIs, there may be some support for shorter observation periods than what are currently recommended.

Risk factors of having a protracted or biphasic response include severe asthma and previous protracted or biphasic responses. Unfortunately, these risk factors are not a fail-safe system either. Previous severity of reactions is not a predictor of future reactions; patients who have had mild reactions in the past are not immune to having anaphylactic responses next time with a biphasic pattern.[36] Other medical comorbidities, such as chronic pulmonary or cardiac disease, and higher-risk patient populations (poor outpatient follow-up or unreliable patient subsets), also should warrant a prolonged observation period.

Before the patient leaves the department, he or she must be well educated on the myriad of symptoms that can comprise an anaphylactic reaction, how to properly administer an EAI, how to call an emergency medical system provider, and when to follow up with an allergist-immunologist. He or she also must be discharged with a prescription for at least 2 EAI devices: one to carry on his or her person at all times, and one to have at home/school/work or any other area in which it may be needed on a regular basis.[36] Surprisingly, these recommendations are not well followed, with large discrepancies in practice styles, ranging from no EAI pen prescriptions, to education of how they work, or not getting proper follow-up for patients who are able to be discharged from the department on the same day.[39]

Admission to the hospital should be considered with any patient who has a history of severe anaphylaxis (requiring previous intensive care unit admission, intubation, central venous access with vasopressor medications), has ingested a potential allergen, has required more than 1 dose of epinephrine, has had progression of symptoms despite treatment, or has any laryngeal edema. Other patients who may be considered for admission are those who would likely need, and not be able to get, close follow-up with an allergist-immunologist. These patients may have new allergens that have not been identified, difficult to manage in the emergency department, or may have difficulty adhering to an outpatient treatment regimen.[36]

SUMMARY

Anaphylaxis is a rapidly progressing, life-threatening disease state that requires early recognition, appropriate treatment, and close monitoring. Because of its high degree of variance in presentation, it is imperative to consider anaphylaxis in the differential diagnosis of a multitude of presenting chief complaints. The mainstay of treatment for anaphylaxis is epinephrine; this is typically given as an IM injection in the anterolateral thigh. For patients in extremis, epinephrine also may be administered via the IV or intraosseous route. Adjunctive therapies, such as antihistamines, IV fluids, and steroids, also may be given, but should never replace epinephrine as the treatment for anaphylaxis. All patients who are treated for anaphylaxis in the emergency department should receive EAIs at the time of discharge to allow for self-administration of epinephrine in the event of future anaphylactic episodes.

REFERENCES

1. Portier P, Richet C. The anaphylactic effect of certain venoms. Comptes Rendus Des Seances De La Societe De Biologie Et De Ses Filiales 1902;54:170–2.
2. Ring J, Grosber M, Brockow K, et al. Anaphylaxis. Chem Immunol Allergy 2014; 100:54–61.
3. Sampson HA, Munoz-Furlong A, Campbell RL, et al. Second symposium on the definition and management of anaphylaxis: summary report–Second National Institute of Allergy and Infectious Disease/Food Allergy and Anaphylaxis Network symposium. J Allergy Clin Immunol 2006;117(2):391–7.
4. Simons FE, Ardusso LR, Bilo MB, et al. World Allergy Organization guidelines for the assessment and management of anaphylaxis. World Allergy Organ J 2011; 4(2):13–37.
5. Strayer R. Strayerisms: anaphylaxis rebuttal. [Internet]. Podcast. 2016. Available at: www.emrap.org.
6. Simons FE. Anaphylaxis. J Allergy Clin Immunol 2010;125(2 Suppl 2):S161–81.
7. Wood RA, Camargo CA Jr, Lieberman P, et al. Anaphylaxis in America: the prevalence and characteristics of anaphylaxis in the United States. J Allergy Clin Immunol 2014;133(2):461–7.
8. Panesar SS, Javad S, de Silva D, et al. The epidemiology of anaphylaxis in Europe: a systematic review. Allergy 2013;68(11):1353–61.
9. Tejedor Alonso MA, Moro Moro M, Mugica Garcia MV. Epidemiology of anaphylaxis. Clin Exp Allergy 2015;45(6):1027–39.
10. Tintinalli JE, Cline D, American College of Emergency Physicians. Tintinalli's emergency medicine manual. 7th edition. New York: McGraw-Hill Medical; 2012.
11. Stone CK, Humphries RL. Current diagnosis & treatment emergency medicine. 6th edition. New York: McGraw-Hill; 2008.
12. Wolfson AB, Hendey GW, Harwood-Nuss A. Harwood-Nuss' clinical practice of emergency medicine. 6th edition. Philadelphia: Lippincott Williams & Wilkins; 2016.
13. Peavy RD, Metcalfe DD. Understanding the mechanisms of anaphylaxis. Curr Opin Allergy Clin Immunol 2008;8(4):310–5.
14. Khoueiry G, Abi Rafeh N, Azab B, et al. Reverse Takotsubo cardiomyopathy in the setting of anaphylaxis treated with high-dose intravenous epinephrine. J Emerg Med 2013;44(1):96–9.
15. Tole JW, Lieberman P. Biphasic anaphylaxis: review of incidence, clinical predictors, and observation recommendations. Immunol Allergy Clin N Am 2007;27(2): 309–26, viii.
16. Irani AM, Akl EG. Management and prevention of anaphylaxis. F1000Res 2015;4.
17. Goodman LS, Gilman A, Brunton LL, et al. Goodman & Gilman's the pharmacological basis of therapeutics. 11th edition. New York: McGraw-Hill; 2006.

18. Lieberman P, Nicklas RA, Oppenheimer J, et al. The diagnosis and management of anaphylaxis practice parameter: 2010 update. J Allergy Clin Immunol 2010; 126(3):477–80.e1-42.
19. Simons FE, Gu X, Simons KJ. Epinephrine absorption in adults: intramuscular versus subcutaneous injection. J Allergy Clin Immunol 2001;108(5):871–3.
20. Kanwar M, Irvin CB, Frank JJ, et al. Confusion about epinephrine dosing leading to iatrogenic overdose: a life-threatening problem with a potential solution. Ann Emerg Med 2010;55(4):341–4.
21. Rawas-Qalaji MM, Simons FE, Simons KJ. Sublingual epinephrine tablets versus intramuscular injection of epinephrine: dose equivalence for potential treatment of anaphylaxis. J Allergy Clin Immunol 2006;117(2):398–403.
22. Rawas-Qalaji MM, Simons FE, Simons KJ. Epinephrine for the treatment of anaphylaxis: do all 40 mg sublingual epinephrine tablet formulations with similar in vitro characteristics have the same bioavailability? Biopharm Drug Dispos 2006;27(9):427–35.
23. Joint Task Force on Practice Parameters, American Academy of Allergy, Asthma and Immunology, American College of Allergy, Asthma and Immunology, Joint Council of Allergy, Asthma and Immunology. The diagnosis and management of anaphylaxis: an updated practice parameter. J Allergy Clin Immunol 2005; 115(3 Suppl 2):S483–523.
24. Lin RY, Curry A, Pesola GR, et al. Improved outcomes in patients with acute allergic syndromes who are treated with combined H1 and H2 antagonists. Ann Emerg Med 2000;36(5):462–8.
25. Sheikh A, Ten Broek V, Brown SG, et al. H1-antihistamines for the treatment of anaphylaxis: Cochrane systematic review. Allergy 2007;62(8):830–7.
26. Choo KJ, Simons E, Sheikh A. Glucocorticoids for the treatment of anaphylaxis: Cochrane systematic review. Allergy 2010;65(10):1205–11.
27. Simons FE, Ebisawa M, Sanchez-Borges M, et al. 2015 update of the evidence base: World Allergy Organization anaphylaxis guidelines. World Allergy Organ J 2015;8(1):32.
28. Stark BJ, Sullivan TJ. Biphasic and protracted anaphylaxis. J Allergy Clin Immunol 1986;78(1 Pt 1):76–83.
29. Jacobs RL, Rake GW Jr, Fournier DC, et al. Potentiated anaphylaxis in patients with drug-induced beta-adrenergic blockade. J Allergy Clin Immunol 1981; 68(2):125–7.
30. Newman BR, Schultz LK. Epinephrine-resistant anaphylaxis in a patient taking propranolol hydrochloride. Ann Allergy 1981;47(1):35–7.
31. Awai LE, Mekori YA. Insect sting anaphylaxis and beta-adrenergic blockade: a relative contraindication. Ann Allergy 1984;53(1):48–9.
32. Toogood JH. Beta-blocker therapy and the risk of anaphylaxis. CMAJ 1987; 137(7):587–8, 590–1.
33. Berkelman RL, Finton RJ, Elsea WR. Beta-adrenergic antagonists and fatal anaphylactic reactions to oral penicillin. Ann Intern Med 1986;104(1):134.
34. Hamilton G. Severe adverse reactions to urography in patients taking beta-adrenergic blocking agents. Can Med Assoc J 1985;133(2):122.
35. Zaloga GP, DeLacey W, Holmboe E, et al. Glucagon reversal of hypotension in a case of anaphylactoid shock. Ann Intern Med 1986;105(1):65–6.
36. Lieberman P, Nicklas RA, Randolph C, et al. Anaphylaxis–a practice parameter update 2015. Ann Allergy Asthma Immunol 2015;115(5):341–84.

37. Grunau BE, Li J, Yi TW, et al. Incidence of clinically important biphasic reactions in emergency department patients with allergic reactions or anaphylaxis. Ann Emerg Med 2014;63(6):736–44.e2.
38. Swaminathan A. Biphasic anaphylactic reactions—How long should we observe? 2013. Available at: http://www.emlitofnote.com/2013/12/biphasic-anaphylactic-reactions-how.html. 2016.
39. Russell WS, Farrar JR, Nowak R, et al. Evaluating the management of anaphylaxis in US emergency departments: Guidelines vs. practice. World J Emerg Med 2013;4(2):98–106.

Back Pain Emergencies
Easily Missed Diagnoses

Cary J. Stratford, PA-C*

KEYWORDS

- Back pain • Epidural abscess • Cauda equina syndrome • Aortic dissection
- Abdominal aortic aneurysm

KEY POINTS

- Back pain emergencies are frequently missed on the initial presentation to the emergency department (ED).
- A focused and careful history with attention toward identifying "red flags" is critical.
- The presence of saddle anesthesia should raise suspicion for cauda equina syndrome.
- Many patients with a spinal epidural abscess are afebrile with a normal white blood cell count on initial presentation to the ED.
- A vascular catastrophe should be considered in any patient with the acute onset of maximal intensity back pain.

INTRODUCTION

Back pain is a common presenting complaint to the emergency department (ED). Twenty-five percent of all adults in the United States report 1 day of back pain within the proceeding 3-month period.[1] In 2008, there were 7.3 million visits to EDs for back pain.[2] The overwhelming majority of back pain complaints are owing to mechanical or musculoskeletal etiologies, and require only symptomatic treatment.

With chief complaints that imply urgent conditions, such as chest pain, dyspnea, and abdominal pain, the emergency clinician is focused on potentially serious causes. However, in the case of back pain, the clinician is often initially focused on more benign causes. A further challenge to the physician assistant (PA) is that, in EDs, urgent care centers, and other acute care environments, triage systems often assign back pain as a low-acuity complaint. As such, potentially serious etiologies are directed toward lower acuity locations. These patients are often evaluated later, after complaints such as chest pain, or in the case of scheduled systems, be given a less time-sensitive appointment than another, more worrisome chief complaint. This article

Disclosure Statement: The author has nothing to disclose.
Emergency Services of New England Inc, 25 Ridgewood Road, Springfield, VT 05156, USA
* 25 Ridgewood Road, Springfield, VT 05156.
E-mail address: carystratford@myfairpoint.net

Physician Assist Clin 2 (2017) 357–369
http://dx.doi.org/10.1016/j.cpha.2017.02.013
2405-7991/17/

discusses the "can't miss" etiologies of acute back pain, including cauda equina syndrome (CES), spinal epidural abscess (SEA), and aortic catastrophes.

HISTORY AND PHYSICAL EXAMINATION

The most available and most useful investigative tool for patients with back pain is a detailed history. The presence, or absence, of certain historical features should aid the seasoned clinician in having a heightened concern. These features should also be important and pertinent points for inclusion in the medical record. The greatest tool the PA has is not the magnetic resonance imaging study, but rather the ability to extract a good history that directs one toward the right differential diagnosis, and then in turn the right workup. "Worst first" is a very appropriate way for emergency medicine providers to approach all patients. When formulating a differential diagnosis for acute back pain, it may not be feasible to routinely explore all the possible life-threatening etiologies in all patients. What is needed then is to focus the differential diagnosis on historical features that suggest the possibility of serious disease.

History of Present Illness

It is common for patients to associate any antecedent trauma to the cause of back pain. Patients can elaborate a cause and effect history that can be misleading to the PA. When an injury is assumed to be the cause, the PA's differential diagnosis often rapidly shrinks and excludes more serious causes. As with gastrointestinal complaints, where patients often associate the meal immediately prior, patients with back pain attempt to understand symptoms in relationship to something they must have done right before the onset of pain. They will recall poor positioning or lifting and connect that event to their pain. Patients with back pain are rarely aware that back pain has a number of potentially serious causes. This potential bias can be overcome by asking about the timing of events and obtaining details of the mechanical circumstances. It is important for the PA to ensure that the onset of symptoms fit with timing of the trauma and that the trauma itself is a plausible source for the patient's pain. Although it is very true that musculoskeletal pain may have its onset delayed by hours, the PA should be careful to scrutinize any delays in the onset of pain, because this can be a suggestion of a more serious etiology.

Pain that begins immediately after a particular injury and is reproduced consistently by position or by palpation are reassuring features. However, if parts of the history do not fall into place for a benign cause, the PA should avoid the temptation to trivialize or disregard these details. Patients often do not make associations with fever or neurologic symptoms with their back pain. Thus, it is critical in the evaluation of ED patients with acute back pain to inquire about the presence of "red flags" for more serious conditions.

Red Flags for Back Pain

The Agency for Healthcare Research and Quality practice guidelines identified several historical features that were considered indicators of potential serious underlying pathology.[3] These red flags are listed in Box 1.

The presence of any back pain red flag should raise suspicion for malignancy, fracture, or infection as the cause of back pain. In addition, age over 50 years increases the likelihood of serious disease. In patients with back pain who report sciatica or lower limb pain or weakness, it is important to consider CES. The PA should question the patient on signs and symptoms of CES, which are listed in Box 2.

Box 1
Back pain red flags

- History of cancer
- Unexplained weight loss
- Immunosuppression
- Intravenous drug use
- History of urinary infection
- Pain increased by rest
- Presence of fever

Critically important sources of life-threatening back pain not included in the Agency for Healthcare Research and Quality guidelines are aortic disasters. Catastrophic vascular events, such as a ruptured or leaking abdominal aortic aneurysm (AAA) and aortic dissection, warrant consideration in the differential diagnosis of back pain. In these cases, back pain is often a predominant feature among other clinical signs and symptoms. Consider a vascular catastrophe as the etiology of acute back pain when patients describe the sudden onset of maximal intensity pain or report pain, weakness, or sensory changes in an extremity in association with abrupt back pain.

It is outside the scope of this article to discuss spinal fracture and fracture management. However, when obtaining a history in patients with acute back pain, it is routine to elicit any fall or injury circumstances. Antecedent trauma can be obvious in the case of a motor vehicle collision or occult in case of a spontaneous compression fracture in an elderly patient. It is critical to appreciate the historical features associated with likelihood of spinal fracture, which are listed in **Box 3**.

A final comment on focused history should be made about duration of symptoms. The majority of patients with musculoskeletal back pain will improve within 4 to 6 weeks.[3] Consider infection, occult fracture, or malignancy in patients where back pain has persisted or worsened beyond 4 weeks.

Physical Examination

Specific physical examination components, laboratory studies, and imaging options will be discussed in detail in this article. Regarding physical examination, it is important to perform a detailed neurologic examination, including an assessment of lower extremity strength and sensation, gait, great toe dorsiflexion, saddle anesthesia, and a straight leg raise test. Gait assessment is often omitted from the ED neurologic

---

Box 2
Signs and symptoms of cauda equina syndrome

- Bladder dysfunction (incontinence or more commonly retention)
- Saddle paresthesias
- Weakness of lower legs
- Loss of anal sphincter tone or frank fecal incontinence
- Bilateral sciatica

> **Box 3**
> **Red flags for spinal fracture**
>
> - History of significant trauma (a fall from a height, motor vehicle collision)
> - Direct blow or point source injury to the back for a young adult,
> - Minor fall or heavy lift in a potentially osteoporotic or elderly individual
> - History of prolonged use of steroids
> - Age >70 years

examination, but is an essential component of the evaluation. Great toe dorsiflexion is a quick way to evaluate L5, the most common nerve root seen with nerve root compression. Straight leg raising that reproduces radicular pain pattern is seen in herniated disc disease and contralateral positive straight leg raising (elevating 1 leg causing radicular symptoms down the other leg) is even more specific. A rectal examination should be done in patients reporting bowel or bladder incontinence.

In addition to a focused neurologic examination, it is also important to perform and document an abdominal examination, vascular examination with attention to peripheral pulses, and an examination of the back. Examination of the back should include inspection and palpation for the presence of midline tenderness, paraspinal tenderness, or costovertebral angle tenderness.

CAUDA EQUINA SYNDROME

CES refers to a characteristic pattern of neuromuscular and urogenital symptoms resulting from the compression of multiple lumbosacral nerve roots below the level of the conus medullaris. CES is most commonly caused by a large lumbar disc herniation. It is very important to note that in patients with preexisting spinal stenosis, it can occur with smaller disc herniations. As with most of the high-risk syndromes presenting with back pain, a high index of clinical suspicion is required to identify CES during its early stages.

No established risk factors exist for the development of CES. The demographics of disease match the ages at which herniated nucleous pulposus presents. In cases of CES, 70% occur in patients with a history of low back pain. In 30% of patients, CES is the first symptom of lumbar disk herniation.[4] Approximately 50% to 70% of patients with CES have a rapid onset of symptoms, but in those with gradual onset disease early detection and timely referral is just as critical.[4]

It is critical to note that, although CES is usually thought of in terms of an acute and dramatic onset, it can also be seen in patients with chronic back pain and sciatica. Patients can even present gradually over weeks or even months.[5] It is important to inquire about any saddle paresthesias or early urinary symptoms even in patients with chronic sciatica. CES should be considered in patients with acute back pain and any of the symptoms listed in (see Box 2). Saddle paresthesias involve the S3 to S5 dermatomes including the perineum, external genitalia, and anus[4] (Fig. 1). It is reported typically as numbness or a "pins-and-needles" sensations of the groin and inner thighs (areas that would contact a saddle when riding a horse).

Physical examination findings in CES include decreased pinprick light touch sensation in the S3 to S5 (saddle area) regions, hyporeflexia of ankle jerk (maybe unilateral), decreased rectal tone, increased postvoid residual urine, and absence of the normal bulbocavernous reflex. The bulbocavernous reflex is not a commonly performed test

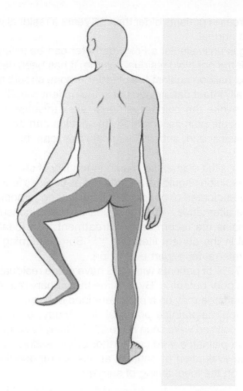

Fig. 1. Distribution of "saddle paresthesias" (S3-S5 dermatomes). (*From* Herkowitz H, Garfin SR, Eismont FJ, et al, editors. Rothman-Simeone the spine. Philadelphia: Saunders-Elsevier; 2006; with permission.)

for the emergency medicine practitioner, but is easy and can be incorporated into the rectal examination. The reflex is normally present, and absent in CES (also in spinal shock), and should be tested when suspicion is present or when ruling out the patient under consideration for CES. To perform the bulbocavernous reflex test, the examiner places a finger in the patient's rectum while simultaneously compressing the base of the penis or the clitoris. An increase is rectal tone is noted in a normal response. The absence of increasing rectal tone represents the absence of the reflex and suggests CES.[6]

Prognosis is better when urinary retention has not developed. Therefore, recognition at the earliest stages when pain and saddle paresthesias are present can improve outcomes. This subset is often referred to as CES-I (I for incomplete). This is in distinction to CES-R (R for retention). Although urinary incontinence is often the most common symptom in CES, the pathophysiology is actually urinary retention with resultant overflow incontinence. Equally important, and in distinction to most cases of urinary retention, the urinary retention is painless. Because the patient does not experience the typical discomfort of a distended bladder, the patient often reports only incontinence, and not the inability to void. Understanding this concept allows one to do an evaluation of postvoid residual urine volume as an easy and valuable screening tool. This can be done by having the patient void fully and using bladder scanning ultrasound technology to detect any residual urine. In patients under age 65 years, a volume of less than

50 mL is normal, whereas in patients older than 65 years a residual volume of less than 100 mL is considered normal.

If bladder scanning is unavailable, a Foley catheter can be inserted after voluntary voiding to evaluate for the postvoid residual volume. It has been described that gentle traction on the inflated balloon against the bladder trigone should produce an urge to void in the neurologically intact patient and not in the patient with CES.[6] This maneuver can also be used to evoke the bulbocavernous reflex (discussed elsewhere in this article). Because the acute pain associated with sciatica can cause urinary retention (as can some analgesics and anticholinergics), this can be a potentially useful discriminator.

MRI without contrast is the diagnostic imaging modality of choice for CES and in the patient with clinical suspicion should be undertaken as soon as feasible.[7] In patients in whom an MRI is contraindicated or not practical, computed tomography (CT) myelography is a reasonable alternative.[7] Emergent neurosurgical consultation for decompression surgery remains the recommended treatment. The ideal timing of surgery remains controversial in the current literature.[8–10] Surgical timing issues should not delay immediate ED referral for expert evaluation.

Between 50% and 70% of patients with CES have some residual neurologic deficit; as many as 20% have poor outcome. By the time that urinary retention is present, the postdecompression damage may be a predetermined outcome. Not surprisingly, this is a disease with a high malpractice potential. In 1 study, 60% of all CES medical malpractice lawsuits analyzed were seen in the ED.[11] Delay to surgical decompression was the main factor in plaintiff's verdicts, further emphasizing the need for ED providers to expedite the evaluation of patients at risk. Compounding these cases are the differing opinions on the ideal timing of surgery.[9,10]

SPINAL EPIDURAL ABSCESS

SEA is a suppurative infection confined to the epidural space. SEA is truly "a great imitator." It is estimated that 51% of patients with SEA have greater than 2 ED visits before diagnosis.[12,13] Once considered quite rare, the incidence of SEA in the United States is increasing.[12,13] The classic triad of back pain, fever, and neurologic deficit are seen in the minority of patients. Therefore, the "typical" presentation is atypical. Subtle presentations are common. Most SEA patients incorrectly correlate an episode of antecedent trauma as the etiology for the back pain. Of even greater concern is that upwards of 14% of SEA patients have a history of chronic back pain.[13] This creates a pitfall for the clinician who anchors on a previous diagnosis as the explanation for the symptoms of what could be an evolving SEA.

The thoracolumbar area is the most frequent site for SEA.[13] This is felt to be owing to the low venous flow structures of that area. The level of radiculopathy in the thoracolumbar region often presents with chest or abdominal pain, making the clinician focus on different organ systems entirely. Having a high index of suspicion in high-risk groups is important in establishing the correct diagnosis. Risk factors, common symptoms, and common examination findings in SEA are listed in Boxes 4–6, respectively.

It is extremely important to note that patients with SEA may present without fever and without an elevated white blood cell count. The absence of either a fever or elevated white blood cell count does not exclude this diagnosis.[13] Neurologic examination is normal in more than two-thirds of patients during the initial ED visit.[13] As the disease progresses, paresthesias develop and can rapidly progress to paralysis. Therefore, the neurologic examination findings are highly variable depending on the time of presentation.

Box 4
Risk factors for spinal epidural abscess

- Diabetes mellitus
- Trauma
- Intravenous drug use
- Alcoholism
- Epidural procedures (injections anesthesia)
- Diseases of immunosuppression including malignancy

MRI with contrast is the single best imaging modality to diagnose SEA[12,16] (**Fig. 2**). MRI with contrast can also differentiate SEA from osteomyelitis and other structural spine processes that can mimic SEA. CT myelography can be an option for those patients not able to undergo an MRI. Importantly, lumbar puncture is contraindicated when a high suspicion for SEA exists.[5]

Staphylococcus aureus is the most common bacteria implicated, with rates of 57% to 73%. Most SEA infections are monomicrobial.[17] Methicillin-resistant *S aureus* is increasingly implicated, and gram-negative organisms can account for up to 18% of cases.[17] Intravenous antibiotics should be started as soon as possible, with surgical drainage and laminectomy also performed as soon as clinically possible.[5] Broad-spectrum antibiotics should be directed at both gram-positive and gram-negative organisms. Vancomycin plus ceftriaxone or meropenem is one recommended antibiotic regimen. Specific agents will depend on patient factors, prior culture sensitivities, and local resistance patterns. Aspergillus species have been implicated in SEA occurring in patients with AIDS and those with prior disseminated fungal infections.[17] Antibiotics with selective surgical drainage, and hyperbaric oxygen management have been trialed, as has CT-guided needle aspiration.[5]

Mortality from SEA can be as high as 15%, and complete neurologic recovery is seen in a little fewer than one-half of all SEA patients. Residual neurologic deficit is common, and the greater the delay to diagnosis, the poorer the outcome. Early diagnosis despite its great clinical challenges is associated with better neurologic recovery and survival.[16,18,19]

AORTIC CATASTROPHES
Aortic Dissection

Acute aortic dissection (AAD) is a life-threating vascular entity that can present with back pain as a primary symptom. As such, it is important to understand this entity and its presentation and to differentiate it from AAA.

Box 5
Common symptoms of spinal epidural abscess

- Back pain (most common but often have chest or abdominal pain)
- Fever (approximately one-third of patients)
- Pain worse at night
- Radiculopathy (variable and often a later finding)

Box 6
Common findings in spinal epidural abscess

- Elevated erythrocyte sedimentation rate in 98%–100% of patients[14]
- Elevated C-reactive protein (≥50 minimally less sensitive than erythrocyte sedimentation rate)[15]
- Positive blood cultures (upwards of 60% of patients)

AAD is defined as the rapid development of a false, blood-filled channel within the tunica media of the aorta. It has an estimated incidence of 3 per 100,000 persons per year.[20] Typically patients present with back, chest, or abdominal pain. It is uncommon in patients less than 40 years of age, unless underlying pathology is present such as Marfan syndrome or abuse of sympathetic agonists.[21]

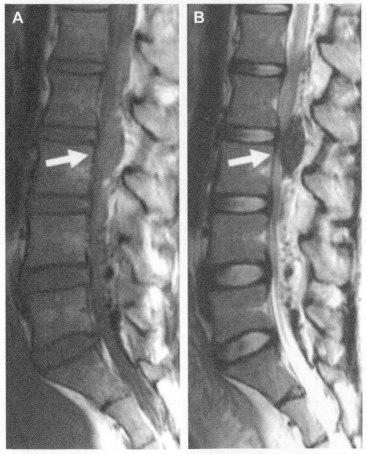

Fig. 2. Sagittal MRI of lumbar spine illustrating epidural abscess. Spinal epidural abscess: appearance on MRI as a guide to surgical management. (*A, B*) Abscess collection in epidural space. (*Data from* Semin Neurol 2011. Thieme Medical Publishers; and *From* JF Parkinson, Sekhon LHS. Spinal epidural abscess: appearance on magnetic resonance imaging as a guide to surgical management. Neurosurg Focus 2004;17(6):130–3; with permission.)

AAD has had a number of classification systems over time. The Stanford classification (types A and B) has become the most common accepted nomenclature. The Stanford classification is valuable because the type is associated with differing therapies. Type A dissections involve the aortic arch, often present with chest pain, and are treated surgically. Type B dissections start below the take off of the left subclavian artery, often present with back pain, and are managed medically. In almost one-half of patients with AAD, the diagnosis is delayed by more than 24 hours, underscoring the importance of remaining vigilant.[20,21]

Studies have examined the accuracy of history and physical in detecting AAD. Most studies, however, are retrospective in design.[20] It is critical to note that no single historical feature or physical examination finding can exclude or secure the diagnosis. Many of the classically associated symptoms and physical examination signs (ie, tearing intrascapular back pain, unilateral pulse or blood pressure deficit, murmur of aortic insufficiency, or widening of the mediastinum on chest radiography) are present less than 50% of the time.[22,23] The abrupt onset of maximal intensity pain at onset is reported in more than 90% of patients with dissection and should alert the clinician.[20]

The presence of chest or upper back pain, combined with neurologic signs and symptoms (ie, weakness, paresthesias) in the extremities, should make one consider an aortic etiology. Because it is unusual to have a patient with chest or upper back pain complain of evolving numbness or weakness, this should be considered a "red flag" complaint and prompt an immediate consideration of aortic dissection.

The diagnosis of AAD is confirmed by CT angiography of the chest and abdomen with intravenous contrast (Fig. 3). MRI along with transesophageal echocardiography can be performed in select patients unable to undergo CT. D-Dimer elevation has been studied in a number of small trials and seems to have a sensitivity of approximately 90% for the diagnosis of AAD, but assigning fixed positive predictive values and prospective evaluation have yet to be completed.[24]

In the case of types A and B AAD, the initial stabilizing management sequence is analgesia, followed by heart rate control, followed by blood pressure control, and

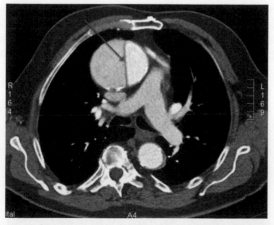

Fig. 3. Contrast computed tomography scan (axial image) demonstrating aortic dissection with intimal flap and false lumen containing contrast. Intimal flap defining false channel (*Arrow*). (*From* JF Parkinson, Sekhon LHS. Spinal epidural abscess: appearance on magnetic resonance imaging as a guide to surgical management. Neurosurg Focus 2004;17(6):130–3; with permission.)

simultaneous surgical consultation.[21] Type A dissections require emergent cardiothoracic surgery consultation for repair, whereas type B dissections are usually managed medically unless there is ischemia of a limb, ischemia of the mesentery, an inability to control hypertension, or frank aortic rupture.

Morphine is an ideal analgesic, because it reduces afterload and sympathetic tone. The heart rate goal is between 60 to 80 bpm and is typically managed with short-acting IV beta blocker medications, such as labetalol or esmolol.[25] Once rate control is established, a blood pressure reduction with a goal systolic blood pressure in the range of 100 to 120 mm Hg can be instituted. This can be accomplished with vasodilator therapy. Nitroprusside and nicardipine are recommended in many texts for blood pressure reduction in AAD.[25]

Abdominal Aortic Aneurysm

A ruptured AAA is a life-threatening event that can present with acute back pain. An aneurysm is defined as a segmental, full-thickness dilation of a blood vessel that is 50% greater than its normal diameter.[26] Although "normal" diameter varies with age, gender, and body habitus, the average diameter of the human infrarenal aorta is about 2.0 cm; the upper limit of normal is typically 3.0 cm.

AAA is 10 times more common in men compared with women of the same age.[27] Age of 65 to 75 years is the peak incidence at rupture. A history of smoking, defined as a consumption of more than 100 cigarettes in a lifetime, is a significant risk factor.[27]

Most AAAs are asymptomatic until the time of rapid expansion or frank rupture. As such, the back pain presentation of an AAA is typically one of rapid onset with pain maximal at onset followed often by rapid clinical deterioration that is unlikely to be missed. Patients may experience unimpressive back, flank, abdominal, or groin pain for some time before rupture. The etiology of that pain is not well-understood. Isolated groin pain is a particularly insidious, and not uncommon, presentation. Retroperitoneal tamponade of an AAA rupture can result in a misleading lack of early findings. Hematuria can be seen. In fact, ureteral colic is a common misdiagnosis in medicolegal cases of missed AAA.

More than one-half of all patients with a ruptured AAA die before reaching the hospital; therefore, only the subset of transiently stable patients will be seen in the ED with back pain as a possible chief complaint. As with AAD, sudden onset of maximal pain is often present, and should be considered a red flag symptom. In contrast, pain of ureteral colic, although sudden in onset, often does not have maximal pain at onset. Only

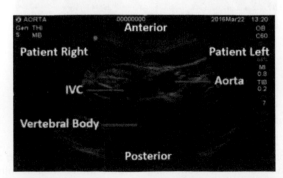

Fig. 4. Normal sonographic landmarks transverse abdominal static image. (*From* CDEM Bedside Ultrasound AA Examination, Gibbons R. Bedside ultrasound AAA examination. Available at: http://cdemcurriculum.com/bedside-ultrasound-aaa-examination/.)

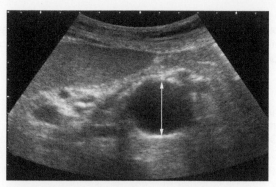

Fig. 5. Transverse (short axis) ultrasound view of abdominal aortic aneurysm. AP outer wall dimension of AAA (*Arrow*). (*From* Emergency ultrasonography resources and tutorials on EM ultrasound. Available at: http://emergencyultrasoundteaching.com/image_galleries/aorta_images/index.hp. Accessed November 24, 2014.)

one-third of AAAs are reported to be palpable on physical examination.[28] The absence of that finding should never be used exclude the diagnosis. The vast majority are found incidentally on screening imaging studies.

The American College of Emergency Physicians has a clinical policy addressing point of care ultrasound. It states that "Patients older than 50 years with the classic presentation of abdominal, back, or flank pain, a pulsatile abdominal mass, should have a bedside aortic ultrasound examination."[28] The same approach should apply to atraumatic abdominal or back pain with unexplained hypotension. Bedside point-of-care ultrasound imaging can be the single most rapid and available screening tool in the ED to evaluate patients at risk (Fig. 4). Although ultrasound imaging does not typically demonstrate the rupture of an AAA (because blood presenting as fluid will remain contained in retroperitoneal space), it will show the presence of the aneurysm (Fig. 5). The accuracy of ultrasound imaging using a diameter of 3.0 cm or less as negative and a diameter of 4.5 cm or greater as positive has been demonstated.[27,28] Most aneurysms rupture at widths in excess of 5.5 cm. Ultrasound visualization can be impeded by bowel gas and by body habitus. In one ED point-of-care ultrasound article, it was noted that up to 17% of scanned ED patients have incomplete visualization of the abdominal aorta.[29]

CT with contrast also defines AAA and provides information on rupture and active blood loss. The major disadvantage to this study is the time involved, and perhaps more important the time out of the ED in a less monitored environment. In stable patients, it does provide a definitive diagnosis.

Treatment for AAA rupture involves immediate surgical repair. Endovascular repair remains an option in the unruptured AAA.

SUMMARY

Back pain is a common presenting complaint to the ED. The overwhelming number of presentations are caused by self-limited mechanical processes, which require only symptomatic treatment. As such, patients with back pain are often assigned a lower acuity triage level. The challenge in emergency medicine is to diagnose the ominous etiologies when they present. Vigilance for the nuances in presentations of the serious causes must be applied to all patients. A careful history that screens for the presence of historical and examination "red flags" is essential. In conjunction, applying an appropriate focused physical examination, can direct the provider to expand the evaluation when needed. Selective imaging and laboratory studies can screen and often define serious etiologies. Virtually all of the serious etiologies have time sensitive windows for treatment and management, so efficiency in the workup is also a critical function for the provider.

REFERENCES

1. Deyo RA, Mirza SK, Martin BI. Back pain prevalence and visit rates: estimates from U.S. national surveys, 2002. Spine (Phila Pa 1976) 2006;31:2724–7.
2. Centers for Disease Control and Prevention, National Center for Health Statistics, Preliminary Data from NAMCS and NHAMCS Top 5 Diagnosis to office based and hospital outpatient departments 2008. Available at: www.cdc.gov/nchs/data/ahcd/preliminary2008/table02.pdf.
3. Bigos S, Bowyer O, Braen G, et al. Acute low back problems in adults. Clinical Practice Guideline No. 14. AHCPR Publication No. 95–0642. Rockville (MD): Agency for Health Care Policy and Research, Public Health Service, U.S. Department of Health and Human Services; 1994.
4. Gardner A, Gardner E, Morely T. Cauda equine syndrome: a review. Eur Spine J 2011;20(5):690–7.
5. Khanna RK, Malik GM, Rock JP, et al. Spinal epidural abscess: evaluation of factors influencing outcome. Neurosurgery 1996;39(5):958–64.
6. Uff CE. Clinical assessment of cauda equina syndrome and the bulbocavernosus reflex. 2009. Available at: http://www.bmj.com/cgi/eletters/338/mar31_1/b396.
7. Wilmink J. Lumbar spinal imaging in radicular pain and related conditions. Springer Science & Business Media 2010. ISBN: 354093829X.
8. Delong WB, Polissar N, Neradilek B. Timing of Surgery is cauda equine syndrome with urinary retention: meta-analysis of observational studies. J Neurosurg Spine 2008;8:305–20.
9. O'Laoire SA, Crockard HA, Thomas DG. Prognosis for sphincter recovery after operation for cauda equina compression owing to lumbar disc prolapse. Br Med J (Clin Res Ed) 1981;282:1852–4.
10. Ahn UM, Ahn NU, Buchowski JM, et al. Cauda equina syndrome secondary to lumbar disc herniation—a meta-analysis of surgical outcomes. Spine 2000; 25(12):1515–22.
11. Daniels E, Gordon Z, French K, et al. Review of medicolegal cases for cauda equina syndrome: what factors lead to an adverse outcome to the provider? Orthopedics 2012;35(3):414–9.
12. Davis DP, Wold RM, Patel RJ, et al. The clinical presentation and impact of diagnostic delays on emergency department patients with spinal epidural abscess. J Emerg Med 2004;26(3):285–91.
13. Curry WT Jr, Hoh BL, Amin-Hanjani S, et al. Spinal epidural abscess: clinical presentation, management, and outcome. Surg Neurol 2005;63(4):364–71.
14. Mehta SH, Shih R. Cervical epidural abscess associated with massively elevated erythrocyte sedimentation rate. J Emerg Med 2004;26(1):107–9.
15. Buensalido J, Reyes M. ESR, CRP and Procalcitonin in the infections of the spine and infections in spinal cord injury patients. Open Infect Dis J 2015;9:1–12.
16. Numaguchi Y, Rigamonti D, Rothman MI, et al. Spinal epidural abscess: evaluation with gadolinium-enhanced MR imaging. Radiographics 1993;13(3):545–60.
17. Mackenzie AR, Laing RB, Smith CC, et al. Spinal epidural abscess: the importance of early diagnosis and treatment. J Neurol Neurosurg Psychiatry 1998; 65:209–12.

18. Koppel BS, Tuchman AJ, Mangiardi JR, et al. Epidural spinal infection in intravenous drug abusers. Arch Neurol 1988;45(12):1331–7.
19. Davis D, Salazar A, Chan TC, et al. Prospective evaluation of clinical decision guideline to diagnose spinal epidural abscess in patient who present to the emergency department with spine pain. J Neurosurg Spine 2011;14(6):765–70.
20. Aldeen A, Rosiere L. Acute aortic dissection. ACEP News 2009.
21. Erbel R, Alfonso F, Boileau C, et al. Task force on aortic dissection, European Society of Cardiology. Diagnosis and management of aortic dissection. Eur Heart J 2001;22:1642–81.
22. Klompas M. Does this patient have an acute thoracic aortic dissection? JAMA 2002;17:2262–72.
23. Hagan PG, Nienaber CA, Isselbacher EM, et al. The international registry of acute aortic dissection (IRAD). JAMA 2000;28(3):897–903.
24. Sutherland A. D-dimer as the sole screening test for acute aortic dissection: a review of the literature. Ann Emerg Med 2008;52(4):339–43.
25. Aldeen A, Rosiere L, Solomon R. Focus on: acute aortic dissection. ACEP News 2009.
26. Meszaros I, Mórocz J, Szlávi J, et al. Epidemiology and clinicopathology of aortic dissection. Chest 2000;117:1271–8.
27. Johnston KW, Rutherford RB, Tilson MD, et al. Suggested standards for reporting on arterial aneurysms. Subcommittee on reporting standards for arterial aneurysms, Ad Hoc Committee on Reporting Standards, Society for Vascular Surgery and North American Chapter, International Society for Cardiovascular Surgery. J Vasc Surg 1991;13:452–8.
28. Wu S, Blackstock U, Lewiss R, et al. Bedside ultrasound of the abdominal aorta clinical and practice management. ACEP News 2010.
29. Blaivas M, Theodoro D. Frequency of incomplete aorta visualization by emergency department bedside ultrasound. Acad Emerg Med 2004;11(1):103–5.

Lethal Rashes

Bartholomew Cambria, PA-C*, Lara West, PA-C

KEYWORDS

- Lethal rash • Staphylococcal toxic shock syndrome • Meningococcemia
- Erythema multiforme minor and major • Toxic epidermal necrolysis
- Stevens–Johnson syndrome

KEY POINTS

- A staphylococcal toxic shock syndrome rash is painless, diffuse, red, macular rash and may be confused with "sunburn" or the flush associated with the fever.
- Aggressive resuscitation, antibiotics, and removal of foreign body are mainstay of treatment.
- Mucosal petechiae may the initial sign of meningococcemia followed by skin rash especially noted on the palms and soles.
- Erythema multiforme target lesion is a characteristic finding, although not present on all patients and herpes simplex is the most common cause.
- Stevens–Johnson syndrome and toxic epidermal necrolysis are differentiated based on body surface area involvement. Early discontinuation of causative medications and aggressive wound care are mainstays of treatment.

STAPHYLOCOCCAL TOXIC SHOCK SYNDROME

Staphylococcus aureus is commonly found on the skin and mucous membranes of healthy adults and children and by age 25, 90% of the general population will have antibodies against the organism.[1] *S aureus* is also known to be the causative agent to several infections that range from folliculitis to abscess and endocarditis. In 1927, a syndrome of fever, myalgias, sore throat, edema, scarlatiniform rash, and desquamation associated with *S aureus* infection was first described.[2] In 1978, Todd and colleagues[3] reported 7 cases in children who presented with similar symptoms as described in 1927 of fever, headache, conjunctival hyperemia, and rash. These cases also presented with acute renal failure, hepatic abnormalities, disseminated intravascular coagulation, and shock: "One patient died, one had gangrene of the toes, and all have had fine desquamation of affected skin and peeling of palms and soles." *S aureus* was isolated from mucosal (nasopharyngeal, vaginal, tracheal) but not from blood and

The authors have nothing to disclose.
Department of Emergency Medicine, Northwell Health, Staten Island University Hospital, 475 Seaview Avenue, Staten Island, NY 10305, USA
* Corresponding author.
E-mail address: BCAMBRIA@NORTHWELL.EDU

Physician Assist Clin 2 (2017) 371–384
http://dx.doi.org/10.1016/j.cpha.2017.02.003

the term toxic shock syndrome (TSS) was coined.[2,3] The peak incidence of S aureus–related illness was seen in 1980 when 890 cases were reported, 91% of which were related to the use of superabsorbent tampons.[4] Similar to the findings from Fernandez-Frackelton,[4] S aureus was isolated from the vagina or cervix of 98% of women with menstrual TSS. The organism produces enzymes that generate propagation of an inflammatory response and exotoxins but, because the organism is often not invasive, the blood cultures are usually negative.[4] Nonmenstrual TSS has also been observed in postoperative and postpartum wounds infections, mastitis, sinusitis, osteomyelitis, burns, respiratory infections after influenza, and enterocolitis.[1] Risk factors are listed in Box 1.

Diagnosis

A clinical criterion for diagnosis of staphylococcal TSS was created by the United States Centers for Disease Control and Prevention. Clinical criteria for diagnosis of staphylococcal TSS are listed in Box 2. A confirmed case is defined by a case, which meets the laboratory criteria, and in which all 5 of the clinical criteria described below are present, (with or without desquamation, because patient death may occur before the desquamation occurs). A probable case meets the laboratory criteria and 4 of the 5 clinical criteria described.[5,6]

The isolation of S aureus is not required for the diagnosis of staphylococcal TSS. The symptoms usually develop rapidly in usually well appearing patients, so admission to an intensive care unit (ICU) should be considered. In evaluating a patient for staphylococcal TSS, serologic testing for Rocky Mountain spotted fever, measles, and leptospirosis in endemic areas should be considered. The rash related to staphylococcal TSS is characterized as a painless, diffuse, red, macular rash resembling "sunburn" or the flush associated with a fever. The rash involves both the skin (including palms and sole) as well as mucous membranes and develops over the first few days of symptoms onset (Fig. 1). Mucosal involvement includes conjunctival and scleral hemorrhage, oropharyngeal hyperemia known as "strawberry tongue" and hyperemia of the vaginal and cervical canal (Fig. 2). In severe cases, ulceration on the mucous membranes with petechiae, vesicles, and bullae may be present. One to

---

Box 1
Risk factors for staphylococcal toxic shock syndrome

- Use of superabsorbent tampons
- Postoperative wound infection
- Postpartum wound infection
- Nasal packing
- Alcohol abuse
- Infection with Influenza A
- Infection with Varicella
- Immunosuppressive: diabetes mellitus, human immunodeficiency virus, cancer
- Chronic cardiac or pulmonary disease
- Nonsteroidal antiinflammatory drugs (not confirmed)

Data from Fernandez-Frackelton M. Bacteria. In: Marx JA, Hockberger RS, Walls RM, et al, editors. Rosen's Emergency Medicine: Concepts and Clinical Practice. Philadelphia: Mosby/Elsevier; 2010.

Box 2
Clinical criteria for diagnosis of staphylococcal toxic shock syndrome

- Fever: temperature ≥102.0°F
- Rash: diffuse macular erythroderma
- Desquamation: 1 to 2 weeks after onset of rash
- Hypotension: systolic blood pressure ≤90 mm Hg for adults or <5th% by age for children aged <16 years
- Multisystem involvement (≥3 of the following organ systems):
    - Gastrointestinal: vomiting or diarrhea
    - Muscular: myalgia or creatine phosphokinase level at least twice the upper limit of normal
    - Mucous membrane: vaginal, oropharyngeal, or conjunctival hyperemia
    - Renal: blood urea nitrogen or creatinine at least twice the upper limit of normal for laboratory or urinary sediment with pyuria (≥5 leukocytes per high-power field) in the absence of urinary tract infection
    - Hepatic: total bilirubin, alanine aminotransferase enzyme, or aspartate aminotransferase enzyme levels at least twice the upper limit of normal for laboratory
    - Hematologic: platelets <100,000/mm³
    - Central nervous system: disorientation or altered mental status

Laboratory findings
- Blood or cerebrospinal fluid cultures blood culture *may* be positive for *Staphylococcus aureus*)
- Negative serologies for Rocky Mountain spotted fever, leptospirosis, or measles

Data from Ref.[5]

2 weeks after the initial onset of symptoms, a fine flaking desquamation occurs on the face, trunk, and extremities followed by full-thickness peeling of the palms, soles, and fingers. Desquamation occurs in the late stages of TSS.[7,8]

Treatment

Patients should be placed in a monitored setting, with aggressive fluid resuscitation and supplemental oxygen, regardless of initial pulse oximetry to reduce acidosis.[4] Assisted ventilation may be necessary. Look for, remove, and culture for a possible source of infection. Remember to remove any foreign bodies from vaginal canal such as tampons and contraceptive sponges, as well as of nasal packing if present. Obtain a surgical consult for wound debridement. Mupirocin is recommended for

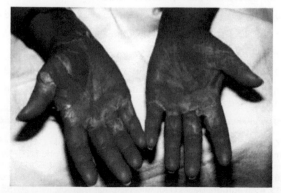

Fig. 1. Staphylococcal toxic shock syndrome.

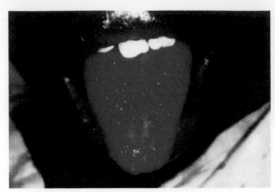

Fig. 2. Staphylococcal toxic shock syndrome. Strawberry tongue.

the eradication of the carrier state if nasal cultures are positive. If vasopressors needed, consider using dopamine and/or norepinephrine. Treatment with intravenous immune globulin (1 g/kg in a single dose administered over several hours on day 1 with a repeat dose of 0.5 mg/kg on days 2 and 3) is recommended in severe cases of TSS in patients that do not respond to intravenous fluids and vasopressors. Box 3 provides recommendations for antibiotic therapy.

"The overall case fatality rate for TSS is 4.1%, with higher rates in non menstrual TSS (5%) compared to menstrual TSS (3%)."[7] Death associated with TSS usually occurs within the first few days of hospitalization but may occur as late as 2 weeks secondary to arrhythmias, cardiomyopathies, respiratory failure, and bleeding. Staphylococcal TSS needs to be differentiated from streptococcal TSS, as noted on Box 4. Streptococcal TSS is associated with more severe soft tissue infections such as necrotizing fasciitis, peritonitis and osteomyelitis. Streptococcal TSS remains a highly fatal disease with a mortality rate of 30% to 70%.[7]

MENINGOCOCCEMIA

Meningococcemia is a potentially fatal infectious illness caused by an aerobic gram-negative diplococcus *Neisseria meningitidis*. Approximately 5% to 10% of the general

---

Box 3
Antibiotic therapy for staphylococcal toxic shock syndrome

Confirmed methicillin-susceptible Staphylococcus aureus

- Clindamycin 600 mg IV every 8 hours (children: 25–40 mg/kg/d in 3 divided doses)
- Plus oxacillin or nafcillin 2 g IV every 4 hours (children: 100–150 mg/kg/24 h IV in 4 divided doses)

Concern for or confirmed methicillin-resistant S aureus

- Clindamycin 600 mg IV every 8 hours (children: 25–40 mg/kg/d in 3 divided doses)
- Plus vancomycin 30 mg/kg/d IV in 2 divided doses (not to exceed 2 g per dose; children: 40 mg/kg/d IV in 4 divided doses)
- Or linezolid, 600 mg IV every 12 hours (children: 10 mg/kg IV every 12 hours)

Data from Liang SY. Toxic shock syndromes. In: Tintinalli JE, Stapczynski J, Ma O, et al, editors. Tintinalli's emergency medicine: a comprehensive study guide, 8e. New York: McGraw-Hill; 2016. Available at: http://accessmedicine.mhmedical.com/content.aspx?bookid=1658&Sectionid=109435589. Accessed July 02, 2016; and Gilbert D, Chambers H, Eliopoulos G, et al. The Sanford guide to antimicrobial therapy 2015. 45th edition. Dallas (TX): Antimicrobial Therapy, Inc.,. 2015.

Box 4
Staphylococcal toxic shock syndrome and streptococcal toxic shock syndrome

	Toxic Shock Syndrome	Streptococcal Toxic Shock Syndrome
Organism	*Staphylococcus aureus* (including MRSA)	Group A *Streptococcus* (*Streptococcus pyogenes*)
Presence of rash	"Sunburn," "fever flushed" followed by desquamation	Necrotizing fasciitis but usually uncommon
Blood culture positivity	Usually negative	High likelihood
Mortality (%)	≤ 5	30–70

Abbreviation: MRSA, methicillin-resistant *S aureus*.

Adapted from Liang SY. Toxic Shock Syndromes. In: Tintinalli JE, Stapczynski J, Ma O, et al, editors. Tintinalli's emergency medicine: a comprehensive study guide, 8e. New York: McGraw-Hill; 2016. Available at: http://accessmedicine.mhmedical.com/content.aspx?bookid=1658&Sectionid=109435589. Accessed July 02, 2016.

population are considered carriers as the *N meningitidis* attaches to epithelial cells in the nasopharynx.[9] In high-risk populations, such as military recruits, the organism can be found in almost one-half of the people without evidence of active disease.[10] If the bacteria enters the bloodstream, symptoms can range from a mild upper respiratory infection and localized infections such as epiglottitis, conjunctivitis, and arthritis to bacteremia, and sepsis progressing to death. Meningitis was first described in 1805 by Vieusseux in Geneva and the causative bacteria identified 1887.[11] In 1963, an outbreak of resistant meningococcal disease occurred in the United States, spurring efforts to develop a vaccine for the infection.[11] Approximately 1400 to 2800 cases of meningococcal infection are reported to the Centers for Disease Control and Prevention annually.[12,13] There are 13 serogroups of which groups A, B, C, Y, and W-135 cause most of the infection. In the United States, outbreaks are usually owing to serogroup B, C and Y. Outbreaks usually occur in daycare centers, schools (especially among freshman in colleges), and army barracks. More than one-half of the cases in infants are caused by serogroup B, for which there is no effective vaccine. A quadrivalent vaccine is available for groups A, C, Y, and W-135 and is recommended for children 11 to 18 years of age and for other high-risk patients. The incidence of meningococcal disease peaks in the winter and decreases in the summer. About every 10 years, massive outbreaks of serogroup A have occurred in sub-Saharan Africa, which is also known as the meningitis belt. The last recorded outbreak occurred in 2007.[12] Waterhouse–Friderichsen syndrome is the most severe form of meningococcemia, characterized by high fever, widespread purpura, disseminated intravascular coagulation, and adrenal failure. Risk factors are listed in Box 5.

Diagnosis

Initial presentations of patients to the emergency department are complaints consistent of fever, headache, irritability, lethargy, myalgias, emesis, diarrhea, or symptoms consistent of an upper respiratory infections, such as cough or rhinorrhea. Only 60% of patients have the classic signs of fever and petechiae or purpura; therefore, the provider must have a high suspicion for this disease. Diagnosis is based on clinical findings and confirmed by the isolation of *N meningitidis* from blood cultures, cerebrospinal (Box 6), synovial, pleural, or pericardial fluid. Polymerase chain reaction is the gold standard for diagnosis.

Box 5
Risk factors for meningococcemia

- Military recruits
- College freshman
- Overcrowding
- Close contact with infected patient
- Asplenia
- Alcohol abuse
- Corticosteroid use
- Recent respiratory illness
- Smoking
- Complement deficiency

Data from Andersen J, Berthelsen L, Bech JB, et al. Dynamics of the meningococcal carrier state and characteristics of the carrier strains: a longitudinal study within three cohorts of military recruits. Epidemiol Infect 1998;121:85.

Mucosal petechiae may appear first, followed by skin petechiae.[10] The skin findings result from the bacteria's invasion and destruction of the endothelium. The rash is initially pink, blanching, and maculopapular, and found on the extremities and trunk, although it may also be noted on the palms, soles, and head. The rash then becomes hemorrhagic petechiae and evolves into a palpable purpura with gray necrotic centers (**Fig. 3**), which are pathognomonic for meningococcal infection.[9]

Treatment

Patients should receive broad spectrum antibiotics until a narrower spectrum agent can be selected based on identification of the organism and its sensitivities.[11] See the treatment regimen for meningococcemia described on **Box 7**. Because these patients can decompensate rapidly and without warning, all patients with possible or confirmed meningococcal should be admitted to the ICU under respiratory isolation for at least 24 hours. Close contacts should receive prophylaxis including those in the household, nursery, and daycare center. Recommendations for prophylaxis for health care providers are indicated for those who may have potentially become exposed during endotracheal intubation and/or manipulation of endotracheal tube.

Box 6
Findings of meningitis on cerebrospinal fluid

- Elevated opening pressure
- Increased protein level
- Decreased glucose
- Polymorphonuclear leukocytosis
- Gram-negative diplococci on Gram stain

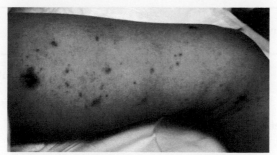

Fig. 3. Petechiae and purpura on the left lower limb in MenC septicemia. (*Courtesy of* David Pace, Paediatric Infectious Diseases Clinic, Mater Dei Hospital, Malta.)

ERYTHEMA MULTIFORME

Erythema multiforme (EM) is an acute, immune-mediated condition hallmarked by the presence of targetlike lesions on the skin. Erosions or bullae involving the mucosal lining of the oral, genital and/or ocular areas often accompanying lesions. EM is divided between major and minor forms (Box 8).

Major EM is defined by mucosal involvement, whereas minor EM spares the mucosa.[16] There has been debate regarding EM and Stevens–Johnson syndrome

---

Box 7
Treatment regimen for meningococcemia

First-line antibiotic therapy[14,15]

- Cefotaxime: 100 mg/kg/day IV in divided doses every 6 hours (up to a maximum of 12 g)
- Ceftriaxone: 100 mg/kg IV, followed by daily dosage of 50 mg/kg every 12 hours (up to a maximum of 4 g)[a]
- Penicillin G: 4 MU (children: 250,000 U/kg/24 h) IV q4h

Second-line antibiotic therapy

- Ampicillin: 2 to 3 g (children: 200–400 mg/kg/24 h) IV q6h
- Chloramphenicol: 50 to 100 mg/kg/24 h IV q6h (max 4 g/d)
- Prophylaxis therapy
  ○ Single-dose ceftriaxone:
    ■ 125 mg IM for age <15 y
    ■ 250 mg IM for age >15 y
  ○ Ciprofloxacin: 500 mg po (adults)
  ○ Rifampin: 600 mg (children: 5–10 mg/kg) po bid for 2 days
  ○ Azithromycin 500 mg po single dose (not routinely used)

Additional therapy

- Dexamethasone: 0.15 mg/kg IV for pediatric meningitis
- Hydrocortisone (Solu-Cortef): 100 mg (children: 2 mg/kg) bolus IV for adrenal insufficiency q8h

[a] Ceftriaxone is not recommended for neonates who have jaundice. Use Cefotaxime instead.
Data from Barlam TF, Kasper DL. Approach to the acutely ill infected febrile patient. In: Kasper D, Fauci A, Hauser S, et al, editors. Harrison's principles of internal medicine, 19e. New York: McGraw-Hill; 2015. Available at: http://accessmedicine.mhmedical.com/content. aspx?bookid51130&Sectionid566320817. Accessed July 03, 2016 and Schaider J. Meningococcemia. Rosen & Barkin's 5-Minute Emergency Medicine Consult. 2015. Available at: http://www. r2library.com/Resource/Title/1451190670/ch0013s10895. Accessed July 15, 2016.

Box 8		
Summary of findings in EM major/minor		
	EM Major	EM Minor
Prodromal	50% influenza-like illness	Usually absent or upper respiratory infection–like symptoms
Onset of rash	1–14 d	3 d
Location of rash	Acral spreading	Extremities with centripetal spreading
Pruritus	Can be present	Absent
Mucosal involvement	Yes	No

Abbreviation: EM, erythema multiforme.

Data from Sokumbi O, Wetter DA. Clinical features, diagnosis, and treatment of erythema multiforme: a review for the practicing dermatologist. Int J Dermatol 2012;51(8):889–902.

(SJS) primarily owing to the close clinical appearance of cutaneous lesions and mucosal erosions found in both conditions. Evidence suggests that SJS has a different disease processes and causes; therefore, EM major should not be used to describe SJS.[17] The exact incidence of EM in the United States is unknown. It is estimated that 1% of dermatologic outpatient visits yearly are secondary to EM. Globally, EM is estimated at approximately 1.2 to 6.0 cases per million individuals per year.[18] EM is usually self-limited, with most cases resolving in weeks. Reoccurrence can occur; however, it is uncommon.[16]

Clinical Manifestations

The term "multiforme" describes the abundance of clinical manifestations that may be observed. Target lesions (Fig. 4) are associated with EM; however, absence of the lesion does not rule out the disease. The rash typically progresses from round erythematous papules that evolve into classic target lesions. Target lesions commonly are made up of 3 components:

- A dusky central area or blister,
- A dark inflammatory zone surrounded by a pale ring of edema, and
- An erythematous ring on the outside of the lesion.

Lesions can involve the oral, ocular, and/or genital mucosa, and commonly manifest as diffuse areas of mucosal erythema, painful erosions, and/or bullae. Seventy percent of patients with EM have oral involvement, specifically the vermilion border and mucosal surfaces, including the buccal mucosa, labial mucosa, gingiva, and tongue.[16]

Diagnosis

Diagnosis is based primarily on clinical appearance; biopsy is rarely necessary. EM has a very long differential diagnosis, which includes essential urticaria, vasculitis, bullous pemphigoid, pemphigus, linear immunoglobulin A dermatosis, acute febrile neutrophilic dermatosis, and dermatitis herpetiformis. Oral lesions present a challenge and must be differentiated from aphthous stomatitis, pemphigus, herpetic stomatitis, and hand–foot–mouth disease. Patients with widely disseminated purpuric macules and blisters and prominent involvement of the trunk and face are likely to have SJS, caused by medication reaction rather than EM.[19,20]

Treatment

EM is usually self-limited, with most cases resolving in weeks.[5,18] Reoccurrence can occur; however, it is uncommon. Symptomatic therapy is the main focus based on

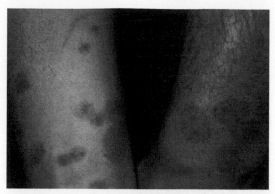

Fig. 4. Erythema multiforme minor. (*Courtesy of* Barry Hahn, MD, Department of Emergency Medicine, Staten Island University, Norwell Health.)

presenting symptoms and location of rash. These therapies include oral antihistamines, topical corticosteroids, analgesics, local skin care, and soothing mouthwashes (eg, oral rinsing with warm saline or a solution of diphenhydramine, xylocaine, and bismuth subsalicylate [Kaopectate]).

For more severe cases, wound care and use of Burrow or Domeboro solution dressings may be necessary. The use of liquid antiseptics, such as 0.05% chlorhexidine, during bathing helps to prevent superinfection. Topical treatment with hydrocolloid and gauze dressing may be used for genital involvement. Local supportive care for eye involvement is important and includes topical lubricants for dry eyes, sweeping of conjunctival fornices, and removal of fresh adhesions. Suppression of herpes simplex virus can prevent herpes simplex virus–associated EM, but antiviral treatment started after the eruption of EM has no effect on the course of the disease.

STEVENS–JOHNSON SYNDROME/TOXIC EPIDERMAL NECROLYSIS

SJS and toxic epidermal necrolysis (TEN) are severe mucocutaneous reactions, most commonly triggered by medications. The disorder is characterized by fever and extensive necrosis and detachment of the epidermis. Incidence for SJS, TEN, and SJS/TEN overlap range from 2 to 7 cases per million people per year. The diseases overlap as noted on **Box 9**. SJS/TEN and are considered to be related disorders and are differentiated based on the body surface area of epidermal involvement and detachment.[21]

Risk Factors

- Medications[22];
- Infection, including mycoplasma pneumonia, cytomegalovirus infections; and
- Idiopathic.

Medications are the major causative agents. Numerous medications have been implicated including antibiotics, antiepileptic drugs, nonsteroidal anti-inflammatory

Box 9 Overlap between SJS and TEN			
	SJS	SJS/TEN Overlap	TEN
Body surface area (%)	<10	10–30	>30
Mortality (%)	5	5–25	25–50

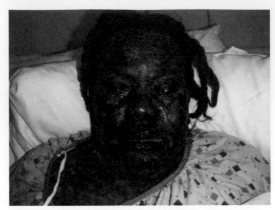

Fig. 5. Toxic epidermal necrolysis. (*Courtesy of* Barry Hahn, MD, Department of Emergency Medicine, Staten Island University, Norwell Health.)

drugs, ampicillin, allopurinol, corticosteroids (topical and systemic), and the antiretroviral drugs nevirapine and abacavir.[22]

Clinical Features

The majority of patients experience symptoms of fever, general malaise, and upper respiratory illness for 1 to 3 days before rash is appreciated. The eyes could be involved before skin manifestations. Skin lesions can present with a wide range of appearances, occurring on the upper torso, limbs, and face (Fig. 5). The palms and soles are commonly involved. Skin lesions typically begin with ill-defined, erythematous macules with purpuric centers, although many cases of SJS/TEN may present with diffuse erythema.[23] The Nikolsky sign, which is easy removal of the epidermal surface with gentle pressure, is present. The Nikolsky sign is a helpful clinical indicator, although it is not specific for SJS/TEN. The skin could be tender to touch before lesions appear.[24,25] The mucosa is involved 90% of the cases. Locations of mucosal lesions include[23]:

- Oral cavity: lips and vermillion border causing issues with dietary intake.
- Ocular: severe conjunctivitis, corneal ulcerations anterior uveitis.
- Genital: urethritis can develop, and may lead to urinary retention.
- Pharyngeal mucosa is affected in nearly all patients.
- Tracheal, bronchial, and esophageal membranes are less frequently involved.
- Intestinal involvement is rare.

Diagnosis

The diagnosis is typically made based on the classic skin findings as described, as well as specific histologic findings. Histologic workup of immediate cryosections reveals widespread necrotic epidermis involving all layers. Differential diagnoses are noted in Box 10.

Treatment

Supportive care with discontinuation of causative agent is the main stay treatment. The SCORTEN score may be used to determine which clinical setting is appropriate for care of patients with SJS/TEN: the ICU, a burn unit, or a regular floor bed. Generally, SCORTEN scores of greater than 2 should be admitted to the ICU or a burn unit.

Box 10

Differential diagnosis of Stevens–Johnson syndrome

- Linear immunoglobulin A dermatosis
- Paraneoplastic pemphigus
- Pemphigus vulgaris
- Bullous pemphigoid
- Acute generalized exanthematous pustulosis
- Disseminated fixed bullous drug eruption
- Staphylococcal scalded skin syndrome

From Harr T, French LE. Toxic epidermal necrolysis and Stevens-Johnson syndrome. Orphanet J Rare Dis 2010;5:39.

The SCORTEN score is based on 7 independent and easily measured clinical and laboratory variable and has been validated for use on days 1 and 3 of hospitalization for SJS/TEN (Box 11).

Studies indicate that the prognosis is better for patients transferred to a burn care unit or ICU early in the disease process. In a retrospective multicenter review of 199 patients with TEN treated at burn care centers, the overall mortality was 32% compared with 51% among patients initially cared for in other settings and transferred to a burn center more than 1 week after disease onset.[26] There are no mainstay medical therapies for SJS/TEN; however, several therapies have been used in clinical practice, including systemic corticosteroids, intravenous immune globulin, cyclosporine, plasmapheresis, and anti-tumor necrosis factor monoclonal antibodies. These therapies have not been adequately studied, except thalidomide, which was found to be harmful, and their use is based on clinical experience and local guidelines. The most commonly used therapies are presented in this section and summarized in Box 12.

SUMMARY

Although most patients presenting to the emergency department with a complaint of rash are not critical, a minority of those patients will have a life-threatening rash that

---

Box 11

SCORTEN score

SCORTEN Parameter	Individual Score	SCORTEN (Sum of Individual Scores)	Predicted Mortality (%)
Age >40 y	Yes = 1, no = 0	0–1	3.2
Malignancy	Yes = 1, no = 0	2	12.1
Tachycardia (>120/min)	Yes = 1, no = 0	3	35.8
Initial surface of epidermal detachment >10%	Yes = 1, no = 0	4	58.3
Serum urea >10 mmol/L	Yes = 1, no = 0	>5	90
Serum glucose >14 mmol/L	Yes = 1, no = 0		
Bicarbonate >20 mmol/L	Yes = 1, no = 0		

Adapted from Harr T, French LE. Toxic epidermal necrolysis and Stevens-Johnson syndrome. Orphanet J Rare Dis 2010;5:39.

Box 12
Medical therapy for SJS and TEN

Treatment	SJS	TEN
Systemic corticosteroids (short term, high dose)	Results mixed: possible benefit, possible harm	Possible harm owing to increased rates of sepsis and impaired reepithelialization
Intravenous immunoglobulin	Possible benefit	Possible benefit
	No significant evidence of harm	
Cyclosporine	Possible benefit	Possible benefit
Plasmapheresis	No data	Possible benefit
		No evidence of harm
Thalidomide	No data	Harmful
		Contraindicated

Abbreviations: SJS, Stevens–Johnson syndrome; TEN, toxic epidermal necrolysis.

Adapted from Nirken M, High WA. Stevens-Johnson syndrome and toxic epidermal necrolysis: pathogenesis, clinical manifestations, and diagnosis. Uptodate. Available at: http://www.uptodate.com/contents/stevens-johnson-syndrome-and-toxic-epidermal-necrolysis-pathogenesis-clinical-manifestations-and-diagnosis/contributor-disclosure. Accessed August 7, 2016.

requires immediate identification and management. This article has discussed 4 potentially lethal rashes and their respective management: staphylococcal TSS, meningococcemia, EM major and minor, and TEN. Although a large majority of the general population will have antibodies against *S aureus*, this organism is also known to be the causative agent to several infections including TSS. The treatment for TSS includes both antibiotic therapy as well as removal of the offending source of infection. With regard to meningococcemia, not all patients will present with the classic signs of fever and petechiae or purpura; therefore, the provider must have a high suspicion for this disease. Diagnosis is based on clinical findings and confirmed by the isolation of *N meningitides*. However, suspicious cases should prompt the provider to give broad-spectrum antibiotics. All patients with possible or confirmed meningococcal should be admitted to the ICU under respiratory isolation for at least 24 hours. EM is self-limiting, with most cases resolving in weeks. Symptomatic therapy is the main focus based on presenting symptoms and location of rash. There has been debate regarding EM and SJS, primarily owing to the close clinical appearance of cutaneous lesions and mucosal erosions found in both conditions. SJS and TEN are severe mucocutaneous reactions, most commonly triggered by medications. Supportive care with discontinuation of causative agent is the main stay treatment. The SCORTEN score may be used to determine which clinical setting is appropriate for care of patients with SJS/TEN.

REFERENCES

1. Kluytmans J, van Belkum A, Verbrugh H. Nasal carriage of staphylococcus aureus: epidemiology, underlying mechanisms, and associated risks. Clin Microbiol Rev 1997;10(3):505–20.
2. Stevens FA. The occurrence of *Staphylococcus aureus* infection with a scarlatiniform rash. JAMA 1927;88:1957–8.
3. Todd J, Fishaut M, Kapral F, et al. Toxic-shock syndrome associated with phage-group-I Staphylococci. Lancet 1978;2(8100):1116–8.

4. Fernandez-Frackelton M. Bacteria. In: Marx JA, Hockberger RS, Walls RM, et al, editors. Rosen's emergency medicine: concepts and clinical practice. Philadelphia: Mosby/Elsevier; 2010. p. 2096–105.e2.

5. Toxic Shock Syndrome (other than streptococcal) (TSS) 2011 Case Definition. Available at: http://wwwn.cdc.gov/nndss/conditions/toxic-shock-syndrome-other-than-streptococcal/case-definition/2011/. Accessed July 5, 2016.

6. Case definitions for infectious conditions under public health surveillance. Centers for Disease Control and Prevention. MMWR Recomm Rep 1997;46(RR-10): 1–55.

7. Liang SY. Toxic shock syndromes. In: Tintinalli JE, Stapczynski J, Ma O, et al, editors. Tintinalli's emergency medicine: a comprehensive study guide, 8e. New York: McGraw-Hill; 2016. Available at: http://accessmedicine.mhmedical.com/content.aspx?bookid=1658&Sectionid=109435589. Accessed July 02, 2016.

8. Hajjeh RA, Reingold A, Weil A, et al. Toxic shock syndrome in the United States: surveillance update, 1979-1996. Emerg Infect Dis 1999;5(6):807–10.

9. Gilbert D, Chambers H, Eliopoulos G, et al. The Sanford Guide to antimicrobial therapy 2015. 45th edition. Dallas (TX): Antimicrobial Therapy; 2015.

10. Andersen J, Berthelsen L, Bech Jensen B, et al. Dynamics of the meningococcal carrier state and characteristics of the carrier strains: a longitudinal study within three cohorts of military recruits. Epidemiol Infect 1998;121(1):85–94.

11. Jaffe J, Ratcliff T. Infectious disease emergencies. Chapter 42. In: Stone C, Humphries RL, editors. Current diagnosis & treatment emergency medicine, 7e. New York: McGraw-Hill; 2011. Available at: http://accessmedicine.mhmedical.com/content.aspx?bookid=385&Sectionid=40357258. Accessed July 03, 2016.

12. Apicella MA. Neisseria meningitidis. In: Mandell GL, Bennett JE, Dolin R, editors. Mandell, Douglas, and Bennett's Principles and practice of infectious diseases. 7th edition. Philadelphia: Elsevier/Churchill Livingstone; 2010. p. 2737–52.

13. Cushing K, Cohn A. Meningococcal disease. Manual for surveillance of vaccine-preventable diseases. 4th edition. Atlanta (GA): Centers for Disease Control and Prevention; 2008.

14. Barlam TF, Kasper DL. Approach to the acutely ill infected febrile patient. In: Kasper D, Fauci A, Hauser S, et al, editors. Harrison's principles of internal medicine, 19e. New York: McGraw-Hill; 2015. Available at: http://accessmedicine.mhmedical.com/content.aspx?bookid=1130&Sectionid=66320817. Accessed July 03, 2016.

15. Schaider J. Meningococcemia. Rosen & Barkin's 5-Minute Emergency Medicine Consult. 2015. Available at: http://www.r2library.com/Resource/Title/1451190670/ch0013s10895. Accessed July 15, 2016.

16. Huff JC, Weston WL, Tonnesen MG. Erythema multiforme: a critical review of characteristics, diagnostic criteria, and causes. J Am Acad Dermatol 1983; 8(6):763–75.

17. Assier H, Bastuji-Garin S, Revuz J, et al. Erythema multiforme with mucous membrane involvement and Stevens-Johnson syndrome are clinically different disorders with distinct causes. Arch Dermatol 1995;131(5):539–43.

18. Sokumbi O, Wetter DA. Clinical features, diagnosis, and treatment of erythema multiforme: a review for the practicing dermatologist. Int J Dermatol 2012; 51(8):889–902.

19. Rehmus WE. Erythema Multiforme. Merck Manual. Available at: http://www.merckmanuals.com/professional/dermatologic-disorders/hypersensitivity-and-inflammatory-disorders/erythema-multiforme. Accessed June 29, 2016.

20. Schofield JK, Tatnall FM, Leigh IM. Recurrent erythema multiforme: clinical features and treatment in a large series of patients. Br J Dermatol 1993;128:542.
21. Pereira FA, Mudgil AV, Rosmarin DM. Toxic epidermal necrolysis. J Am Acad Dermatol 2007;56:181–200.
22. Thammakumpee J, Yongsiri S. Characteristics of toxic epidermal necrolysis and Stevens-Johnson syndrome: a 5-year retrospective study. J Med Assoc Thai 2013;96(4):399–406.
23. Schwartz RA, McDonough PH, Lee BW. Toxic Epidermal Necrolysis: part I. Introduction, history, classification, clinical features, systemic manifestations, etiology, and immunopathogenesis. J Am Acad Dermatol 2013;69(2):173.e1-13.
24. Creamer D, Walsh SA, Dziewulski P, et al. U.K. guidelines for the management of Stevens–Johnson syndrome/toxic epidermal necrolysis in adults 2016. J Plast Reconstr Aesthet Surg 2016;69(6):736–41.
25. Harr T, French LE. Toxic epidermal necrolysis and Stevens-Johnson syndrome. Orphanet J Rare Dis 2010;5:39.
26. Palmieri TL, Greenhalgh DG, Saffle JR, et al. A multicenter review of toxic epidermal necrolysis treated in US burn centers at the end of the twentieth century. J Burn Care Rehabil 2002;23(2):87–96.

Pregnancy Disasters in the First Trimester

Lynn Scherer, MS, PA-C[a],*, Kayla Zappolo, MS, PA-C[b]

KEYWORDS

- Pregnancy • Ectopic pregnancy • Abortion • Vaginal bleeding • Ultrasonography
- Appendicitis • Hyperemesis gravidarum • β-hCG

KEY POINTS

- A primary goal in pregnant patients complaining of abdominal or pelvic pain with or without vaginal bleeding in the first trimester is to differentiate between ectopic pregnancy and spontaneous abortion.
- Bedside ultrasonography and β–human chorionic gonadotropin (β-hCG) allow emergency medicine clinicians to obtain accurate information faster, improving time to consultation and increasing patient satisfaction.
- Low levels of β-hCG do not reliably exclude an ectopic pregnancy.
- In patients who have undergone assisted reproduction, the finding of an intrauterine pregnancy does not exclude the diagnosis of an ectopic pregnancy.
- All female patients of childbearing age should be considered pregnant until proved otherwise.

INTRODUCTION

Conditions such as abdominal pain, pelvic pain, and vaginal bleeding are common presenting complaints to the emergency department (ED). In short, any female patient of childbearing age is pregnant until proved otherwise. Early complications of pregnancy usually happen in the first trimester, before gestational viability. Pregnant women present a diagnostic challenge to clinicians. Patients' symptoms can be vague and, through a thorough history and methodical approach to pregnant patients, clinicians will be better able to identify those women who are ultimately at risk for death from ectopic rupture and other potential life-threatening obstetric complications.

Disclosure: The authors have nothing to disclose.
[a] Department of Emergency Medicine, Albert Einstein Healthcare Network, Korman B-6, 5501 Old York Road, Philadelphia, PA 19141, USA; [b] Department of Emergency Medicine, Albert Einstein Healthcare Network, 5501 Old York Road, Philadelphia, PA 19141, USA
* Corresponding author.
E-mail address: schererl@einstein.edu

Physician Assist Clin 2 (2017) 385–400
http://dx.doi.org/10.1016/j.cpha.2017.02.004
2405-7991/17/© 2017 Elsevier Inc. All rights reserved.

Once a female patient is determined to be pregnant and is presenting with abdominal pain, pelvic pain, or vaginal bleeding, the emergency medicine clinician is left with 2 primary questions: is the pregnancy intrauterine or ectopic and, if the pregnancy is intrauterine, is the pregnancy viable? With quantitative β–human chorionic gonadotropin (β-hCG) and bedside ultrasonography (US), emergency medicine clinicians are frequently able to make a definitive diagnosis and disposition on the first visit.[1]

There has been an increase in the availability and use of bedside US in EDs. The approach to female patients with pelvic complaints (including pelvic pain, vaginal bleeding, and vaginal bleeding in pregnancy) has been transformed by the use of bedside US. Clinicians familiar with transabdominal US (TAU) and transvaginal US (TVU) examinations can obtain more accurate information faster, thereby improving time to consultation or discharge and achieving an increase in patient satisfaction.[2,3]

THE BASICS

It is important to understand fundamental information about the pregnant patient and be able to articulate those findings with the consultant obstetrician.

First and foremost, as with all patients, it is important to enter into the patient interaction with understanding and empathy and avoid judgment. The patient may, or may not, have known that she was pregnant on entering your department. It is insensitive to assume that the news you are delivering to the patient about her pregnancy status or her diagnosis is either welcome or unwelcome. It is essential to use this opportunity to be patient, sensitive, aware, and if necessary include social work resources during the patient visit. It is important to remember that this could be a pregnancy resulting from sexual abuse and the pregnancy is unwanted, or that this may be a patient who has spent her life savings on fertility treatments and the news that her pregnancy is no longer viable could be devastating.

PHYSIOLOGIC CHANGES IN PREGNANCY

Pregnancy involves a number changes in anatomy, physiology, and biochemistry. These changes can challenge the maternal reserves. Knowledge of these adaptations is critical for understanding normal laboratory measurements, knowing the drugs likely to require adjustments, and recognizing women who are predisposed to medical complications during pregnancy. Table 1 lists the changes that may be seen in early pregnancy.

EMERGENCY DEPARTMENT EVALUATION OF PREGNANT PATIENTS
Triage and Initial Management

Any female patient of childbearing age who presents with abdominal, pelvic pain, or vaginal bleeding and who is hemodynamically unstable should be moved to a major resuscitation area, have 2 large-bore intravenous (IV) lines placed, and receive an initial fluid bolus of an isotonic crystalloid solution. Rapid assessment of pregnancy status and anemia are first priorities. Patients with mild pain and/or bleeding with stable vital signs can be seen in a timely manner; however, it is important to frequently reassess vital signs in these patients to determine whether the patient's clinical course is worsening. The approach to pregnant patients should be handled similarly to that of nonpregnant patients. Determining whether a female patient is pregnant allows clinicians to expand the differential diagnosis and approach the patient in a systematic way, asking key historical questions and formulating the most likely clinical path to achieve the accurate diagnosis.

Table 1 Physiologic changes in pregnancy	
Vital Signs	• Heart rate increases 15–20 bpm • Blood pressure decreases systolic and diastolic (5–10 mm Hg and 10–15 mm Hg, respectively) • Respiratory rate unchanged
Cardiovascular Changes	• Cardiac output increases 30%–50% • Circulating blood volume increases at 6–8 wk gestation (plasma increases more than the RBCs, so the hematocrit decreases) • Systemic vascular resistance decreases
Pulmonary Changes	• Increased tidal volume by 30%–40% • Decreased functional residual capacity • Vital capacity unchanged • Oxygen demands of mother and fetus increase by approximately 20% • Increased ventilation • Decreased arterial Pco_2 (presents as dyspnea) • Arterial blood gas during pregnancy most often reveals a compensated respiratory alkalosis • Changes usually caused by increased progesterone level
Hematology Changes	• Normal leukocytosis is as high as 15,000 cells/μL • The concentrations of clotting factors, including fibrinogen (factor I) and factors VII, VIII, IX, and X, increase in pregnancy • Bleeding time, PT, PTT unchanged • Pregnancy is a hypercoagulable state = increased risk of venous thromboembolism (thromboembolism is the primary cause of maternal mortality)
Renal Changes	• Enlargement and dilation of the kidneys and urinary collecting system = normal • Glomerular filtration rate increased • BUN/Cr decreased • Frequent urination (secondary to enlarged uterus resulting in decreased bladder capacity)
GI Changes	• Decreased GI motility (secondary to increased progesterone level) • Impaired gallbladder contractility • GI changes can cause a variety of symptoms, including early N&V, hyperemesis gravidarum, GERD, and constipation • Itching can be a result of biliary cholestasis
Metabolic Changes	• Postprandial hyperglycemia • Marked hypoglycemia during periods of fasting • Insulin resistance occurs secondary to increasing levels of human placental lactogen
Musculoskeletal Changes	• Back pain: increased incidence (compensation of the lumbar spine results in a lumbar lordosis)

Abbreviations: bpm, beats per minute; BUN/Cr, blood urea nitrogen/creatinine ratio; GERD, gastroesophageal reflux disease; GI, gastrointestinal; N&V, nausea and vomiting; PT, prothrombin tine; PTT, partial thromboplastin time; RBCs, red blood cells.
Data from Refs.[1,4,5]

History of Present Illness

It is crucial to obtain a thorough history of present illness (HPI) and review of symptoms on all pregnant patients. As with all HPIs, be sure to obtain the onset, location, character, and provoking and relieving factors of the abdominal/pelvic pain or vaginal bleeding. It is also important to establish the severity of pain using a pain scale and to determine the severity of bleeding.

In abdominal pain, clinicians may obtain a history of migratory pain that originates around the umbilicus and then further localizes to the right lower quadrant, which is a classic description of acute appendicitis. However, on examination, pregnant patients may not present with classic physical findings of definitive right lower quadrant tenderness, because the enlarging uterus can cause the appendix to migrate. Therefore, right midabdomen and right upper quadrant pains are common complaints in pregnant patients with acute appendicitis, especially in the later portion of pregnancy.

As mentioned, it is important to determine the presence and degree of vaginal bleeding or vaginal discharge. The volume and duration of blood loss should be characterized. A common way to obtain this information is to quantify the number of pads the patient needs to change over a 24-hour period. In addition, it is valuable to obtain any report of passing tissue. It is vital to reassess the amount of bleeding during the patient's stay in the ED to evaluate for increasing hemorrhage and determine whether there is any hemodynamic instability caused by ongoing blood loss. If vaginal discharge has been discussed while obtaining the history, the clinician should ask about the discharge descriptors, such as odor, volume, color, and duration, and any previous treatments.

It is essential to obtain a history of the patient menstrual cycle. The patient's last menstrual period (LMP) should be determined, as should specific cycle information, including number of days and whether the cycles have been regular or irregular. The patient's LMP can be used to establish an estimated gestational age of the fetus.

It is valuable to inquire about any genitourinary complaints the patient may be having, such as urinary frequency, urgency, dysuria, or hematuria. Further essential questions to be asked during the history are whether the patient has had any recent history of trauma or syncope. If the patient is known to be pregnant, be sure to ascertain whether or not the patient has had any obstetrics care, including any US scans performed documenting intrauterine pregnancy (IUP) during the current pregnancy.

The classic triad of ectopic pregnancy is abdominal pain, missed menses, and vaginal bleeding. However, this triad is not sensitive, because up to 25% of patients lack the full triad and up to 10% have no symptoms.[5,6]

Review of Systems

Similar to nonpregnant patients, the most common symptoms of appendicitis include anorexia, nausea, and/or vomiting associated with abdominal pain. Many pregnant patients have atypical presentations of appendicitis and may also complain of symptoms such as heartburn or indigestion, diarrhea, and generalized malaise or fatigue.

Past Medical History

In evaluating any pregnant patient, clinicians must obtain a pregnancy history including gravid and parity status (Table 2); complications with past pregnancies,

Table 2 Common terminology	
G: number of times pregnant, including the current pregnancy	P: subdivided into the mnemonic: Texas Power and Light
$G4P_{1021}$	T: number of term gestations P: number of preterm deliveries/gestations A: number of abortions (spontaneous or voluntary) L: number of living offspring

Abbreviations: G, gravid; P, parity.

including history of spontaneous or elective abortions, preeclampsia, or eclampsia; or gestational diabetes. A thorough sexual history to include history of current concerns for a sexually transmitted infection is valuable and, if present, this should be added to the patient's risk factors for spontaneous abortion or ectopic pregnancy. Additional past medical history of gynecologic surgeries, such as tubal ligation, also increase the risk for ectopic pregnancy. Two other valuable aspects of the past medical history are whether or not a patient is undergoing fertility treatments and what is the Rh status. Rh status is important to determine whether the patient needs RhoGAM.

Physical Examination

Physical examination is essential when trying to determine the diagnosis of any patient. It is important to review the vital signs when the patient presents, along with serial measurements throughout the visit to ensure hemodynamic stability. Tachycardia, with or without hypotension, suggests hypovolemia and possibly ectopic rupture. Importantly, bradycardia can be present with intraabdominal hemorrhage.[7]

On the abdominal examination, note the location of abdominal tenderness and the presence of peritoneal signs (eg, guarding, rigidity), and costovertebral angle tenderness. A thorough pelvic examination should be performed with a chaperone present. Evaluate the external genitalia for causes of vaginal bleeding, such as laceration, lesion, infection, or Bartholin abscess. The speculum examination should provide enough information to document the presence of blood, clots, or products of conception (POC) in the vaginal vault, as well as internal causes of bleeding or issues arising from the cervix (eg, laceration, lesions, masses). The amount of bleeding from the cervical os should be noted and documented. In addition, the bimanual examination should assess whether or not the cervical os is open or closed, the size the uterus (Table 3), the presence of tenderness or any mass on palpation of the uterus and the adnexa, and the possible discovery of cervical motion tenderness.

DIFFERENTIAL DIAGNOSIS

There are various differentials to consider after gathering the history and performing the physical examination. First trimester bleeding occurs in 20% to 25% of all pregnancies.[4] Of that the patients who experience bleeding, approximately 50% end in spontaneous abortion and 50% proceed normally.[8] The differential can be divided into pregnancy-related diagnoses and non–pregnancy-related diagnoses (Table 4).

Ectopic Pregnancy

Ectopic pregnancy is the third leading cause of maternal mortality, with an incidence of 10%.[11] The incidence of ectopic pregnancy has increased steadily and it now

Table 3 Typical uterine size by weeks	
6–8 wk	Size of an orange
10 wk	At symphysis pubis
20 wk	At umbilicus
20+ wk	20+ wk: measure the size of the uterus from the symphysis pubis; each centimeter is equal to 1 wk of pregnancy

From Schofer JM. Emergency medicine: a focused review of the core curriculum. Milwaukee (WI): American Academy of Emergency Medicine Resident and Student Association; 2008.

Table 4	
Differential diagnosis of first trimester pregnancy complications	
Pregnancy Related	**Not Pregnancy Related**
Ectopic pregnancy	Ovarian cysts
Spontaneous abortion	Urinary tract infection/urinary calculus
Hydatidiform mole (gestational trophoblastic disease)	Appendicitis
Normal IUP	Cholelithiasis/cholecystitis
Implantation bleeding (minimal bleeding that occurs at first missed period)	Ovarian torsion
Heterotopic pregnancy	Trauma to the cervix
Corpus luteum cyst	IBD
	Pelvic infection

Abbreviation: IBD, inflammatory bowel disease.
Data from Refs.[4,9,10]

accounts for approximately 2% of all pregnancies. The incidence of ectopic pregnancy among women presenting to the ED with vaginal bleeding or pain in the first trimester is consistently as high as 14%. Only 50% of patients have the classic risk factors (Table 5).[12–14]

Ruptured ectopic pregnancy requires emergent obstetrics (OB)/gynecology (Gyn) consultation and emergent surgical intervention. Nonruptured ectopic pregnancies that are less than 4 cm with β-hCG level less than 5000 mIU/mL may be treated with methotrexate therapy, otherwise the treatment is surgical. Table 6 provides information regarding methotrexate therapy.

There are many diagnostic challenges that can lead to potential misdiagnosis and negative outcomes for patients with ectopic pregnancies. The following items are common pitfalls in the evaluation of patients with suspected ectopic pregnancy.

- Do not over-rely on the history and physical to determine risk for ectopic pregnancy. Approximately 10% of patients with ectopic pregnancy do not have pain at their initial presentations.
- The patient's β-hCG level is too low to be an ectopic. Ectopic pregnancies can happen at any β-hCG level.

Table 5	
Risk factors for ectopic pregnancy	
Previous ectopic pregnancy	History of PID
Current IUD	History of tubal ligation/tubal surgery
Smoking	Advanced age (35–44 y)
Prior spontaneous or induced abortion	Abdominal or pelvic surgery
Assisted reproduction techniques	

Abbreviations: IUD, intrauterine device; PID, pelvic inflammatory disease.
Data from Schofer JM. Emergency medicine: a focused review of the core curriculum. Milwaukee (WI): American Academy of Emergency Medicine Resident and Student Association; 2008; and Heaton HA. Ectopic pregnancy and emergencies in the first 20 weeks of pregnancy. In: Tintinalli JE, Stapczynski JS, Ma OJ, et al, editors. Tintinalli's emergency medicine: a comprehensive study guide. 8th edition. New York: McGraw-Hill Education; 2016. p. 628–6.

Table 6 Methotrexate therapy	
Essential Laboratory Tests Before Initiating Methotrexate Therapy	• CBC with differential, evaluate platelets • Hepatic profile • BMP to evaluate renal function
Absolute Contraindications	• Alcoholism • Immunodeficiency • Peptic ulcer • Active disease of the lungs, liver, kidneys, or hematopoietic system
Relative Contraindications	• Patients with an ectopic gestational sac larger than 3.5 cm or with embryonic cardiac motion observed on US

Serious Complications	• Treatment failure, with rupture of the ectopic pregnancy
	  ○ In several cohort studies, 20% of patients receiving methotrexate required surgery.
	  ○ Ruptured ectopic pregnancy must be considered in the differential diagnosis of patients who present to the ED with concerning symptoms or signs after methotrexate therapy
	  ○ If a patient presents who has had methotrexate treatment with pain or vaginal bleeding, do not perform a pelvic examination and begin the work-up for ectopic rupture and consult OB/Gyn
	• Because treatment failures are common, close follow-up must be arranged before discharge

Abbreviations: BMP, basic metabolic panel; CBC, complete blood count.
Data from Refs.[8,9,15–20]

- Do not let the radiologist talk you out of a US scan. If the β-hCG level is less than 1500 mIU/mL, radiologists may indicate that US is not indicated. Assure them you are concerned clinically for an ectopic pregnancy and are looking for evidence of that or free fluid.
- Be wary of the normal US report. US early in the course of an ectopic pregnancy can be reported as an empty uterus, no adnexal mass, and no free fluid. This finding does not rule out ectopic in patients with concerning historical and examination features.
- A normal increase in β-hCG levels does not exclude ectopic pregnancy. In the setting of an empty uterus this increases the likelihood of an ectopic pregnancy.
- Reassess the patient often. Failure to appreciate the degree of blood loss, or the progression of symptoms, may result in a poor outcome.
- Do not just wait for OB in a hemorrhaging patient who may become unstable. Although most emergency medicine clinicians do not perform uterine evacuation, performing a pelvic examination and removing any POC that may be within the cervical os often makes the uterus contract and may slow the bleeding.
- Remember to consider heterotopic, particularly if the patient has received fertility treatments or is unstable despite an IUP seen on US.
- Be sure to set up appropriate follow-up for the patient and provide good return precautions. Patient with minimal bleeding when being seen can decompensate with increased bleeding or may be evolving ectopic pregnancy.

Spontaneous Abortion

The second question clinicians have to determine is whether or not the pregnancy is viable or not. Spontaneous abortion is the most common serious complication of pregnancy and is defined as the spontaneous termination of pregnancy before 20 weeks of gestation.

Appendicitis

Acute appendicitis, in both pregnant and nonpregnant patients, is one of the most common surgical emergencies that emergency medicine clinicians encounter throughout their careers. Timely and accurate diagnosis is important to initiate proper management and prevent complications, such as perforation. The accurate diagnosis of acute appendicitis in a pregnant woman can present a challenge to clinicians /because of a multitude of factors, such as the anatomic changes related to the gravid uterus as well as the normal abdominal/gastrointestinal discomfort related to pregnancy.

In any patient, independent of pregnancy status, if there is a clinical concern for appendicitis or peritoneal signs on examination, early surgical consultation is important. However, in pregnant patients, early OB consultation should also be obtained, because OB is likely to be part of every pregnant patient's care and needs to monitor the patient throughout the hospitalization. Antibiotic administration should include coverage for both gram-negative and gram-positive bacteria. Include all consultants in the antibiotic selection. There has been recent evidence that medical management alone with antibiotics may be sufficient for select nonpregnant patients with acute appendicitis. However, research has shown that it is not recommended for pregnant patients and is associated with poor outcomes. Surgical appendectomy is considered the standard of care in the treatment of acute appendicitis in pregnant patients.

THE EVALUATION
Laboratory Evaluation

As mentioned, all women of childbearing age are considered pregnant until proved otherwise. Urine pregnancy tests are sensitive to β-hCG levels as low as 20 mIU, and these levels become detectable 9 to 11 days after ovulation and fertilization. Urine specific gravity should be noted, because urine β-hCG testing may be falsely negative if the urine is very dilute. Serum testing of β-hCG levels has a higher level of sensitivity, with quantitative detectability at serum β-hCG levels as low as 5 mIU. In general, β-hCG level doubles every 48 hours for the first 8 weeks. Table 7 lists the estimates of β-hCG levels during pregnancy. A large range is given for each gestational age; note that β-hCG level must be used in conjunction with the rest of the clinical assessment and should not be used as a stand-alone value.

Other considerations must be taken into account in the laboratory evaluation of pregnant women. If the patient's Rh status is unknown and there is no documentation of Rh status from previous pregnancies, clinicians must determine whether pregnant patients are Rh positive or negative. In Rh-negative women, administer 50 μg of anti-D immunoglobulin in all cases of documented first-trimester loss of pregnancy.[22] Consider a complete blood count (CBC) if there is a concern for significant hemorrhage or resultant anemia from blood loss. Leukocytosis with a bandemia is a common finding in acute appendicitis; however, a normal white blood cell count is not sufficient to exclude acute appendicitis. Laboratory evaluation may not be helpful and should not be relied on as the only factor when considering acute

Table 7
Serum beta human chorionic gonadotropin levels compared with gestational age

Gestational Age (wk)	hCG Level (mIU/mL)
3	5–50
4	5–426
5	18–7340
6	1080–56,500
7–8	7, 650–229,000
9–12	25,700–288,000
13–16	13,300–254,000
17–24	4060–165,400
25–40	3640–117,000

Data from Refs.[5,14,21]

appendicitis in a pregnant patient. Consider a basic metabolic panel (BMP) if there is a concern for significant electrolyte abnormalities or dehydration, especially in patients with hyperemesis who have been unable to tolerate oral intake for a prolonged period of time. Consider bedside Accu-Check if there is a concern for hypoglycemia.

Another important laboratory test in pregnant patients is the urinalysis. All pregnant women require treatment of asymptomatic bacteriuria. Asymptomatic bacteriuria has been associated with complications such as pyelonephritis and premature rupture of membranes/preterm labor.

Ultrasonography

With the wide availability of bedside US in EDs, more clinicians are now routinely using US in their evaluation of these patients.[23] The primary indication for bedside US is to evaluate for the presence of an IUP, minimizing the likelihood of an ectopic pregnancy when modifying factors such as infertility treatment (putting patients at risk of heterotopic pregnancy) are not present. The bedside US scan can include either a TAU or TVU to verify the presence of an IUP. The bedside ED US scan may or may not visualize the adnexa well.[23] If the adnexa, uterus, and cul-de-sac cannot be well visualized, a formal US scan should be performed by the radiology department. US has become the modality of choice given the risk of adverse side effects of radiation exposure, and is considered the safest primary imaging modality for both pregnant and nonpregnant patients.[24,25] Tables 8 and 9 provide guides to what is seen on TAU and TVU during pregnancy and how the study may be optimized.

Using US in the evaluation of pregnancy-related complaints in the ED requires each clinician to be aware of the various potential findings. An IUP is typically confirmed by the finding of a double gestational sac with an intrauterine fetal pole or yolk sac. Depending on gestational age, fetal heart activity may also be observed. Normal fetal cardiac activity varies from 120 beats/min (bpm) to 170 bpm during the gestational period. The US findings of an ectopic pregnancy can be divided into findings that are diagnostic, suggestive, or indeterminate of an ectopic pregnancy. Ectopic fetal heart activity or an ectopic fetal pole are findings that are diagnostic of an ectopic pregnancy. Findings that are suggestive of an ectopic gestation include a moderate to large amount of cul-de-sac fluid without an IUP or an adnexal mass without an IUP (usually complex). Often in early gestation there are indeterminate findings that cannot rule out potential ectopic pregnancy. An empty uterus, nonspecific fluid

Table 8	
Ultrasonography findings, approach, and optimization	
TAU	TVU
5–6 wk: gestational sac visible	4–5 wk: gestational sac visible
7–8 wk: fetal pole and fetal heart activity are visible	6–7 wk: fetal pole and fetal heart activity are visible
Optimized if bladder is full	Optimized if bladder is empty

collections, and an abnormal sac are a few of the most common findings in ectopic pregnancies. Even if a single gestational sac is identified, there still may be concern for a heterotopic pregnancy in patients taking fertility medications. The finding of a bunch-of-grapes or snowstorm appearance is characteristic of a hydatidiform mole (gestational trophoblastic disease).[9]

US can also be helpful in identifying other causes of bleeding during pregnancy, such as a hemorrhagic ovarian cyst or subchorionic hemorrhage. It can also be helpful in the initial evaluation of appendicitis. Often, a healthy appendix cannot be visualized on US. However, in acute appendicitis, a tubular noncompressible structure measuring more than 7 mm in diameter without peristalsis can be diagnostic. In nonpregnant patients in whom US either cannot be used or results in an inconclusive study, computed tomography (CT) with IV contrast should be used. In pregnant patients, there is concern for fetal exposure to the ionizing radiation associated with CT of the abdomen and pelvis. MRI is the diagnostic study of choice in pregnant patients when US cannot be obtained or the results are inconclusive.[9]

In addition, with respect to the use of bedside US in the evaluation of pregnant patients, the American College of Emergency Physicians (ACEP) has developed a clinical policy regarding critical issues in the initial evaluation and management of patients presenting to the ED in early pregnancy.[22] Within the clinical policy are recommendations for use of US and quantitative β-hCG levels. Clinical findings and strengths of recommendations regarding patient management were made according to the following criteria:

- Level A recommendations: generally accepted principles for patient management that reflect a high degree of clinical certainty (based on strength of evidence class I or overwhelming evidence from strength of evidence class II studies that directly address all of the issues).

Table 9	
β–Human chorionic gonadotropin levels and associated ultrasonography findings	
β-hCG Level (mIU/mL)	Associated Findings
>1500	IUP typically visible by TVU Cardiac activity typically visible on TVU
2000	Level typically expected time of missed menses
>3000	IUP typically visible by TAU
>6500	Cardiac activity typically visible on TAU
Undetectable	Typically 3–4 wk postpartum

Data from Sohoni A, Bosley J, Miss JC. Bedside ultrasonography for obstetric and gynecologic emergencies. Crit Care Clin 2014;30(2):207–26, v.

- Level B recommendations: may identify a particular strategy or range of management strategies that reflect moderate clinical certainty (based on strength of evidence class II studies that directly address the issue, decision analysis that directly addresses the issue, or strong consensus of strength of evidence class III studies).
- Level C recommendations: strategies for patient management that are based on class III studies, or, in the absence of any adequate published literature, based on panel consensus.

The ACEP recommendations on the use of US in early pregnancy include the following clinical questions:

1. Should emergency physicians obtain pelvic US scans in clinically stable pregnant patients who present to the ED with abdominal pain and/or vaginal bleeding and a β-hCG level below a discriminatory threshold?
   - Level A recommendations: none
   - Level B recommendations: none
   - Level C recommendations: perform or obtain a pelvic US scan for symptomatic pregnant patients with β-hCG levels below any discriminatory threshold.
2. In patients who have an indeterminate transvaginal US scan, what is the diagnostic utility of β-hCG for predicting possible ectopic pregnancy?
   - Level A recommendations: none specified
   - Level B recommendations: do not use the β-hCG value to exclude the diagnosis of ectopic pregnancy in patients who have an indeterminate US scan
   - Level C recommendations: obtain specialty consultation or arrange close outpatient follow-up for all patients with an indeterminate pelvic US scan

The treatment of patients in early pregnancy requires a sense of urgency, a methodical process, and attention to detail. Fig. 1 provides an algorithmic approach to the incorporation of US into the evaluation and management of pregnant patients.

SPECIAL CIRCUMSTANCES OF EARLY PREGNANCY
Hyperemesis Gravidarum

Nausea with or without vomiting is so common in early pregnancy that mild symptoms may be considered part of the normal physiology of the first trimester. Some degree of nausea with or without vomiting occurs in up to 90% of pregnancies. The incidence of women with severe symptoms is not well documented and reports vary from 0.3% to 3% of pregnancies.[26] The mean onset of symptoms is 5 to 6 weeks' gestation, symptoms peak at about 9 weeks, and usually resolve during the middle of the second trimester. However, symptoms may continue all the way until delivery.[27–29] Sixty percent of women are asymptomatic 6 weeks after onset of nausea.[28] Although the lay term for mild pregnancy-related nausea and vomiting is morning sickness, the symptoms may occur at any time of day and often (80%) persist throughout the day.

Hyperemesis gravidarum is considered a severe form of nausea and vomiting, although there is no clear demarcation between common pregnancy-related morning sickness and this infrequent pathologic disorder. The diagnosis can be made in women with pregnancy-related vomiting that occurs more than 3 times

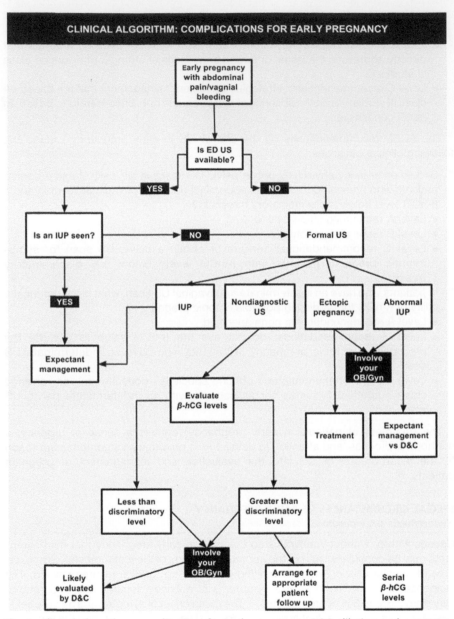

CLINICAL ALGORITHM: COMPLICATIONS FOR EARLY PREGNANCY

Fig. 1. Clinical algorithm: complications for early pregnancy. D&C, dilation and curettage. (*Adapted from* Houry D. Complications in pregnancy part I: early pregnancy. Emergency Medicine Practice 2007;9(6):16.)

per day with weight loss greater than 3 kg or 5% of body weight and ketonuria.[30] In contrast with women with mild disease, women with hyperemesis have orthostatic hypotension, laboratory abnormalities, and physical signs of dehydration.

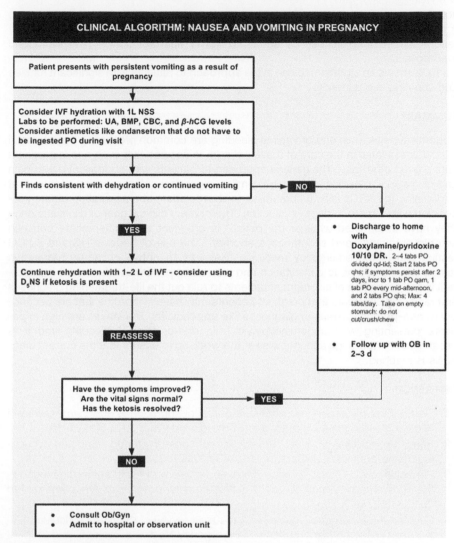

Fig. 2. Clinical algorithm: nausea and vomiting in pregnancy. D₅NS, 5% dextrose in normal saline; DR, distribution ratio; IVF, intravenous fluid; Max, maximum; NSS, normal saline solution; PO, by mouth; qd, every day; qam, every morning; qhs, at bedtime; tabs, tablets; tid, 3 times a day; UA, urinalysis. (*Adapted from* Houry D. Complications in pregnancy part I: early pregnancy. Emergency Medicine Practice 2007;9(6):17.)

Although there are scoring systems for the diagnosis of hyperemesis gravidarum, they have not been validated for guiding management. The standard initial evaluation of pregnant women with persistent nausea and vomiting includes measurement of weight, orthostatic blood pressure, heart rate, laboratory tests, and an obstetric US examination (if not previously performed). The fetal heart rate should be determined to confirm viability.

Patients who present with severe symptoms of nausea but seem hydrated can be managed as outpatients; however, if they present with persistent or prolonged vomiting or have symptoms of dehydration, rehydration with IV fluids should occur. If the patient has ketonuria suspected from starvation metabolism, it is generally recommended that glucose be added to the IV fluid solution to reverse ketotic metabolism.

Fig. 2 shows an algorithm to use in the approach to patients with significant nausea and vomiting in pregnancy.

SUMMARY

Abdominal/pelvic pain and/or vaginal bleeding are common presenting symptoms in EDs. It is essential in the care of these patients to assume that everyone is pregnant until proved otherwise. The general approach to patients with abdominal/pelvic pain and/or vaginal bleeding should be similar regardless of pregnancy status, first addressing the ABCs (airway, breathing, and circulation) of resuscitation before proceeding with a more in-depth evaluation. The primary clinical goal of clinicians once they have determined whether the patient is pregnant is to differentiate between ectopic pregnancy and spontaneous abortion. The use of bedside US and β-hCG testing allows the emergency medicine clinicians to obtain accurate information faster, improving time to consultation and increasing patient satisfaction. It is important in the evaluation of all pregnant patients to rule out the life-threatening diagnoses first, and stay cognizant that pregnant patients may have symptoms that are secondary to non–pregnancy-related diagnoses like appendicitis. The stakes are high in patients presenting with abdominal/pelvic pain and/or vaginal bleeding and it is essential to be thorough and stepwise in the work-up to ensure that the correct diagnosis is reached.

REFERENCES

1. Dart R. First-trimester emergencies: a practical approach to abdominal pain and vaginal bleeding in early pregnancy. Emerg Med Pract 2003;5(11):1–15.
2. Sohoni A, Bosley J, Miss JC. Bedside ultrasonography for obstetric and gynecologic emergencies. Crit Care Clin 2014;30(2):207–26.
3. Panebianco NL, Shofer F, Fields JM, et al. The utility of transvaginal ultrasound in the ED evaluation of complications of first trimester pregnancy. Am J Emerg Med 2015;33(6):743–8.
4. Schofer JM. Emergency medicine: a focused review of the core curriculum. Milwaukee (WI): American Academy of Emergency Medicine Resident and Student Association; 2008.
5. Beckman C, Ling F, Barzansky B, et al. Obstetrics and gynecology. 6th edition. Philadelphia, PA: Lippincott Williams & Wilkins; 2010.
6. Ectopic pregnancy, Medscape. 2016. Available at: http://emedicine.medscape.com/article/2041923-overview. Accessed July 12, 2016.
7. Snyder HS. Lack of a tachycardic response to hypotension with ruptured ectopic pregnancy. Am J Emerg Med 1990;8(1):23–6.
8. Episode 23: Vaginal bleeding in early pregnancy, emergency medicine cases. 2012. Available at: https://emergencymedicinecases.com/episode-23-vaginal-bleeding-in-early-pregnancy. Accessed August 1, 2016.
9. Houry D. Complications in pregnancy part I: early pregnancy. Emerg Med Pract 2007;9(6):1–22.
10. Heaton HA. Ectopic pregnancy and emergencies in the first 20 weeks of pregnancy. In: Tintinalli JE, Stapczynski JS, Ma OJ, et al, editors. Tintinalli's

emergency medicine: a comprehensive study guide. 8th edition. New York: McGraw-Hill Education; 2016. p. 628–36.

11. Morrison LJ, Toma A, Gray S. General approach to the pregnant patient. In: Marx J, Hockberger R, Walls R, editors. Rosen's emergency medicine concepts and clinical practice. 8th edition. Philadelphia: Elsevier Saunders; 2014. p. 2271–81.

12. van Mello NM, Mol F, Ankum WM, et al. Ectopic pregnancy: how the diagnostic and therapeutic management has changed. Fertil Steril 2012;98(5):1066–73.

13. Stovall TG, Kellerman AL, Ling FW, et al. Emergency department diagnosis of ectopic pregnancy. Ann Emerg Med 1990;19(10):1098.

14. Tulandi T. Ectopic pregnancy: clinical manifestations and diagnosis. Netherlands: Wolters Kluwer, Alphen aan den Rijn, Uptodate; 2016. Available at: http://www.uptodate.com/contents/ectopic-pregnancy-clinical-manifesta tions-and-diagnosis?source=see_link. Accessed July 25, 2016.

15. American College of Obstetricians and Gynecologists. Medical management of ectopic pregnancy. ACOG Practice Bulletin No. 94. Washington, DC: ACOG; 2008.

16. Periti E, Comparetto C, Villanucci A, et al. The use of intravenous methotrexate in the treatment of ectopic pregnancy. J Chemother 2004;16:211–5.

17. Ransom MX, Garcia AJ, Bohrer M, et al. Serum progesterone as a predictor of methotrexate success in the treatment of ectopic pregnancy. Obstet Gynecol 1994;83:1033–7.

18. Tawfiq A, Agameya A-F, Claman P. Predictors of treatment failure for ectopic pregnancy treated with single-dose methotrexate. Fertil Steril 2000;74:877–80.

19. Rozenberg P, Chevret S, Camus E, et al. Medical treatment of ectopic pregnancies: a randomized clinical trial comparing methotrexate-mifepristone and methotrexate-placebo. Hum Reprod 2003;18:1802–8.

20. Kumtepe Y, Kadanali S. Medical treatment of ruptured with hemodynamically stable and unruptured ectopic pregnancy patients. Eur J Obstet Gynecol Reprod Biol 2004;116:221–5.

21. Bernstein D, Hahn S. Critical issues in the initial evaluation and management of patients presenting to the emergency department in early pregnancy. Available at: www.ACEP.org: http://www.acepnow.com/article/critical-issues-initial-evaluation-management-patients-presenting-emergency-department-early-pregnancy/?singlepage=1. Accessed July 18, 2016.

22. Hahn S, Lavonas E, Mace S, et al. Clinical policy: critical issues in the initial evaluation and management of patients presenting to the emergency department in early pregnancy. Ann Emerg Med 2012;60:381–90. Available at: https://www.acep.org/MobileArticle.aspx?id=48489&coll_id=618&parentid=740.

23. Moore CL, Molina AA, Lin H. Ultrasonography in community emergency departments in the United States: access to ultrasonography performed by consultants and status of emergency physician–performed ultrasonography. Ann Emerg Med 2006;47:147–53.

24. Barnhart KT, Simhan H, Kamelle SA. Diagnostic accuracy of ultrasound above and below the beta-hCG discriminatory zone. Obstet Gynecol 1999;94(4):583.

25. Jammal M, Josh Ennis J, Gharahbaghian L. Tips for trans-abdominal pelvis imaging in first trimester pregnancy. ACEP.org. Available at: https://www.acep.org/content.aspx?id=98218. Accessed July 18, 2016.

26. Matthews A, Haas DM, O'Mathúna DP, et al. Interventions for nausea and vomiting in early pregnancy. Cochrane Database Syst Rev 2015;(9):CD007575.

27. Association of Professors of Gynecology and Obstetrics. Nausea and vomiting of pregnancy. Washington, DC: Association of Professors of Gynecology and Obstetrics; 2001.

28. Goodwin TM. Hyperemesis gravidarum. Obstet Gynecol Clin North Am 2008;35: 401.

29. Fell DB, Dodds L, Joseph KS, et al. Risk factors for hyperemesis gravidarum requiring hospital admission during pregnancy. Obstet Gynecol 2006;107:277.

30. Golberg D, Szilagyi A, Graves L. Hyperemesis gravidarum and *Helicobacter pylori* infection: a systematic review. Obstet Gynecol 2007;110:695.

Current Concepts in the Evaluation of the Febrile Child

Michelle Lynn Seithel, BS, MSPAS, PA-C*,
Krysta Jade Arnold, BS, MSPAS, PA-C

KEYWORDS

- Fever • Serious bacterial infection • Thermometer • Immunizations
- Yale Observation Scale • Rochester criteria • Philadelphia criteria • Boston criteria

KEY POINTS

- Pediatric fever is a common and challenging presenting complaint.
- A thorough history and physical examination and correct method of temperature measurement are crucial.
- Immunization rates remain high, but some vaccine-preventable diseases are on the rise.
- Clinical decision tools and diagnostic evaluation are used to risk stratify febrile children.
- All children who appear ill or are under 28 days should be hospitalized.

INTRODUCTION

Febrile children account for a substantial proportion of emergency department (ED) visits. Most children who present with fever are less than 3 years of age.[1] Patients presenting with fever can be among of the more daunting challenges that providers face. Determining the source of the fever, the child's associated risks of serious illness or complication, offering assurances to worried parents, and creating a treatment plan that brings all of those things together can be difficult for even the most experienced ED provider. Throughout this article, the authors will discuss pediatric fever, and the current concepts in evaluation and management of the febrile child. The authors will discuss how certain factors must influence ED provider approach and management of febrile children, as well as the approach to febrile children within certain age cohorts. A discussion on immunizations and the way they have shaped current evaluation of fever in children will occur. The authors will also discuss how to incorporate evidence-based clinical decision rules into ED provider practice.

Disclosure Statement: The authors have nothing to disclose.
Emergency Department, University of Missouri Hospitals and Clinics, One Hospital Drive, 1E10, DC0 29.00, Columbia, MO 65212, USA
* Corresponding author.
E-mail address: seithelm@health.missouri.edu

Physician Assist Clin 2 (2017) 401–420
http://dx.doi.org/10.1016/j.cpha.2017.02.005
2405-7991/17/Published by Elsevier Inc.

physicianassistant.theclinics.com

FEVER

Fever is a controlled increase in body temperature over the normal values for an individual.[2] Several different definitions of fever exist, but most experts define fever as a rectal temperature of 38°C or above.[3] The hypothalamus regulates body temperature in response to changes in blood temperature, as well as neural connections to receptors in skin and muscle. Fever results when the body's thermostat has been reset to a higher temperature in response to increased circulating endogenous pyrogens. There are a variety of conditions that can cause fever (Box 1).[2,3] Contrary to popular belief, a single normal body temperature does not exist. Every person exhibits diurnal variation in body temperature, with lower body temperatures in the morning, and temperatures up to 1°C higher in the afternoon or early evening. Healthy individuals have been known to have a mean rectal body temperature between 36.1 C and 37.4 C.[4]

EVALUATION OF THE FEBRILE CHILD
Method of Fever Measurement

There are many methods of body temperature measurement that can be used to evaluate febrile children. Choice of oral, rectal, axillary, temporal, or tympanic thermometer should vary among patient population. And, since the method of temperature measurement varies among EDs, the ED provider should also know the benefits and limitations to each method of temperature measurement (Table 1).[5] For example, tympanic measurement may give false readings if the instrument is not properly positioned or the external ear canal is occluded by wax, regardless of the age group in

---

Box 1
Conditions that can cause fever in pediatric patients

Viral infections

Bacterial infections

Malignancy

Rheumatic diseases

Autoimmune disease

Metabolic diseases

Vaccine administration

Medications

Biologic agents

Tissue injury

Central nervous system abnormalities

Inflammatory diseases

Granulomatous diseases

Endocrine disorders

Genetic disorders

Excess exposure to environmental heat

From Behrman RE, Kliegman RM, Jenson HB. Nelson's textbook of pediatrics. 18th edition. London: W. B. Saunders; 1999; and Hay WW. Current pediatric diagnosis & treatment. 18th edition. New York: Lange Medical Books/McGraw-Hill, Medical Pub. Division; 2007.

Table 1
Methods of temperature measurement

Thermometer Type	Benefits of Use	Limitations to Use
Axillary	• Least invasive • Recommended by American Academy of Pediatrics for all infants	• Least accurate • Requires placement in axilla for 4 min
Oral	• Easily accessed site • More accurate than axillary measurement	• Altered by eating or drinking within 15 min of measurement • Not recommended under age 2 • Requires closed mouth for 3–4 min
Rectal	• Most accurate	• Variable readings depending on depth of insertion and stool in rectum • Discomfort • Risk of rectal perforation in infants
Temporal	• Easily accessed site • Fast • Second most accurate site	• Insulation of site by clothing or other coverings may affect readings • Diaphoresis may affect readings
Tympanic	• Fast • Easily accessed site	• Poor accuracy • Affected by environmental temperature, cerumen impaction, and otitis media • Not recommended in patients under 6 mo of age

From Ward MA. Patient information: fever in children (beyond the basics). Fever in infants and children: pathophysiology and management. 2016. Available at: http://www.uptodate.com/contents/fever-in-children-beyond-the-basics. Accessed July 26, 2016.

which the device is used.[3] The ED provider should be cautious not to dismiss parent claims of fever prior to ED arrival regardless of method used to measure temperature, or the child's temperature upon ED presentation. Studies have verified that mothers are able to reliably indicate presence or absence of a fever without the use of a thermometer.[6] Neonates that have a historical fever but no fever on presentation have been found to have an 8.4% rate of serious bacterial infection (SBI).[7]

Collection of the Clinical History

Preverbal patients presenting to the ED for evaluation of fever require careful and complete clinical history collection. ED providers should take care to ask parents and/or caregivers about the following

- Duration of fever
- Maximum temperature recorded at home
- Chronic medical conditions and past medical history
- Immunization status of the child
- Potential exposure to known infectious agents including sick contacts within the home
- Recent travel
- Observed associated symptoms (**Box 2**)[3]

Box 2
Associated symptoms of fever

Ear pulling

Cough

Vomiting

Diarrhea

Inconsolable crying

Crying when moved or even touched

Neck stiffness

Purple spots or dots on the skin

Rashes

Drooling or inability to swallow

Difficulty awakening child

Labored breathing

Crying with urination

From Hay WW. Current pediatric diagnosis & treatment. 18th edition. New York: Lange Medical Books/McGraw-Hill, Medical Pub. Division; 2007.

- Medications given
- Fluid intake
- Urine output
- Group B Strep and herpes simplex virus (HSV) status of the mother in neonates
- Complications of pregnancy, delivery, and puerperal period

Physical Examination

The physical examination of a febrile child is extremely important and should be thorough. A careful review of the vital signs, including respiratory rate, oxygen saturation, and heart rate should also be completed. Physical examination assessment should include

- Appearance and hydration status (including evaluation of the fontanelle)
- Breathing
- Head, ears, eyes, nose, and throat (HEENT) evaluation
- Abdominal and genitourinary (GU) evaluation
- Musculoskeletal evaluation
- Skin inspection
- Neurologic evaluation

Abnormalities should be noted, and if consistent with history, deemed as the possible source of the fever. For a brief review on physical examination abnormalities worth noting in evaluation of the febrile child, see **Table 2**.[2,3]

Diagnostic Evaluation

In certain circumstances, diagnostic testing should be completed when evaluating the febrile child. Those circumstances include

- Age of patient less than 90 day old
- Fever of unknown origin

Table 2
Physical examination abnormalities

Appearance and Hydration Status	• Dry mucous membranes • Sunken, bulging, or flat fontanelles
Breathing	• Evaluation of oxygen saturation • Accessory muscle use or retractions • Respiratory rate • Auscultation of crackles, wheezes, or rhonchi
HEENT	• Conjunctivitis • Swelling of eyelid or presence of eyelid lesions • Cutaneous oral lesions • Pharyngeal erythema or swelling • Inflammation of the ear canal • Ear canal or nasal foreign body • Inflammation or rupture of the tympanic membrane • Nasal congestion or rhinorrhea
Abdominal and GU	• Presence of peritonitis • Hyperactive bowel sounds • Distention • Presence of a mass or organomegaly • GU skin lesions • GU area hygiene
Musculoskeletal	• Joint swelling • Joint erythema • Limited range of motion of one or more joints
Skin	• Rash • Open wounds • Cellulitis or abscess formation
Neurologic	• Regression of previous developmental milestones • Inconsolable crying • Irritable or odd behavior • Abnormal alertness or attentiveness • Abnormal responses to noise, light, and touch • Poor muscle tone or posturing

From Behrman RE, Kliegman RM, Jenson HB. Nelson's textbook of pediatrics. 18th edition. London: W. B. Saunders; 1999; and Hay WW. Current pediatric diagnosis & treatment. 18th edition. New York: Lange Medical Books/McGraw-Hill, Medical Pub. Division; 2007.

- Physical examination findings that are concerning for pathologic processes that require further diagnostic testing
- Ill-appearing

Routine use of diagnostic testing is not recommended in febrile children. A well-appearing, well-hydrated, low-risk, immunized child over a certain age threshold with evidence of a routine viral infection can be safely sent home with symptomatic treatment and careful return precautions. Many focal bacterial infections can also be treated on an outpatient basis with appropriate oral antibiotics.[2] Routine diagnostic testing often ordered for evaluation of the febrile child includes, but is not limited to

- Complete blood count
- C-reactive protein (CRP)
- Procalcitonin
- Blood culture

- Urinalysis
- Urine culture
- Chest radiograph (CXR)
- Cerebral spinal fluid analysis
- Respiratory viral testing

Complete Blood Cell Count

A complete blood count, including the absolute number of neutrophils (ANC) or band formation, can be helpful in predicting occult bacteremia in a febrile child. Although this test lacks both specificity and sensitivity, research does suggest that the higher the white blood cell (WBC) count and number of band forms, the greater the risk of bacteremia.[1] Most clinical practice guidelines suggest using a total WBC of at least 15,000 as a determining factor between patients who can be observed and those who need empiric antibiotic therapy.[8]

C-Reactive Protein

CRP is an acute phase reactant that is released in response to inflammation. Elevated CRP levels are more sensitive and specific than WBC in distinguishing febrile children with SBI from those without bacterial illness.[9] CRP has been studied numerous times in an effort to provide a better laboratory predictor of SBI. Studies suggest that a CRP less than 5 mg/dL effectively rules out SBI in the febrile child.[9]

Procalcitonin

Procalcitonin is released from all tissues in response to a bacterial infection. An increase in circulating procalcitonin associated with bacterial infection or sepsis is reported to be more rapid and more specific than WBC elevation. An elevated procalcitonin level has a sensitivity between 73% and 96% and specificity between 50% and 94% in predicting SBI in the febrile child.[10]

Blood Culture

A single large volume blood culture is recommended if the child appears ill, if the degree of illness is uncertain, or if antibiotic therapy is to be initiated immediately.[4] Bacteria isolated from culture, as well as sensitivity to antibiotic classes, allows the provider to tailor therapy for the child. Outpatient therapy is still possible, as long as the parents have a reliable method to be reached and the ability to return if the culture should return positive.

Urinalysis and Urine Culture

All children without identifiable source of fever, particularly female children and uncircumcised male children under the age of 2 years, should have a urine sample collected by urethral catheterization or suprapubic aspiration.[9] A urinalysis (UA) showing greater than 10 WBC per high power field (hpf) is considered positive and warrants treatment. A urine culture is the definitive test to establish or exclude the diagnosis of a urinary tract infection. A Gram-stained smear of urine sediment may be used to obtain immediate information, as approximately 40% of young children with a urinary tract infection have a normal UA.[1]

Chest Radiograph

A chest radiograph is helpful in children with evidence of pulmonary disease and fever. Evidence of pulmonary disease includes[8]

- Respiratory rate greater than 50 breaths per minute
- Rales, rhonchi, retractions, or wheezing on lung auscultation
- Grunting, retractions, or nasal flaring
- Cough
- Coryza
- Stridor

Most nontoxic-appearing children with infiltrates on chest radiograph are presumed to have viral, not bacterial, infection, because they almost always have negative blood cultures.[1] If there is consolidation and air bronchograms suggestive of aveolar disease or diffuse bilateral small fluffy infiltrates with increased peribronchial markings suggestive of bronchopneumonia; a bacterial process is more likely.[8]

Cerebral Spinal Fluid Analysis

Lumbar puncture and cerebral spinal fluid analysis are the only tests to exclude the diagnosis of meningitis.[1] Febrile children that meet the following criteria should always undergo lumbar puncture as part of their diagnostic evaluation

- Less than 28 day old
- Ill or toxic appearance
- High risk of bacterial infection, as outlined by clinical decision guides listed later in this article
- Evidence of invasive infection
- New seizure during a fever-free period
- Meningeal signs on physical examination

It is ideal to complete the lumbar puncture prior to administration of empiric antibiotics.[8] However, a delay in being able to preform a lumbar puncture should not prevent the patient from quickly receiving antibiotics.

Respiratory Virus Testing

A multitude of respiratory viruses can cause fever in childhood. Influenza, parainfluenza, and respiratory syncytial virus (RSV) are among a few of the most common respiratory viruses to affect children. Local community and seasonal outbreak trends should be considered when evaluating febrile children for respiratory viruses, and clinical diagnosis can be as accurate as most laboratory testing, especially with RSV.[3] Common complications of most respiratory virus infections are more likely when secondary bacterial infection is present.[3] There is significant risk of the febrile child to have concomitant urinary tract infection (UTI) in cases of bronchiolitis caused by RSV, as well as a high risk of SBI with parainfluenza.[11] With the risk of SBI being high in the presence of positive respiratory viral testing, febrile children with respiratory viruses should have additional diagnostic testing. In the setting of positive laboratory or clinical diagnosis of RSV, at least a UA and urine culture should also be completed. In the setting of parainfluenza, the child should also have a UA, urine culture, CBC count, and blood culture.[11]

DIAGNOSTIC TESTING IN THE FUTURE-RNA BIOSIGNATURE ANALYSIS

RNA biosignatures are responses found within the leukocytes of hosts infected with microbial pathogens, and the approach of analyzing those biosignatures has already demonstrated value in distinguishing between viral and bacterial infections in older children and adults.[12] A recent study looking at the use of RNA biosignature analysis in children 60 days old or younger suggests that the use of this analysis may reduce the need for blood, urine, and cerebrospinal fluid (CSF) cultures in the future.[12]

FEVER BY AGE

As children age, many factors change the likelihood, circumstance, and severity of illness associated with fever. Special consideration should be given to the age of the child presenting with fever.

0 to 28 Days Old

Because of their susceptibility to serious disease, including sepsis, children present-ing with fever at this age should be treated conservatively.[2] The risks and conse-quences associated with unrecognized and untreated SBI is high within this group. SBI involves the presence of bacteremia, UTI, pneumonia, meningitis, osteomyelitis, or septic arthritis.[10] In addition to community-acquired infections, children in this age group may also have been exposed to perinatal bacteria (ie, group B *Strepto-coccus*) and viruses (ie, HSV). SBI is present in 10% to 15% of previously healthy full-term infants presenting with rectal temperatures of at least 38°C.[2] The Rochester Criteria, outlined later in this article, are used to stratify patients into risk groups within this age range. A full diagnostic evaluation, as outlined previously, and hospital admis-sion for parental antibiotics, should be strongly considered in all circumstances within this age group. Common organisms that cause febrile illness and SBI in neonates include

- Group B *Streptococcus*
- *Escherichia coli* and other gram-negative rods
- *Enterococcus*
- *Listeria monocytogenes*
- *Streptococcus pneumoniae*
- *Haemophilus influenzae*
- *Neisseria meningitidis*
- HSV

29 to 90 Days Old

Children in this age group are at risk for invasive infection from perinatal organisms as well as from community sources. Several risk stratification tools are available in this age group, and are outlined later in this article. If the child appears ill, or if there is any uncertainty regarding the child's condition or risk status, diagnostic studies are recommended.[8] Because children less than 90 day old are not fully immunized against pneumococcus and *H influenzae* type b, even well-appearing children in this age group may need to undergo diagnostic testing. Diagnostic testing in this age group should include at least a CBC, a UA, as well as blood and urine cultures. A lumbar puncture should be considered for children in this age group who present with fever with meningeal signs, rash characteristic of meningitis, or neurologic symptoms. Stool cultures may be useful in evaluation of children who have fever and diarrhea that may be consistent with colitis.[8] Common organisms that cause febrile illness and SBI in this age group include

- Group B *Streptococcus*
- *E coli* and other gram-negative rods
- *Enterococcus*
- *L monocytogenes*

- *S pneumoniae*
- *H influenzae*
- *N meningitidis*
- Respiratory syncytial virus
- Influenza and parainfluenza viruses

90 Days to 36 Months Old

It is difficult to estimate the risk of SBI in children of this age group because of the increased immunization coverage of the most common invasive organisms. The Yale Observation Scale (YOS), outlined later in this article, can be used for risk stratification to determine which febrile children in this age group should undergo diagnostic testing and possible hospital admission for parenteral antibiotics. Ill-appearing, febrile children in this age group should undergo diagnostic testing to include at least a CBC, UA, and blood and urine cultures.

In well-appearing, previously healthy immunized children in this age group who have a fever less than 39°C, clinical evaluation without diagnostic testing or antibiotic therapy can occur if the patient is able to have outpatient follow-up in 2 to 3 days.[13] Use of diagnostic testing within this age group should be tailored to the symptoms with which the patient presents if the source of fever is not identified by physical examination findings. The most common organisms causing fever and SBI in children of this age group include

- *E coli*
- Group A *Streptococcus*
- *Salmonella*
- *S pneumoniae* (in unimmunized children)
- *H influenzae* (in unimmunized children)
- *N meningitidis*
- *S aureus*
- RSV
- Influenza and parainfluenza viruses

IMMUNIZATIONS

The immunization of children against a multitude of preventable diseases has changed the way that children presenting with fever are assessed and treated. Immunizations have decreased the morbidity and mortality of many infectious diseases, and are touted as one of the greatest achievements in public health.[14] For example, cases of *H influenzae* type B in children less than 5 year old were the leading cause of bacterial meningitis and SBI in the prevaccine era.[15] These cases have now decreased by 99%.[16] Prior to having a vaccine against them, over 700 cases of meningitis, 5 million ear infections, and 200 deaths could be blamed pneumococcal infections. Severe pneumococcal infections in children have been reduced by 88% through vaccination.[17] Even children who are partially immunized, those who have not had the 12- to 15-month booster series, are considered at much lower risk for SBI.[18] Currently, there are immunizations for 16 common vaccine-preventable diseases (VPDs) that are recommended by the US Centers for Disease Control and Prevention in children from birth to 18 years of age (Box 3).[19]

It is imperative that the ED provider questions the parents regarding immunization history in any child presenting with fever. If the parents have elected not to immunize or delay immunization, VPDs must be considered as the potential fever source. Nationally, the number of children who are vaccinated remains high, with a median

---

Box 3
Immunizations recommended for children from birth to 18 years of age

Diphtheria, tetanus, pertussis (DTap)

Haemophilus influenzae type b (Hib)

Hepatitis A (HepA)

Hepatitis B (HepB)

Human papillomavirus (2vHPV, 4vHPV, 9vHPV)

Inactivated poliovirus (IPV)

Influenza (IIV, LAIV)

Measles, mumps, rubella (MMR)

Meningococcal (Hib-MenCY, MenACWY-D, MenACWY-CRM, MenB)

Pneumococcal conjugate (PCV13)

Rotavirus (RV)

Varicella (VAR)

From Birth-18 Years & "Catch-up" Immunization Schedules. Centers for Disease Control and Prevention. 2016. Available at: http://www.cdc.gov/vaccines/schedules/hcp/child-adolescent.html. Accessed July 10, 2016.

---

exemption rate for school aged children only 1.7%.[20] However, there has recently been a resurgence of some VPDs secondary to parental vaccination hesitancy, including pertussis and measles.[14] This reluctance to fully immunize children has also threatened the herd immunity that has previously protected children that were unable to be immunized due to age or other health problems. In 2014, there were 644 cases of measles (as opposed to 32 in 2004) and 17,325 cases of pertussis in the United States.[20] Both of these VPDs can cause SBI and lead to severe complications. All health care providers should be knowledgeable of the safety and efficacy of immunizations. ED providers should feel compelled to use this knowledge to discuss immunizations with vaccine hesitant parents. Provider resources on ways to discuss vaccinations with parents can be found online at www.cdc.gov/vaccinations/conversations.

CLINICAL DECISION GUIDES

There are several clinical decision guides available to help risk stratify children presenting with fever. With the exception of the YOS, most utilize diagnostic studies to classify patients into risk groups. The YOS has been shown, with a high negative predictive value, to be a reasonably accurate test to predict bacteremia.[21] The YOS, described in **Table 3**,[21] can be easily learned and used as a triage tool for ED providers attempting to determine the necessity of further diagnostic testing in febrile children. A child with a positive YOS, with a score of 10 or above, must be further investigated for possible SBI.[21] Other clinical decision guides include the Philadelphia Protocol, Rochester Criteria, and the Boston Criteria. Each of these criteria requires diagnostic testing to risk stratify febrile children. The choice on which criteria to use should be based on patient age cohort as well as provider preference and experience. Recent research has also indicated that a new clinical decision guide, the "Step by Step"

Table 3 Yale Observation Scale	
Cry	Strong or no cry = 1 Whimper or sob = 3 Weak cry, moaning, or high pitched cry = 5
Parental reaction	Content or brief cry = 1 Cries off and on = 3 Persistent cry = 5
State variation	Awakens quickly = 1 Difficult to awaken = 3 No arousal or falls asleep = 5
Color	Pink = 1 Acrocyanosis = 3 Pale, cyanotic, mottled = 5
Hydration	Eyes, skin, and mucus membranes moist = 1 Mouth slightly dry = 3 Eyes sunken and/or mucus membranes dry = 5
Social responses	Alert or smiles = 1 Alert or brief smile = 3 No smile, anxious, or dull = 5

Yale Observation Scale: Score ≤10 SBI risk 2.7%; Score = 11 to 15 SBI risk 26%; Score >16 SBI risk 92.3%.

From Bang A, Chaturvedi P. Yale Observation Scale for prediction of bacteremia in febrile children. Indian J Pediatr 2009;76(6):599–604.

approach, may also be a reliable way to risk stratify febrile children. **Table 4**[22–25] outlines each of these guides.

Philadelphia Protocol

Originally developed from a study seeking to reduce empiric antibiotic use and hospitalizations in infants less than 2 months old who presented with fever, the Philadelphia Protocol has become an invaluable stratification tool. With a 98% sensitivity, the Philadelphia Protocol can safely identify febrile infants with a temperature of at least 38.0°C who can be discharged home.[22] Unique to this and the Rochester Criteria, febrile infants who are low risk may be discharged home without antibiotics.[23] The Philadelphia Protocol requires that all of the following be met in order for the infant to fall into the low-risk group

- Well-appearing infant 29 day old to 60 day old
- Reassuring physical examination
- WBC count less than 15,000/mm^3
- Band-to-neutrophil ratio less than 0.2
- UA with less than 10 WBC/hpf
- Urine Gram stain negative
- CSF less than 8 WBC/mm^3
- CSF Gram stain negative
- CXR without infiltrate (if obtained)
- Stool without blood and few to no fecal leukocytes on smear (if indicated)

If one or more of the previously mentioned criteria are not met, the patient is considered to be high risk and should be admitted with initiation of empiric antibiotics.[22]

Table 4
Clinical decision guides

	Rochester Criteria	Philadelphia Criteria	Boston Criteria	Step-By-Step
Age-Group	≤60 d old	29–60 d old	28–89 d old	0–90 d old Note: Infants <21 d old automatically are high risk
Medical History	• Term infant • No antibiotics in the perinatal period • Not hospitalized longer than mother • No prior antibiotics • No history of hyperbilirubinemia • No past medical history		• No antibiotics in the preceding 48 h • No immunizations in the preceding 48 h	
Physical Examination Findings	• Well-appearing • No ear, soft tissue, or bone infection	Well-appearing without abnormalities on examination	• No signs of dehydration • Well-appearing infant • No skeletal, soft tissue, skin, or ear infections on physical examination	• Well appearing • Normal airway, breathing, and circulation findings
Laboratory Findings	• CBC: WBC <15,000/mm^3 • Band neutrophils <1500/mm^3 • UA: <10 WBC/hpf • Stool: fecal leukocytes <5 WBC/hpf	• CBC: WBC <15,000/mm^3 • Band to neutrophil ratio <0.2 • Urinalysis: <10 WBC/hpf. Urine Gram stain-negative • CSF: <8 WBC/mm. CSF Gram stain negative • CXR: without infiltrate (if obtained) • Stool: negative for blood and few to no fecal leukocytes on smear (if indicated)	• CBC: WBC <20,000/mm^3 • CSF: <10 cells/mm^3 • UA: <10 WBC/hpf • CXR: no infiltrate	• CBC: ANC <10,000/mm^3 • CRP: <20 mg/L • UA: no leukocytes • Procalcitonin: ≤0.5 ng/mL
Disposition				
High-Risk	Hospitalize with antibiotics	Hospitalize with antibiotics	Hospitalize with antibiotics	Hospitalize with antibiotics
Low-Risk	Discharge without antibiotics but with close follow-up	Discharge without antibiotics but with close follow-up	Discharge with antibiotics and close follow-up	Discharge without antibiotics and close follow-up
Sensitivity	92%	98%	—	92%
Specificity	50%	42%	94.6%	—

From Dagan R, Powell KR, Hall CB, et al. Identification of infants unlikely to have serious bacterial infection although hospitalized for suspected sepsis. J Pediatrics 1985;107(6):855–60; and Gomez B, Mintegi S, Bressan S, et al. Validation of the "step-by-step" approach in the management of young febrile infants. Pediatrics 2016;138(2):http://dx.doi.org/10.1542/peds.2015-4381.

Rochester Criteria

The Rochester Criteria also support discharge home of low-risk infants with close follow-up and without antibiotics. It can be used in infants from ages 0 to 60 days presenting with fever of at least 38.0°C. If all reassuring criteria are met, the febrile infant has a less than 1% risk of SBI.[23] The reassuring Rochester Criteria include

- Well-appearing infant
- No skeletal, soft tissue, skin, or ear infections noted on physical examination
- Full-term birth
- No prior illness
  - No prior hospitalization
  - Not hospitalized longer than mother after delivery
  - No prior antibiotics
  - No hyperbilirubinemia
  - No chronic or underlying illness
- CBC count less than 15,000/mm³
- Band neutrophils less than 1500/mm³
- UA with less than 10 WBC/hpf
- If diarrhea is present then fecal leukocytes less than 5 WBC/hpf

Boston Criteria

The Boston Criteria can be used to risk stratify febrile infants up to 89 days of age who present with a fever of at least 38.0°C. Unlike the Philadelphia Protocol and Rochester Criteria, the Boston Criteria recommend empiric antibiotic therapy for both high-risk and low-risk infants.[24] Low-risk infants may still be discharged home using these criteria, but antibiotics are recommended in addition to close follow-up. The Boston Criteria include

- Well-appearing infant
- No skeletal, soft tissue, skin, or ear infections on physical examination
- No signs of dehydration
- No antibiotics in the preceding 48 hours
- No immunizations in the preceding 48 hours
- WBC count less than 20,000/mm³
- CSF less than 10 cells/mm³
- UA less than 10 WBC/hpf
- CXR without infiltrate

"Step by Step" Approach

This approach was recently validated as a tool to identify infants who present with fever without a source at risk for an invasive bacterial infection, and to identify those who can safely be discharged home without lumbar puncture or empiric antibiotic therapy. This tool was found to have a sensitivity and negative predictive value for ruling out invasive bacterial infection of 92.0% and 99.3%, respectively.[25] Using this method, both clinical and laboratory criteria are applied in a sequential order, starting with the general appearance of the infant, then the age and results of the UA, and finally blood, testing including procalcitonin, CRP and absolute neutrophil count. According to the findings of the study, the febrile child can safely be discharged home without lumbar puncture or antibiotics if the following criteria are met

- Well-appearing child with normal airway, breathing, and circulation
- Older than 21 days

- No leukocytes on UA
- Procalcitonin no more than 0.5 ng/mL
- CRP less than 20 mg/L or ANC less than 10,000/mm^3

The authors do recommend a period of close observation in children who present with very short fever duration, as some blood biomarkers such as procalcitonin can take longer than a few hours to rise. The authors do recommend a period of close observation in children who present with very short fever duration as some blood biomarkers, such as procalcitonin, can take longer than a few hours to rise.[25]

TREATMENT, DISPOSITION, AND FOLLOW-UP OF THE FEBRILE CHILD

All children who appear clinically ill, are unable to maintain hydration, or who do not have appropriate follow-up after discharge should be admitted for further evaluation and management. Choices for antibiotics are based on age, local susceptibilities, and the type of infection thought to be the cause of the fever.[11]

Fever is treated with acetaminophen or ibuprofen. Aspirin should never be used in treatment of fever in infants and children less than 16 years of age because of the risk of Reye syndrome.[11] Acetaminophen, which can be given orally or rectally, has the following recommended dosing regimen

- 15 mg/kg/dose every 6 to 8 hours up to a maximum daily dose of 60 mg/kg for neonates
- 15 mg/kg/dose every 4 to 6 hours up to a maximum daily dose of 75 mg/kg for infants and children
- 1 g per dose up to 4 g maximum per day in children greater than 65 kg

Ibuprofen's recommended dosing regimen for all children over 6 months of age is

- 10 mg/kg/dose orally every 6 to 8 hours with a maximum daily dose of 40 mg/kg
- Children who weigh over 60 kg should not receive more than 2400 mg/d of ibuprofen

For ibuprofen, the lowest effective dose and the shortest effective treatment duration should be used to decrease risk of gastrointestinal (GI) upset. Caregivers should be cautioned that when calculating dosages of acetaminophen and ibuprofen for children, all sources of these medications should be considered, as many over the counter cough and cold medications contain acetaminophen and ibuprofen, and accidental overdose can occur.

The practice of alternating acetaminophen and ibuprofen is quite commonly recommended. However, a practical application of an alternating dosing regimen is not readily apparent, and confusion about dosing schedule may also lead to accidental overdose. Studies have consistently found that an alternating regimen provides little to no benefit when compared with monotherapy.[26]

Treatment 0 to 28 Days Old

In this age group differentiating between sick and well neonates is difficult and the risk of SBI is high, varying from 12% to 26%.[27] The Rochester Criteria is available for risk stratification in this age group. However, because of the high incidence of SBI, a full diagnostic evaluation including lumbar puncture, and hospital admission for intravenous antibiotics are considered the standard management for all infants in this age group presenting with fever of 38.0°C or above.[9] Antibiotic regimens in this age group commonly include ampicillin and cefotaxime, or ampicillin and gentamicin. Acyclovir is not routinely used, but should also be initiated in those infants who have mucocutaneous vesicles, a maternal history of genital HSV, or who have seizures or other neurologic symptoms suggestive of HSV encephalitis. Ceftriaxone should not be given to children this age because of the risk of increased hyperbilirubinemia secondary to bilirubin displacement.[11] For information about empiric antibiotic treatment in this age group, refer to **Box 4**.[8]

Treatment 29 to 90 Days Old

Even well-appearing infants 29 to 90 days with a rectal temperature of 38.0°C or above should undergo laboratory testing to further investigate possible sources of fever.[9]

For infants aged 29 to 60 days, the Philadelphia Protocol is commonly utilized to risk stratify those infants who may be at risk for SBI. If the low risk criteria for the Philadelphia Protocol are met, and reliable follow-up can be arranged within 24 hours, then the infant may be discharged home with or without empiric antibiotic therapy depending on provider preference and experience. Infants who do not meet these criteria should be admitted and treated appropriately. The Boston Criteria can also be applied in this age group. If the infant is deemed low risk by the Boston Criteria, empiric antibiotic therapy is recommended if the infant is discharged home. Currently there is no specific standard of care for management of well-appearing infants in this age group, and practice among providers is variable. However, most well-appearing infants should receive the same evaluation as the ill-appearing infants. Hospital admission with empiric antibiotic treatment with cefotaxime or ceftriaxone should be initiated if application of any of the clinical decision guides places the child into the high-risk group.[9] Consideration should be given for adding ampicillin, if there is concern for *Listeria*, or vancomycin, if there is concern for soft tissue infections or meningitis.[9]

Lumbar puncture may not be necessary in the well-appearing infant with reliable caregivers and close follow-up.[9] If a lumbar puncture is performed, a single dose of ceftriaxone should be administered prior to discharge.[8] The decision whether to discharge home a well-appearing infant in this age group is difficult and should be made after careful evaluation of the infant and consideration of the diagnostic results. Consideration for the availability of prompt re-evaluation and follow-up must also be given. Consultation with the infant's primary care provider or pediatrician should be made.

Box 4
Recommended antibiotic regimen for infants 0 to 28 days old

- Ampicillin: 50 mg/kg/dose every 8 hours
  and
- Gentamicin: 2.5 mg/kg/dose
  or
- Ampicillin: 50 mg/kg/dose every 8 hours
  and
- Cefotaxime: 50 mg/kg/dose every 8 hours

If ED providers are concerned for HSV infection, acyclovir should be added.

- Acyclovir: 60 mg/kg/d divided in 3 doses

From Smithermann HF, Macias CG. Evaluation and management of the febrile young infant (7 to 90 days of age). UpToDate; 2015. Available at: http://www.uptodate.com/home. Accessed May 23, 2016.

Clinical evaluation and management of a well-appearing infant aged 61 to 90 days is similar to well-appearing infants 29 to 60 days, and is also challenging due to the lack of definitive clinical guidelines. The Boston Criteria are helpful to risk stratify infants in this age group. Hospital admission and empiric antibiotic therapy for high-risk infants aged 61 to 90 days follow the same regimen as high-risk infants aged 29 to 60 days. This age group may also be safely discharged home if the Boston Criteria are met and follow-up can be established in 24 hours.[24]

For the recommended antibiotic regimen in this age group, refer to **Box 5**.[8]

Treatment 90 Days to 36 Months of Age

In this age group, clinical assessment starts to become more reliable. As discussed previously, the YOS is a triage tool used to risk stratify those in this age group for SBI. Those children with a score of 10 or above or children who appear ill or have unstable vital signs should undergo complete diagnostic evaluation. Children who appear ill should also be admitted to the hospital with antibiotics treating the common pathogens for this age group.

Children within this age group who have fever without a source, and have not been completely immunized should undergo a CBC count and UA with culture regardless of appearance. If the WBC count is 20,000/μL or greater, then a chest radiograph is also recommended even in the absence of pulmonary symptoms. If the WBC is 15,000/μL or greater, a single dose of ceftriaxone 50 mg/kg intramuscularly is recommended pending culture result, with follow-up in 24 hours.[9]

Healthy girls ages 6 to 24 months, circumcised boys less than 6 month old, and uncircumcised boys less than 12 months old who have been completely immunized, and do not have a source for infection should have UA and urine culture completed.[9] If the UA is positive, the patient may still safely be discharged home for outpatient treatment as long as the child appears well and is tolerating oral intake.

A significant proportion of children who present with fever will have a self-limited viral infection or a focal source of infection.[18] Well-appearing, immunized children who are felt to have a virus as the source of their symptoms should not be given antibiotics. Parents should be educated on symptomatic treatment and return precautions for the associated viral illness. Symptomatic treatments include: cool mist humidified air, fever control, and nasal suctioning. When the decision is made to start antibiotic therapy the provider must take great care in assuring that the antibiotic is appropriately prescribed, as up to 50% of the time antibiotics are not optimally

---

Box 5
Recommended antibiotic regimen in infants 29 to 90 days old

- Cefoxatime: 50 mg/kg/dose every 8 hours
  or,
- Ceftriaxone: 50 mg/kg
  with or without
- Ampicillin (if concerned for *Listeria*): 50 mg/kg/dose every 8 hours
- Vancomycin (if concerned for soft tissue infections or meningitis): 15 mg/kg every 6 hours
- Ceftriaxone (if discharged home after lumbar puncture): 50 mg/kg

From Smithermann HF, Macias CG. Evaluation and management of the febrile young infant (7 to 90 days of age). UpToDate; 2015. Available at: http://www.uptodate.com/home. Accessed May 23, 2016.

Box 6
Recommended antibiotic regimen for infants 90 days to 36 months old

Uncomplicated urinary tract infections:

- Cefixime 8 mg/kg oral daily for 7 to 10 days
- Trimethoprim/sulfamethoxazole 5 mg/kg (based on trimethoprim component) oral twice a day for 7 to 10 days

Otitis media:

- Children with acute otitis media who have not received amoxicillin within the last 30 days and who do not have concurrent conjunctivitis are treated with:
  - High-dose amoxicillin 40 to 45 mg/kg 2 times daily:
    - 10 days for children under 2 with severe symptoms
    - 7 days for children 2 to 5 with mild-to-moderate symptoms
    - 5 to 7 days for children over 6 with mild-to-moderate symptoms
  - Penicillin allergic:
    - Cefdinir 14 mg/kg once daily
    - Cefpodoxime 5 mg/kg 2 times daily
    - Ceftriaxone 50 mg/kg (max 1 g) every 24 hours × 3 days
- For those who have received antibiotics within the last 30 days or who have associated conjunctivitis:
  - Amoxicillin–clavulanate 40 to 45 mg/kg 2 times daily
- Children who do not improve after 48 to 72 hours of amoxicillin should be given:
  - Amoxicillin–clavulanate 40 to 45 mg/kg 2 times daily
  - Ceftriaxone 50 mg/kg (max 1 g) every 24 hours × 3 days

Pharyngitis:

- Benzathine penicillin G <27 kg 600,000 units intramuscularly, ≥27 kg 1.2 million units intramuscularly once
- Penicillin VK <27 kg 250 mg by mouth 2 to 3 times daily, ≥27 kg 500 by mouth twice daily for 10 days
- Amoxicillin 25 mg/kg by mouth 2 times daily (max 500 mg/dose) or 50 mg/kg once daily (maximum of 1000 mg) for 10 days
- Cephalexin 20 mg/kg by mouth 2 times daily (max 500 mg/dose) for 10 days
- Azithromycin 12 mg/kg by mouth daily for 5 days (max 500 mg/dose)
- Clindamycin 7 mg/kg by mouth 3 times daily (max 300 mg/dose) for 10 days

Pneumonia:

- Outpatient community-acquired pneumonia in children less than 5 is treated with:
  - High-dose amoxicillin 40 to 45 mg/kg 2 times daily for 10 days
    - ± Azithromycin 10 mg/kg day 1(max 500 mg), 5 mg/kg days 2 to 5 (max 250 mg) for atypical coverage
- Inpatient treatment options for presumed bacterial pneumonia in children who have been fully immunized with conjugate vaccines for *Haemophilus influenzae* type B and *Streptococcus pneumoniae*, and in areas where penicillin-resistance in invasive strains of pneumococcus is low, include the following:
  - Ampicillin 50 mg/kg intravenously 4 times daily
  - Ceftriaxone 50 mg/kg intravenously 2 times daily
  - Cefotaxime 50 mg/kg intravenously 3 times daily
- If there is suspected methicillin-resistant *S aureus* (MRSA), providers should add
  - Clindamycin 10 mg/kg intravenously 4 times daily or
  - Vancomycin 15 mg/kg intravenously 4 times daily
- Inpatient treatment options for presumed bacterial pneumonia in children who have not been fully immunized with conjugate vaccines for *H influenzae* type B and *S pneumoniae*

or in areas where penicillin resistance in invasive strains of *Pneumococcus* is significant, include the following:
  ○ Ceftriaxone 50 mg/kg intravenously 2 times daily
  ○ Cefotaxime 50 mg/kg intravenously 3 times daily

- If there is suspected MRSA, providers should add
  ○ Clindamycin 10 mg/kg intravenously 4 times daily or
  ○ Vancomycin 15 mg/kg intravenously 4 times daily

- In addition to beta lactam antibiotics, if the diagnosis of atypical infection is, one of the following options should be added
  ○ Azithromycin 10 mg/kg intravenously once daily for days 1 and 2, then 5 mg/kg days 3 to 5
  ○ Clarithromycin 7.5 mg/kg by mouth 2 times daily for 7 to 14 days
  ○ Doxycycline 1 to 2 mg/kg intravenously by mouth 2 times daily (children over 7)
  ○ Levofloxacin 16 to 20 mg/kg/d intravenously/by mouth (by mouth preferred) divided every 12 hours (only for children 6 months to 4 years who cannot tolerate macrolides or have reached growth maturity)

From Flerlage J, Hospital JH, Engorn B. The Harriet Lane handbook. 20th edition. Mosby; 2015; and Bradley JS, Byington CL, Shah SS, et al. The management of community-acquired pneumonia in infants and children older than 3 months of age: clinical practice guidelines by the Pediatric Infectious Diseases Society and the Infectious Diseases Society of America. Clin Infect Dis 2011;53(7): http://dx.doi.org/10.1093/cid/cir531.

prescribed, often being given when not necessary and at the incorrect dose or duration. This has led to over 2 million antibiotic-resistant illnesses and 23,000 deaths per year.[28]

Children within this age group who have a likely bacterial source for their fever should be treated according to local susceptibilities and likely pathogen. Common causes of fever in children in this age group may include the following: urinary tract infection, otitis media, pharyngitis, and pneumonia. For otitis media, a wait-and-see approach with symptomatic treatment can be taken when the child is 6 to 23 months and has unilateral nonsevere symptoms or when the child is over 2 and has nonsevere symptoms.[28] For recommended antibiotic treatment regimens for common causes of fever in this age group, refer to **Box 6**.[29,30]

SUMMARY

Fever is a common, yet challenging symptom of pediatric patients presenting to the ED. Although most of those presenting with fever have a benign viral illness or a bacterial infection that can be managed with outpatient treatment, it is crucial for the ED provider to identify and treat those who are at risk for an SBI.[31–35] In order to identify fever source, a careful history collection and thorough physical examination must be completed on all children presenting with fever. Patient age and immunization status are two of the main factors that influence management and treatment of the febrile child. Diagnostic evaluation is needed in all children less than 90 day old presenting with fever. Clinical decision guides are available and are useful in helping to risk stratify patients in whom the ED provider is unsure of management and disposition. The ED provider should have a low threshold to hospitalize any child who appears ill, is unable to maintain hydration, or has unstable vital signs. Well-appearing children over 28 day old who have fever without a source, who meet low risk criteria as outlined by the clinical decision guides discussed previously may be safely discharged home. Well-appearing febrile children over 28 day old with identifiable source of infection should be placed on the appropriate antibiotic regimen. In all cases in which a febrile child will be sent home, ensuring close outpatient follow-up is imperative.

REFERENCES

1. Baraff LJ, Lee SI. Fever without source. Pediatr Infect Dis J 1992;11(2):146–51.
2. Behrman RE, Kliegman RM, Jenson HB. Nelson's textbook of pediatrics. 18th edition. London: W. B. Saunders; 1999.
3. Hay WW. Current pediatric diagnosis & treatment. 18th edition. New York: Lange Medical Books/McGraw-Hill, Medical Pub. Division; 2007.
4. Blackwell J, Goolsby MJ. Fever of unknown source: outpatient evaluation and management for children 2 months to 36 months of age. J Am Acad Nurse Pract 2002;14(2):51–4.
5. Ward MA. Patient information: Fever in children (Beyond the Basics). Fever in infants and children: Pathophysiology and management. 2016. Available at: http://www.uptodate.com/contents/fever-in-children-beyond-the-basics. Accessed June 26, 2016.
6. Graneto JW, Soglin DF. Maternal screening of childhood fever by palpation. Pediatr Emerg Care 1996;12(3):183–4.
7. Yarden-Bilavsky H, Bilavsky E, Amir J, et al. Serious bacterial infections in neonates with fever by history only versus documented fever. Scand J Infect Dis 2010;42(11–12):812–6.
8. Smithermann HF, Macias CG. Evaluation and management of the febrile young infant (7 to 90 days of age). UpToDate; 2015. Available at: http://www.uptodate.com/home. Accessed May 23, 2016.
9. Pulliam PN, Attia MW, Cronan KM. C-reactive protein in febrile children 1 to 36 months of age with clinically undetectable serious bacterial infection. Pediatrics 2001;108(6):1275–9.
10. Manzano S, Bailey B, Girodias J-B, et al. Impact of procalcitonin on the management of children aged 1 to 36 months presenting with fever without source: a randomized controlled trial. The Am J Emerg Med 2010;28(6):647–53.
11. Tintinalli JE, Stapczynski JS. Tintinalli's emergency medicine: a comprehensive study guide. 7th edition. New York: McGraw-Hill; 2011.
12. Mahajan P, Kuppermann N, Suarez N, et al. RNA transcriptional biosignature analysis for identifying febrile infants with serious bacterial infections in the emergency department. JAMA 2016;316(8):846–57.
13. Kuzmanovic S, Roncevic N, Stojadinovic A. Fever without a focus in children 0-36 months of age. Medicinski Pregled Med Pregl 2006;59(3–4):187–91.
14. Barrows MA, Coddington JA, Richards EA, et al. Parental vaccine hesitancy: clinical implications for pediatric providers. J Pediatr Health Care 2015;29(4):385–94.
15. Vaccination. Centers for Disease Control and Prevention. 2014. Available at: http://www.cdc.gov/hi-disease/vaccination.html. Accessed June 26, 2016.
16. For clinicians. Centers for Disease Control and Prevention. 2016. Available at: http://www.cdc.gov/hi-disease/clinicians.html. Accessed June 26, 2016.
17. Pneumococcal conjugate (PCV13) VIS. Centers for Disease Control and Prevention. 2015. Available at: http://www.cdc.gov/vaccines/hcp/vis/vis-statements/pcv13.html. Accessed September 17, 2016.
18. Allen CH, Fleisher GR, Kaplan SL, et al. Fever without a source in children 3 to 36 months of age. Fever without a source in children 3 to 36 months of age. 2016. Available at: http://www.uptodate.com/contents/fever-without-a-source-in-children-3-to-36-months-of-age/contributors. Accessed June 29, 2016.
19. Birth-18 years & "catch-up" immunization schedules. Centers for Disease Control and Prevention; 2016. Available at: http://www.cdc.gov/vaccines/schedules/hcp/child-adolescent.html. Accessed July 10, 2016.

20. Seither R, Calhoun K, Knighton CL, et al. Vaccination coverage among children in kindergarten—United States, 2013–14 school year. Centers for Disease Control and Prevention; 2014. Available at: http://www.cdc.gov/mmwr/preview/mmwrhtml/mm6333a2.htm. Accessed July 22, 2016.
21. Bang A, Chaturvedi P. Yale Observation Scale for prediction of bacteremia in febrile children. Indian J Pediatr The Indian J Pediatr 2009;76(6):599–604.
22. Baker MD, Bell LM, Avner JR. Outpatient management without antibiotics of fever in selected infants. New Engl J Med N Engl J Med 1993;329(20):1437–41.
23. Dagan R, Powell KR, Hall CB, et al. Identification of infants unlikely to have serious bacterial infection although hospitalized for suspected sepsis. The J Pediatr 1985;107(6):855–60.
24. Baskin MN, O'rourke EJ, Fleisher GR. Outpatient treatment of febrile infants 28 to 89 days of age with intramuscular administration of ceftriaxone. The J Pediatr 1992;120(1):22–7.
25. Gomez B, Mintegi S, Bressan S, et al. Validation of the "step-by-step" approach in the management of young febrile infants. Pediatrics 2016;138(2). http://dx.doi.org/10.1542/peds.2015-4381.
26. Shortridge L, Harris V. Alternating acetaminophen and ibuprofen. Paediatrics Child Health 2007;12(2):127–8.
27. Schwartz S, Raveh D, Toker O, et al. A week-by-week analysis of the low-risk criteria for serious bacterial infection in febrile neonates. Arch Dis Child 2008; 94(4):287–92.
28. About antimicrobial resistance. Centers for Disease Control and Prevention. 2015. Available at: http://www.cdc.gov/drugresistance/about.html. Accessed June 29, 2016.
29. Flerlage J, Hospital JH, Engorn B. The Harriet Lane handbook. 20th edition. Mosby; 2015.
30. Bradley JS, Byington CL, Shah SS, et al. The management of community-acquired pneumonia in infants and children older than 3 months of age: clinical practice guidelines by the Pediatric Infectious Diseases Society and the Infectious Diseases Society of America. Clin Infect Dis 2011;53(7):e25–76.
31. Bruel AVD, Bruyninckx R, Vermeire E, et al. Signs and symptoms in children with a serious infection: a qualitative study. BMC Fam Pract BMC Fam Pract 2005;6(1).
32. Thompson M, Bruel AVD, Verbakel J, et al. Systematic review and validation of prediction rules for identifying children with serious infections in emergency departments and urgent-access primary care. Health Technology Assess Health Technol Assess 2012;16(15). http://dx.doi.org/10.3310/hta16150.
33. Family practice notebook. Philadelphia Criteria for febrile infant 29-60 days. Available at: http://www.fpnotebook.com/legacy/id/exam/phldlphcrtrfrfbrlinfnt960dys.htm. Accessed July 1, 2016.
34. Rochester Criteria for Febrile Infant 0 to 60 days. Available at: http://www.fpnotebook.com/id/exam/rchstrcrtrfrfbrlinfnt0t60dys.htm. Accessed July 1, 2016.
35. Boston Criteria for febrile infant 28-89 days. Available at: http://www.fpnotebook.com/id/exam/bstncrtrfrfbrlinfnt889dys.htm. Accessed July 1, 2016.

Skin and Soft Tissue Infections: Causes and Treatments

Clint Kalan, MMSc, PA-C*, Jon Femling, MD, PhD

KEYWORDS

- Abscess • Cellulitis • Necrotizing skin and soft tissue infection
- Incision and drainage • Loop drainage • Staphylococcus • Streptococcus • MRSA

KEY POINTS

- Skin and soft tissue infections are most commonly caused by *Streptococcus* spp and *Staphylococcus aureus*, with an increasing prevalence of MRSA.
- Cellulitis is best treated with antibiotic coverage for *Streptococcus* species.
- Abscess and other purulent infections have a predominance of MRSA, and are best treated with incision and drainage.
- Necrotizing soft tissue infections carry a high mortality and warrant emergent surgical consultation and broad-spectrum antibiotics.

INTRODUCTION

Skin and soft tissue infections (SSTIs) are a frequent cause of visits to the emergency department, with diseases of the skin and subcutaneous tissues accounting for 3.9% of all emergency department visits nationwide.[1] Physician assistants in emergency medicine are seeing an increase in disease prevalence and a changing pattern of disease in the last decade.[2–5] The breadth and scope of infections that confront an emergency medicine provider are large. Providers must be prepared to deal with spontaneous infections, intravenous (IV) drug use–associated infections, infected traumatic wounds, diabetic ulcers, surgical site infections, parasites, fungal infections, and animal bites. Although the diversity of infections is large, most cases seen by a physician assistant in the emergency department are bacterial in nature.[6–8] Bacterial skin infections are purulent or nonpurulent, and further differentiated by severity.[9]

Disclosure Statement: C. Kalan has no relevant financial disclosures. J. Femling has been funded by the Emergency Medicine Foundation to study Skin and soft tissue infections, has enrolled subjects in a clinical trial (but not personally received funds from) for Cubist Pharmaceuticals, and intends to enroll subjects in a clinical trial (but has not personally received funds from) for Cempra Pharmaceuticals.
Department of Emergency Medicine, University of New Mexico School of Medicine, #1 University of New Mexico, MSC 11 6025, Albuquerque, NM 87131, USA
* Corresponding author.
E-mail address: Cpkalan@salud.unm.edu

Necrotizing infections, an important subset of acute bacterial skin infections, have exceedingly high morbidity and mortality and require prompt evaluation and treatment.[10] This article describes the microbiology, clinical findings, diagnosis, and treatment of acute bacterial SSTIs focusing on emergency department diagnosis, management, and disposition.

MICROBIOLOGY

Streptococcus species and *Staphylococcus aureus* are the primary organisms of concern in most acute bacterial SSTIs. Importantly, the incidence of SSTIs presenting for emergency care has risen dramatically[3,8,11–15] with a concomitant increase in the prevalence of community-acquired methicillin-resistant *S aureus* (CA-MRSA).[4,5,7,16,17] The dramatic increase in CA-MRSA has impacted the presentation of SSTIs with a greater proportion of infections presenting with a purulent abscess rather than pure cellulitis. Traditional risk factors for MRSA infection, such as recent hospital admission, antibiotic use, IV drug abuse, diabetes, and age,[18] have become less reliable as the incidence of purulent SSTIs in young, healthy populations has increased (generally thought to be CA-MRSA infections).[19] In general, MRSA should be considered in all patients with a purulent infection.

Although most nonpurulent SSTIs have historically been thought to be caused by streptococcal species,[20–22] a recent study using advanced microbial identification techniques questions this assertion and implicates *S aureus* in many of these infections.[23] Current clinical trials focused on identifying optimal treatment strategies for pure cellulitis in the setting of recent microbial changes are needed.

In contrast to cellulitis, the predominant cause of purulent infections is easier to identify and is most commonly *S aureus* with CA-MRSA representing a crucial cause that must be addressed in SSTIs presenting to the emergency department.[4,5,8,16,19,24–26] Importantly, methicillin resistance is reported in around 50% or more of most *S aureus* isolates[7,27] and is a crucial consideration when choosing antimicrobial therapies. Necrotizing infections are often polymicrobial, although single infections with group A β-hemolytic streptococci and clostridial species are important etiologies to consider. Consistent with the other acute SSTIs described in this article *S aureus* has shown an increased contribution to these infections.[28,29]

CELLULITIS AND ERYSIPELAS (NONPURULENT SKIN AND SOFT TISSUE INFECTIONS)
Clinical Presentation

Cellulitis has classically been defined as an infection of the deeper dermis and subcutaneous tissues, whereas erysipelas has been considered a well-demarcated infection of the upper dermis. Current guidelines do not differentiate the treatment of these entities,[9] therefore they are discussed together under the term of cellulitis.

Cellulitis is generally a painful, erythematous, warm and edematous area of skin, without any signs of purulent drainage, furunculous, carbunculosis, or fluctuance. A "peau de orange" appearance can occur with edema surrounding the follicles (Fig. 1). Sometimes streaking lymphangitis can occur. Risk factors for cellulitis are listed in Box 1.[30]

Diagnosis

Although the diagnosis of cellulitis is a clinical one, careful attention must be paid to excluding the possibility of a purulent infection requiring incision and drainage. Clinical examination is not sensitive enough to detect small areas of purulence or some deeper abscesses in certain patients.[31–34] Bedside point-of-care ultrasound should be used

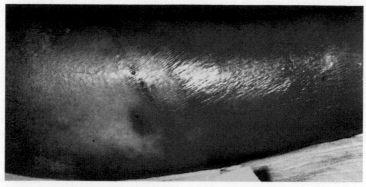

Fig. 1. Clinical presentation of cellulitis. Streptococcal cellulitis complicating a leg wound (wound not shown). (*From* Leaper DJ. Traumatic and surgical wounds. BMJ 2006;332(7540):532–5; with permission.)

routinely in patients with concern for an abscess. Importantly, learning and using this diagnostic modality requires little time investment.[35] Deep venous thrombosis must be considered in the differential diagnosis of cellulitis, and screening ultrasonography should be considered in cases of lower extremity cellulitis. Laboratory investigations, blood cultures, and/or biopsies are not recommended in patients with simple cellulitis[9] because of their low yield.[36,37] Even advanced microbial detection techniques are insufficient to clearly diagnose the bacterial cause of cellulitis.[23] Blood cultures and laboratory investigations should be considered in patients with signs of systemic illness (ie, fever, tachycardia, hypotension, altered mental status).[9]

Treatment and Disposition

Cellulitis should be treated with antibiotics. The specific choice of antimicrobial therapy depends on clinical severity and must be modified as needed depending on clinical response to treatment. A guide for differentiating mild, moderate, and severe infection and empiric antimicrobial choices for nonpurulent infections is shown in **Fig. 2.**[9] Although the Infectious Diseases Society of America recommendations do not generally include MRSA coverage for nonpurulent infections, recent studies have highlighted the importance of considering MRSA as a cause of pure cellulitis,[23,27] especially in cases of IV drug abuse or other penetrating traumatic wounds.[9]

Box 1
Risk factors for cellulitis

- Extremity edema
- Venous insufficiency
- History of cellulitis
- Obesity
- Tinea pedis

Data from Chlebicki MP, Oh CC. Recurrent Cellulitis: risk factors, etiology, pathogenesis and treatment. Curr Infect Dis Resp 2014;16(9):422.

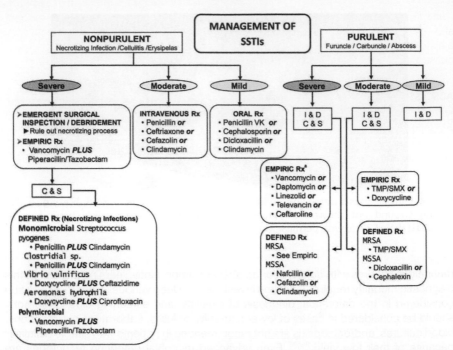

Fig. 2. Skin and soft tissue infection differentiation and treatment. (1) Purulent SSTIs. Mild infection: for purulent SSTI, incision and drainage is indicated. Moderate infection: patients with purulent infection with systemic signs of infection. Severe infection: patients who have failed incision and drainage plus oral antibiotics or those with systemic signs of infection, such as temperature greater than 38°C, tachycardia (heart rate >90 beats per minute), tachypnea (respiratory rate >24 breaths per minute), or abnormal white blood cell count (<12,000 or <400 cells/μL), or immunocompromised patients. (2) Nonpurulent SSTIs. Mild infection: typical cellulitis/erysipelas with no focus of purulence. Moderate infection: typical cellulitis/erysipelas with systemic signs of infection. Severe infection: patients who have failed oral antibiotic treatment or those with systemic signs of infection (as defined previously under purulent infection), or those who are immunocompromised, or those with clinical signs of deeper infection, such as bullae, skin sloughing, hypotension, or evidence of organ dysfunction. Two newer agents, tedizolid and dalbavancin, are also effective agents in SSTIs, including those caused by MRSA, and may be approved for this indication by June 2014. C & S, culture and sensitivity; I & D, incision and drainage; MSSA, methicillin-susceptible *Staphylococcus aureus*; Rx, treatment; TMP/SMX, trimethoprim-sulfamethoxazole. [a] Because daptomycin and televancin are not approved for use in children, vancomycin is recommended; clindamycin may be used if clindamycin resistance is <10%–15% at the institution. (*From* Stevens DL, Bisno AL, Chambers HF, et al. Practice guidelines for the diagnosis and management of skin and soft tissue infections: 2014 update by the Infectious Diseases Society of America. Clin Infect Dis 2014;59:147–59; with permission.)

Many patients with a mild nonpurulent SSTI are discharged home on oral antibiotics. Fever, chronic ulcers or edema, wound infections, and recurrent cellulitis have all been shown to be predictors of outpatient failure,[38] as have elevated lactate values and hand infections.[39] The duration of treatment necessary has not been definitively shown; however, some studies have shown a 5-day course sufficient in selected populations.[40] Close follow-up is recommended, as is marking the leading edge of the cellulitis to evaluate disease progression. Marking the leading edge allows the patient and providers to easily assess the response to treatment.

In moderate and severe cases, parenteral antibiotics and admission to the hospital should be pursued. This treatment pathway should also be considered in patients with a history of immunosuppression or risk factors in Fig. 2. Necrotizing infections, as discussed next, should always be a consideration in patients with severe disease.

ABSCESS (PURULENT SKIN AND SOFT TISSUE INFECTIONS)
Clinical Presentation

Purulent SSTIs include cutaneous abscesses, carbuncles, furuncles, infected sebaceous cysts, or any cellulitis with a discharge. Many abscesses present with some drainage, although closed abscesses with palpable fluctuance is also common (Fig. 3). Some deeper abscesses may only be identified with the assistance of ultrasound. Although purulent and nonpurulent infections have similar etiologies, some differences exist. Breaks in the skin, either intentionally or accidentally are important considerations to evaluate. Location of the abscess has important implications in the treatment and cause. Infected Bartholin glands and pilonidal cysts raise the possibility for atypical organisms and polymicrobial infections.

Diagnosis

Differentiating cellulitis from abscess clinically can sometimes be challenging.[31] Ultrasound can serve an important role in cases where diagnosis is unclear.[32,33,35] The typical features of abscess on ultrasound are seen in Fig. 4.[41]

Radiography is generally unnecessary, although it can be considered to evaluate for a subcutaneous foreign body or osteomyelitis, and may incidentally reveal subcutaneous air, a rare but specific finding for a necrotizing infection. Septic arthritis and bursitis should be considered with either a purulent or nonpurulent SSTI that overlies a joint, and appropriate diagnostic evaluation and consultation pursued. Wound cultures are recommended by guidelines when antibiotics are to be administered for cutaneous abscess, but not infected epidermoid cysts.[9] In practice, most simple purulent SSTIs are caused by S aureus,[4,12,15,28] with many isolates being resistant to methicillin.[12,13,18,19,24,25,27] Empiric treatment is frequently performed and may be acceptable in mild cases. As in nonpurulent conditions, blood cultures are recommended in the setting of systemic illness.[9]

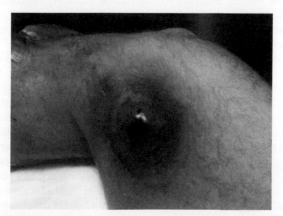

Fig. 3. Clinical presentation of abscess. Abscess in a 49-year-old man with history of intravenous drug use. (*Courtesy of* the authors.)

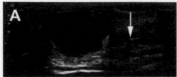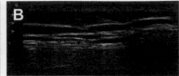

Fig. 4. Ultrasonographic findings of abscess. Soft tissue induration. Ultrasound images of an abscess cavity with surrounding induration (A) and images of the same patient's contralateral normal soft tissue and no induration (B). Normal soft tissue is characterized by horizontal white lines parallel to the skin surface. The edge of induration is visualized lateral (arrow) and deep to the abscess cavity. (From Gaspari RJ, Blehar D, Polan D, et al. The Massachusetts abscess rule: a clinical decision rule using ultrasound to identify methicillin-resistant Staphylococcus aureus in skin abscesses. Acad Emerg Med 2014;21(5):558–67; with permission.)

Treatment and Disposition

Incision and drainage is a mainstay of the treatment of any abscess. Needle drainage of cutaneous abscesses is typically insufficient, with a reported cure rate of only 26%.[42] Thorough exploration of the abscess and breaking down internal loculations is key to successful resolution of the abscess. In the special circumstance of breast abscess, small studies have proposed a trial of needle aspiration and antibiotics before incision and drainage in this cosmetically sensitive area.[43–45] Consultation with a breast surgeon is recommended in these cases.

Although packing of abscesses has long been standard practice in many emergency departments, recent data have shown it to be unnecessary in immunocompetent patients and significantly more painful.[46–48] This is true even in perianal abscesses,[49] which are thought to be a higher risk for contamination and polymicrobial infection. The standard practice of irrigating abscesses does not improve outcomes in simple abscesses[50] and increases the likelihood of aerosolizing infected tissues.

An alternative to packing of abscesses in cosmetically sensitive areas, complex abscesses, or in patients with risk factors for treatment failure who do not wish to undergo repeated dressing changes (eg, children) is the loop-drainage technique. This technique is demonstrated in Fig. 5. The drain is typically left in place until resolution of drainage and surrounding cellulitis. This technique showed similar outcomes with cosmetically better results secondary to the small incisions needed.[47,51,52] Primary closure of abscesses after incision and drainage has been studied in small trials[53] with some success. However, there are no current recommendations for this in the emergency department setting.

There is some debate regarding the use of antibiotics to treat patients with drained abscesses. For complicated infections with systemic signs of illness, there is general consensus for initiating antimicrobial therapy (see Fig. 2),[9] with coverage for MRSA being paramount. Guidelines also recommend the use of broad-spectrum, parenteral antibiotics for severe disease. A recent study[54] questions previous recommendations for a drainage alone strategy in small cutaneous abscesses with little surrounding cellulitis. Multiple previous studies and a meta-analysis had only shown a risk of recurrence, and no improvement in cure rate[55–58] with antibiotic treatment. However, the recent paper by Talan and colleagues[57] had significantly more subjects than the previous literature combined and showed a number needed to treat of 15 when comparing trimethoprim-sulfamethoxazole to placebo with a 7-day regimen. It is notable that incision and drainage alone has shown cure rates greater than 80%[54,57,59] and that rare, but serious, side-effects of antimicrobial therapy do occur.[60]

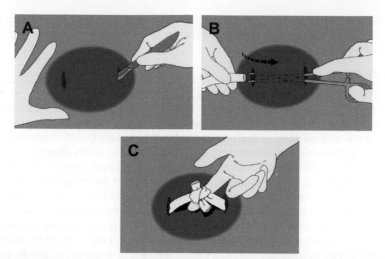

Fig. 5. Loop drainage technique. (*A*) Make two incisions of at least 5 mm in length at least 1 cm apart. Express all purulent material and break down loculations. (*B*) Pass a 0.25-inch Penrose drain between the two incision sites. (*C*) Tie the Penrose drain loosely, ensuring that there is no skin tension to avoid tissue necrosis. One should be able to easily slip a finger underneath the drain.

NECROTIZING INFECTION
Clinical Presentation

Necrotizing SSTIs (NSSTIs) are a rare but incredibly serious type of infection that emergency medicine physician assistants may encounter. The mortality for these infections ranges from 10% to 38%,[10,28,61–63] although does seem to be decreasing with early recognition.[64] These infections generally involve the deep subcutaneous tissue and the superficial muscle fascial layer. Patients generally have a history of some trauma, which could be minor, for the pathogens to seed the deep subcutaneous tissues. This trauma could be as simple as a minor abrasion or as complex as a perforated viscous. Because these conditions track along deeper tissues, skin findings can be minimal to absent at the onset of the disease. These patients often have pain and tachycardia out of proportion to fever and findings.[62,65] More specific skin findings include bullae, subcutaneous emphysema, or woody induration of the affected area, although these are often absent.[65] Patients can have extensive skin changes, fevers, and signs of systemic toxicity, although NSSTIs often present without these findings. Clinicians must maintain a high index of suspicion for NSSTI in any patient presenting with cellulitis or abscess, especially in the setting of severe pain or pain extending beyond the obvious border of the infection.

Many different classification schemata have been used to classify NSSTIs; however, typing by causative organism is the most oft-used. In general, polymicrobial infections are considered type I and the most common. Type II NSSTIs are defined as monomicrobial infections, generally Group A *Streptococcus* infections, and less common than type I. Systems differ on classifying clostridial gas gangrene, gram-negative (generally *Vibrio* sp) monomicrobial infections, fungal, and MRSA infections. The most common risk factor for developing an NSSTI is diabetes mellitus, although peripheral vascular disease, renal dysfunction, IV drug abuse, and recent surgical infection all have been seen as common comorbidities.[63,64,66] Some type II infections may occur with a minor break in the skin and no obvious comorbidities. Given that, it is unlikely for an emergency clinician to be able to distinguish between the types of necrotizing infection in the acute setting.

Diagnosis

The diagnosis of NSSTI in the emergency department remains a clinical one, based predominantly on examination and clinical suspicion. The true gold standard for diagnosis is accomplished by visualization of the affected fascia in the operating room, and because early surgical intervention has been shown to greatly benefit mortality,[67] early surgical consultation is recommended. Laboratory testing, such as white blood cell count, electrolytes (including sodium), lactate, blood cultures, and reactive markers, should be pursued, but is insufficiently sensitive to clinch the diagnosis. Because of the often subtle nature of the disease entity, a large proportion of NSSTIs are initially misdiagnosed. In one study in 2003, Wong and coworkers found that only 14.6% of patients with NSSTIs admitted to the hospital carried the diagnosis at time of admission.

Because of the invasive nature of surgical diagnosis and high rate of misdiagnosis, many have sought to evaluate laboratory diagnostics and imaging modalities to aid in the diagnosis of this disease entity. Although contrasted MRI is highly sensitive and specific,[68,69] the delay in surgical management often makes this ill-advised. There is an emerging body of literature that both soft tissue ultrasound[70,71] and contrasted computed tomography scanning[72,73] could be of benefit in the diagnosis of NSSTI; however, there is not enough validated prospective data that either are sensitive enough to exclude NSSTI and neither should delay surgical consultation.

Wong and coworkers[66] published a laboratory risk index in 2004 to help distinguish NSSTIs from other SSTIs, which is often used to evaluate patients with suspected NSSTI. This score comprised various laboratory values often ordered in the evaluation of necrotizing infection, such as white blood cell count, C-reactive protein, serum sodium, serum glucose, and hemoglobin. Multiple attempts at validating this score have shown sensitivity less than 70% for these life-threatening infections.[63,74] As such, although these laboratory tests and blood cultures can be considered and interpreted in the proper clinical context, they should not be used as a basis to exclude an NSSTI.

Treatment and Disposition

Any patient with a suspected NSSTI should be given broad-spectrum IV antibiotic parenteral coverage (see **Fig. 2**) and receive appropriate fluid resuscitation and supportive therapy for sepsis and septic shock, if needed. Antibiotic coverage should address the potential for polymicrobial infection, given its high prevalence in these infections. Although antibiotics may be later refined, emergency department coverage should be broad spectrum and at an appropriate loading dose. The previously widely used 1 g of vancomycin is often insufficient for MRSA coverage, and weight-based loading and maintenance dosing should be applied.

Emergent surgical consultation is highly recommended. Early surgical debridement is considered gold standard therapy and has been the only intervention proven to benefit mortality.[10] These patients may likely require intensive care postoperatively. Although IV immunoglobulin has been studied in a few small patient cohorts, its widespread use is not recommended at this time.[9]

SUMMARY

SSTIs are an incredibly common and sometimes dangerous presentation to the emergency department. Simple cellulitis can likely be treated as an outpatient with appropriate therapy. Purulent infections should raise suspicion for CA-MRSA, and although some abscesses can be treated with incision and drainage alone, signs of systemic illness should prompt antibiotic coverage with an agent effective against MRSA. NSSTIs carry high morbidity and mortality, are difficult to diagnose, and should prompt emergent surgical consultation and broad-spectrum antimicrobials.

REFERENCES

1. National Hospital Ambulatory Medical Care Survey: 2011 Emergency Department Summary Tables. 2011. Available at: http://www.cdc.gov/nchs/data/ahcd/nhamcs_emergency/2011_ed_web_tables.pdf. Accessed June 19, 2016.
2. Guillamet CV, Kollef MH. How to stratify patients at risk for resistant bugs in skin and soft tissue infections? Curr Opin Infect Dis 2016;29(2):116–23.
3. Suaya JA, Mera RM, Cassidy A, et al. Incidence and cost of hospitalizations associated with Staphylococcus aureus skin and soft tissue infections in the United States from 2001 through 2009. BMC Infect Dis 2014;14:296.
4. Moran GJ, Krishnadasan A, Gorwitz RJ, et al. Methicillin-resistant S. aureus infections among patients in the emergency department. N Engl J Med 2006;355(7):666–74.
5. Talan DA, Krishnadasan A, Gorwitz RJ, et al. Comparison of Staphylococcus aureus from skin and soft-tissue infections in US emergency department patients, 2004 and 2008. Clin Infect Dis 2011;53(2):144–9.
6. Dryden MS. Skin and soft tissue infection: microbiology and epidemiology. Int J Antimicrob Agents 2009;34(Suppl 1):S2–7.
7. Moet GJ, Jones RN, Biedenbach DJ, et al. Contemporary causes of skin and soft tissue infections in North America, Latin America, and Europe: report from the SENTRY Antimicrobial Surveillance Program (1998-2004). Diagn Microbiol Infect Dis 2007;57(1):7–13.
8. Ray GT, Suaya JA, Baxter R. Microbiology of skin and soft tissue infections in the age of community-acquired methicillin-resistant Staphylococcus aureus. Diagn Microbiol Infect Dis 2013;76(1):24–30.
9. Stevens DL, Bisno AL, Chambers HF, et al. Practice guidelines for the diagnosis and management of skin and soft tissue infections: 2014 update by the Infectious Diseases Society of America. Clin Infect Dis 2014;59(2):147–59.
10. McHenry CR, Piotrowski JJ, Petrinic D, et al. Determinants of mortality for necrotizing soft-tissue infections. Ann Surg 1995;221(5):558–63 [discussion: 563–5].
11. Ray GT, Suaya JA, Baxter R. Incidence, microbiology, and patient characteristics of skin and soft-tissue infections in a U.S. population: a retrospective population-based study. BMC Infect Dis 2013;13:252.
12. Qualls ML, Mooney MM, Camargo CA, et al. Emergency department visit rates for abscess versus other skin infections during the emergence of community-associated methicillin-resistant Staphylococcus aureus, 1997-2007. Clin Infect Dis 2012;55(1):103–5.
13. Pallin DJ, Egan DJ, Pelletier AJ, et al. Increased US emergency department visits for skin and soft tissue infections, and changes in antibiotic choices, during the emergence of community-associated methicillin-resistant Staphylococcus aureus. Ann Emerg Med 2008;51(3):291–8.
14. Hersh AL, Chambers HF, Maselli JH, et al. National trends in ambulatory visits and antibiotic prescribing for skin and soft-tissue infections. Arch Intern Med 2008;168(14):1585–91.

15. Taira BR, Singer AJ, Thode HC, et al. National epidemiology of cutaneous abscesses: 1996 to 2005. Am J Emerg Med 2009;27(3):289–92.
16. Adam HJ, Allen VG, Currie A, et al. Community-associated methicillin-resistant *Staphylococcus aureus*: prevalence in skin and soft tissue infections at emergency departments in the Greater Toronto Area and associated risk factors. CJEM 2009;11(5):439–46.
17. Singer AJ, Talan DA. Management of skin abscesses in the era of methicillin-resistant *Staphylococcus aureus*. N Engl J Med 2014;370(11):1039–47.
18. Stenstrom R, Grafstein E, Romney M, et al. Prevalence of and risk factors for methicillin-resistant *Staphylococcus aureus* skin and soft tissue infection in a Canadian emergency department. CJEM 2009;11(5):430–8.
19. Stryjewski ME, Chambers HF. Skin and soft-tissue infections caused by community-acquired methicillin-resistant *Staphylococcus aureus*. Clin Infect Dis 2008;46(Suppl 5):S368–77.
20. Bernard P, Bedane C, Mounier M, et al. Streptococcal cause of erysipelas and cellulitis in adults. A microbiologic study using a direct immunofluorescence technique. Arch Dermatol 1989;125(6):779–82.
21. Jeng A, Beheshti M, Li J, et al. The role of beta-hemolytic streptococci in causing diffuse, nonculturable cellulitis: a prospective investigation. Medicine (Baltimore) 2010;89(4):217–26.
22. Eriksson B, Jorup-Rönström C, Karkkonen K, et al. Erysipelas: clinical and bacteriologic spectrum and serological aspects. Clin Infect Dis 1996;23(5):1091–8.
23. Crisp JG, Takhar SS, Moran GJ, et al. Inability of polymerase chain reaction, pyrosequencing, and culture of infected and uninfected site skin biopsy specimens to identify the cause of cellulitis. Clin Infect Dis 2015;61(11):1679–87.
24. Wu D, Wang Q, Yang Y, et al. Epidemiology and molecular characteristics of community-associated methicillin-resistant and methicillin-susceptible *Staphylococcus aureus* from skin/soft tissue infections in a children's hospital in Beijing, China. Diagn Microbiol Infect Dis 2010;67(1):1–8.
25. Frazee BW, Lynn J, Charlebois ED, et al. High prevalence of methicillin-resistant *Staphylococcus aureus* in emergency department skin and soft tissue infections. Ann Emerg Med 2005;45(3):311–20.
26. Borgundvaag B, Ng W, Rowe B, et al, EMERGency Department Emerging Infectious Disease Surveillance NeTwork (EMERGENT) Working Group. Prevalence of methicillin-resistant *Staphylococcus aureus* in skin and soft tissue infections in patients presenting to Canadian emergency departments. CJEM 2013;15(3):141–60.
27. Lee C-Y, Tsai H-C, Kunin CM, et al. Clinical and microbiological characteristics of purulent and non-purulent cellulitis in hospitalized Taiwanese adults in the era of community-associated methicillin-resistant *Staphylococcus aureus*. BMC Infect Dis 2015;15:311.
28. Lee TC, Carrick MM, Scott BG, et al. Incidence and clinical characteristics of methicillin-resistant *Staphylococcus aureus* necrotizing fasciitis in a large urban hospital. Am J Surg 2007;194(6):809–12 [discussion: 812–3].
29. Miller LG, Perdreau-Remington F, Rieg G, et al. Necrotizing fasciitis caused by community-associated methicillin-resistant *Staphylococcus aureus* in Los Angeles. N Engl J Med 2005;352(14):1445–53.
30. Chlebicki MP, Oh CC. Recurrent cellulitis: risk factors, etiology, pathogenesis and treatment. Curr Infect Dis Rep 2014;16(9):422.
31. Marin JR, Bilker W, Lautenbach E, et al. Reliability of clinical examinations for pediatric skin and soft-tissue infections. Pediatrics 2010;126(5):925–30.

32. Marin JR, Dean AJ, Bilker WB, et al. Emergency ultrasound-assisted examination of skin and soft tissue infections in the pediatric emergency department. Acad Emerg Med 2013;20(6):545–53.

33. Tayal VS, Hasan N, Norton HJ, et al. The effect of soft-tissue ultrasound on the management of cellulitis in the emergency department. Acad Emerg Med 2006;13(4):384–8.

34. Squire BT, Fox JC, Anderson C. ABSCESS: applied bedside sonography for convenient evaluation of superficial soft tissue infections. Acad Emerg Med 2005;12(7):601–6.

35. Berger T, Garrido F, Green J, et al. Bedside ultrasound performed by novices for the detection of abscess in ED patients with soft tissue infections. Am J Emerg Med 2012;30(8):1569–73.

36. Perl B, Gottehrer NP, Raveh D, et al. Cost-effectiveness of blood cultures for adult patients with cellulitis. Clin Infect Dis 1999;29(6):1483–8.

37. Duvanel T, Auckenthaler R, Rohner P, et al. Quantitative cultures of biopsy specimens from cutaneous cellulitis. Arch Intern Med 1989;149(2):293–6.

38. Peterson D, McLeod S, Woolfrey K, et al. Predictors of failure of empiric outpatient antibiotic therapy in emergency department patients with uncomplicated cellulitis. Acad Emerg Med 2014;21(5):526–31.

39. Volz KA, Canham L, Kaplan E, et al. Identifying patients with cellulitis who are likely to require inpatient admission after a stay in an ED observation unit. Am J Emerg Med 2013;31(2):360–4.

40. Hepburn MJ, Dooley DP, Skidmore PJ, et al. Comparison of short-course (5 days) and standard (10 days) treatment for uncomplicated cellulitis. Arch Intern Med 2004;164(15):1669–74.

41. Gaspari RJ, Blehar D, Polan D, et al. The Massachusetts abscess rule: a clinical decision rule using ultrasound to identify methicillin-resistant Staphylococcus aureus in skin abscesses. Acad Emerg Med 2014;21(5):558–67.

42. Gaspari RJ, Resop D, Mendoza M, et al. A randomized controlled trial of incision and drainage versus ultrasonographically guided needle aspiration for skin abscesses and the effect of methicillin-resistant *Staphylococcus aureus.* Ann Emerg Med 2011;57(5):483–91.e1.

43. Chandika AB, Gakwaya AM, Kiguli-Malwadde E, et al. Ultrasound guided needle aspiration versus surgical drainage in the management of breast abscesses: a Ugandan experience. BMC Res Notes 2012;5:12.

44. Naeem M, Rahimnajjad MK, Rahimnajjad NA, et al. Comparison of incision and drainage against needle aspiration for the treatment of breast abscess. Am Surg 2012;78(11):1224–7.

45. Schwarz RJ, Shrestha R. Needle aspiration of breast abscesses. Am J Surg 2001; 182(2):117–9.

46. Kessler DO, Krantz A, Mojica M. Randomized trial comparing wound packing to no wound packing following incision and drainage of superficial skin abscesses in the pediatric emergency department. Pediatr Emerg Care 2012;28(6):514–7.

47. Leinwand M, Downing M, Slater D, et al. Incision and drainage of subcutaneous abscesses without the use of packing. J Pediatr Surg 2013;48(9):1962–5.

48. O'Malley GF, Dominici P, Giraldo P, et al. Routine packing of simple cutaneous abscesses is painful and probably unnecessary. Acad Emerg Med 2009;16(5): 470–3.

49. Tonkin DM, Murphy E, Brooke-Smith M, et al. Perianal abscess: a pilot study comparing packing with nonpacking of the abscess cavity. Dis Colon Rectum 2004;47(9):1510–4.

50. Chinnock B, Hendey GW. Irrigation of cutaneous abscesses does not improve treatment success. Ann Emerg Med 2016;67(3):379–83.
51. Tsoraides SS, Pearl RH, Stanfill AB, et al. Incision and loop drainage: a minimally invasive technique for subcutaneous abscess management in children. J Pediatr Surg 2010;45(3):606–9.
52. Ladd AP, Levy MS, Quilty J. Minimally invasive technique in treatment of complex, subcutaneous abscesses in children. J Pediatr Surg 2010;45(7):1562–6.
53. Singer AJ, Thode HC, Chale S, et al. Primary closure of cutaneous abscesses: a systematic review. Am J Emerg Med 2011;29(4):361–6.
54. Talan DA, Mower WR, Krishnadasan A, et al. Trimethoprim-sulfamethoxazole versus placebo for uncomplicated skin abscess. N Engl J Med 2016;374(9): 823–32.
55. Duong M, Markwell S, Peter J, et al. Randomized, controlled trial of antibiotics in the management of community-acquired skin abscesses in the pediatric patient. Ann Emerg Med 2010;55(5):401–7.
56. Hankin A, Everett WW. Are antibiotics necessary after incision and drainage of a cutaneous abscess? Ann Emerg Med 2007;50(1):49–51.
57. Singer AJ, Thode HC. Systemic antibiotics after incision and drainage of simple abscesses: a meta-analysis. Emerg Med J 2014;31(7):576–8.
58. Macfie J, Harvey J. The treatment of acute superficial abscesses: a prospective clinical trial. Br J Surg 1977;64(4):264–6.
59. Rajendran PM, Young D, Maurer T, et al. Randomized, double-blind, placebo-controlled trial of cephalexin for treatment of uncomplicated skin abscesses in a population at risk for community-acquired methicillin-resistant *Staphylococcus aureus* infection. Antimicrob Agents Chemother 2007;51(11):4044–8.
60. Chan HL, Stern RS, Arndt KA, et al. The incidence of erythema multiforme, Stevens-Johnson syndrome, and toxic epidermal necrolysis. A population-based study with particular reference to reactions caused by drugs among out-patients. Arch Dermatol 1990;126(1):43–7.
61. Bilton BD, Zibari GB, McMillan RW, et al. Aggressive surgical management of necrotizing fasciitis serves to decrease mortality: a retrospective study. Am Surg 1998;64(5):397–400 [discussion: 400–1].
62. Wong CH, Chang HC, Pasupathy S, et al. Necrotizing fasciitis: clinical presentation, microbiology, and determinants of mortality. J Bone Joint Surg Am 2003; 85-A(8):1454–60.
63. Bernal NP, Latenser BA, Born JM, et al. Trends in 393 necrotizing acute soft tissue infection patients 2000-2008. Burns 2012;38(2):252–60.
64. Soltani AM, Best MJ, Francis CS, et al. Trends in the incidence and treatment of necrotizing soft tissue infections: an analysis of the National Hospital Discharge Survey. J Burn Care Res 2014;35(5):449–54.
65. Anaya DA, Dellinger EP. Necrotizing soft-tissue infection: diagnosis and management. Clin Infect Dis 2007;44(5):705–10.
66. Wong CH, Khin LW, Heng KS, et al. The LRINEC (Laboratory Risk Indicator for Necrotizing Fasciitis) score: a tool for distinguishing necrotizing fasciitis from other soft tissue infections. Crit Care Med 2004;32(7):1535–41.
67. Hadeed GJ, Smith J, O'Keeffe T, et al. Early surgical intervention and its impact on patients presenting with necrotizing soft tissue infections: a single academic center experience. J Emerg Trauma Shock 2016;9(1):22–7.
68. Brothers TE, Tagge DU, Stutley JE, et al. Magnetic resonance imaging differentiates between necrotizing and non-necrotizing fasciitis of the lower extremity. J Am Coll Surg 1998;187(4):416–21.

69. Schmid MR, Kossmann T, Duewell S. Differentiation of necrotizing fasciitis and cellulitis using MR imaging. AJR Am J Roentgenol 1998;170(3):615–20.
70. Castleberg E, Jenson N, Dinh VA. Diagnosis of necrotizing faciitis with bedside ultrasound: the STAFF Exam. West J Emerg Med 2014;15(1):111–3.
71. Hosek WT, Laeger TC. Early diagnosis of necrotizing fasciitis with soft tissue ultrasound. Acad Emerg Med 2009;16(10):1033.
72. Carbonetti F, Cremona A, Carusi V, et al. The role of contrast enhanced computed tomography in the diagnosis of necrotizing fasciitis and comparison with the laboratory risk indicator for necrotizing fasciitis (LRINEC). Radiol Med 2016;121(2): 106–21.
73. Zacharias N, Velmahos GC, Salama A, et al. Diagnosis of necrotizing soft tissue infections by computed tomography. Arch Surg 2010;145(5):452–5.
74. Liao CI, Lee YK, Su YC, et al. Validation of the laboratory risk indicator for necrotizing fasciitis (LRINEC) score for early diagnosis of necrotizing fasciitis. Tzu Chi Med J 2012;24(2):73–6.

Pitfalls in Wound Management

Dennis Tankersley, MS, PA-C[a],*, Tanya Schrobilgen, MS, PA-C[b]

KEYWORDS

- Wound care • Burn care • Irrigation • Dressings • Antibiotic prophylaxis

KEY POINTS

- Patient factors of compromised healing must be considered.
- Wound irrigation is a significant factor in the prevention of infection.
- Antibiotics are not commonly indicated in the treatment of acute lacerations.
- Understanding burn categorization and referral requirements is important.

INTRODUCTION

The goals of wound repair are hemostasis, restoration of function, and optimal cosmesis. Boxes 1 and 2 list the primary factors that can affect acute wound healing. Although providers can only control a small portion of these factors, it is important to understand the role that each plays in the patient's chances of having a desirable outcome.

METHODS TO PREVENT WOUND INFECTION

Risk of infection in wounds increases with prolonged time to closure.[1] However, wounds may be closed with good success later than the commonly held belief of 8 to 12 hours. Wounds closed up to 19 hours after injury have a higher rate of healing than those closed later than the 19-hour mark.[2] Wounds to areas of high vascularity, such as the face and scalp, may be successfully repaired later than those with less vascularity, like the anterior lower leg. Although cosmetic restoration is always a goal of wound closure, areas of high cosmetic importance, such as the face, should be considered for wound repair even if the timing of closure is not ideal.

Disclosure: D. Tankersley is a SEMPA board member, CEP America employee, San Gorgonio Memorial Healthcare District and Hospital Board Member. T. Schrobilgen is a CEP America employee.
[a] Department of Emergency Medicine, EMPA Fellowship, Arrowhead Regional Medical Center, 400 North Pepper, Suite M107, Colton, CA 92324, USA; [b] EMPA Fellowship, Arrowhead Regional Medical Center, 400 North Pepper, Suite M107, Colton, CA 92324, USA
* Corresponding author.
E-mail address: dennistankersley@CEP.com

Box 1
Risk factors for wound infection or poor healing

Delayed care

Heavy contamination

Retained foreign body

Diabetes mellitus (DM)

Obesity

Peripheral artery disease (PAD)

Chronic steroid use

Other immune-suppressed states

All traumatic wounds are considered contaminated. Heavily contaminated wounds are at greater risk of infection than those that are minimally contaminated. Adequate irrigation is the best method of cleaning a contaminated wound and is discussed in further detail later in this article.

Retained foreign bodies not only increase the risk of infection but are a major area of litigation regarding wound care outcomes.[3] Most foreign bodies in wounds presenting to the emergency department are wood, metal, or glass. Most retained foreign bodies can be found with exploration on physical examination, and nearly 20% are identified by radiographs alone.[4] Therefore, radiographs should be considered for any patients with a mechanism of injury or other history suspicious for foreign bodies within the wound (**Fig. 1**). To ensure adequate exploration and visualization, wounds should be anesthetized and good hemostasis achieved before examination, which should be done in good lighting. If the wound is near a joint, exploration should be performed while ranging the extremity to allow identification of tendon or joint capsule involvement.

Several patient-related factors can have a negative impact on wound healing and place patients at higher risk for infection. Patients with DM may have neuropathy, immune system impairment, and decreased peripheral blood flow. Patients with any PAD or venous stasis also have reduced healing capacity, including obese patients, who also have impaired healing caused by decreased vascularity of adipose tissue. Chronic steroid use or other immune-compromised states may lead to higher rates of infection.[5] Patients with these issues should be followed closely and should have a low threshold for specialist referral.

Common methods of promoting rapid healing and preventing wound infection include irrigation, debridement of devitalized tissue, prophylactic antibiotic administration, use of antimicrobial sutures, proper closure with good wound margin apposition, avoidance of wound dead space, and appropriate suture tension.

Box 2
Techniques to improve wound healing and decrease risk of infection

Irrigation

Debridement

Antibiotic prophylaxis

Wound margin apposition and tension

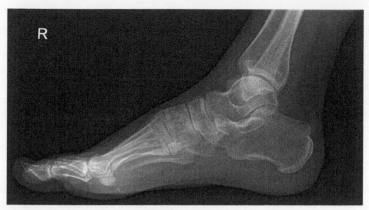

Fig. 1. Radiograph showing a retained foreign body. (*From* Haverstock BD. Puncture wounds of the foot. Clin Podiatr Med Surg 2012;29(2):311–22.)

One of the most important steps to preventing infection of acute wounds is irrigation.[6] Irrigation helps to remove debris and loose, devitalized tissue while decreasing the bacterial load within the wound.

The 3 primary factors that affect wound irrigation efficacy are irrigation solution, pressure of irrigation, and volume of irrigation. Potable tap water works equally well as normal saline or sterile water for the purposes of wound irrigation. Cleansing solutions (eg, Dakin solution, chlorhexidine, hydrogen peroxide, and rubbing alcohol) should be avoided because they can cause harm to local tissue and may not significantly decrease bacterial loads.[7,8] In cases of highly contaminated wounds, a 1% povidone-iodine (Betadine) solution can be used without risk of local tissue damage if an antiseptic solution is desired. This solution can easily be made at the bedside by diluting the standard 10% Betadine with water or saline in a 1:10 ratio.[9] However, this has not been proven to provide significantly more benefit than tap water alone.

More important than the solution used in the process of irrigation are the other 2 factors of pressure and volume. There is little evidence to determine the best pressure for irrigation. However, it is thought that high pressures may cause local tissue damage and dispersion of debris into the surround tissues.[10] Although there are many commercial devices available for wound irrigation, a commonly accepted practice is to use a 60-mL syringe attached to an angiocatheter of 18 to 20 gauge.

Volume of wound irrigation is dictated by wound characteristics such as location and depth, and contamination type and degree, as well as patient risk factors for poor healing. Wounds should be irrigated with a minimum of 200 mL per centimeter of wound, or until all debris is removed from the wound bed.

The goal of wound debridement is to remove permanently devitalized tissues. This removal should be done with a sharp instrument such as a scalpel or scissors. Removing this tissue prevents it from becoming a nidus for infections as it breaks down, and allows the body's normal healing responses to take place without unnecessarily having to phagocytize this necrotic tissue. It is important that the effect of tissue loss on both function and wound tension is considered when preforming debridement. Care must be taken to remove as little tissue as is necessary to provide a healthy wound bed.

The methods by which the wound is repaired also affect its ability to heal efficiently. Common wound closure methods include Steri-Strips, tissue adhesive, staples, and suture. The selection of closure devices is determined based on the characteristics of the wound. Regardless of which is chosen, the goal should be full wound margin approximation and eversion. Although enough tension must be applied to approximate tissue, the sutures must be loose enough to prevent exaggerated patient discomfort, ischemia, and tissue necrosis during healing.[11] In wounds that are deep, superficial closure techniques may not be adequate to approximate the margins of the wound to its full depth. In these cases, it is important that deep sutures are placed to prevent a pocket or potential space know a dead space from being created. Dead spaces allow the accumulation of fluid and may harbor bacteria leading to infection and abscess.

ANTIBIOTIC PROPHYLAXIS

Proper wound healing is expected in clean wounds that are well vascularized and without evidence of infection, devitalized tissue, or foreign bodies.[12] As previously discussed, the most important methods of infection prevention are irrigation and debridement. All wounds are colonized with bacterial microorganisms; however, not all wounds are considered infected. Infected wounds show 1 or more of the following: surrounding erythema and edema, purulent discharge, lymphangitic streaking, and possible foul odor. Systemic signs and symptoms of infection, such as fevers, chills, confusion, leukocytosis and/or hyperglycemia, may also be present. Well-healing wounds should be free from these signs of infection and show epithelialization and granulation tissue. In cases in which signs of infection are present, antibiotic use is a necessity. When infection is not currently present but the patient or wound shows risk factors for poor healing, prophylactic antibiotics are often considered.

The role of antibiotic use for wounds without evidence of infection remains controversial. Further investigation is needed to determine whether use of prophylactic antibiotics is effective in preventing infection. Although the supportive evidence is lacking, it is reasonable to consider their use in high-risk injuries such as contaminated or crushed wounds that need extensive debridement, wounds that are opened for a prolonged time (>8 hours) that may need primary closure, animal bites, marine injuries, injuries through shoes, sites with poor vascular supply, and involvement of vulnerable sites (eg, bone, joint, or cartilage).[13] The literature does not support the routine use of antibiotics in simple and clean wound management. There are too few studies comparing the role of prophylactic antibiotic use with the sole use of irrigation and debridement in high-risk injuries, therefore it is up to the clinician's experience and judgment to determine the need for antibiotics. The consideration for antibiotics should also include the patient's living conditions, access to follow-up, possible morbidity, and cost of complications should an infection occur (Box 3).

Crush injuries are considered high-risk injuries and need extensive debridement. Because of the mechanism, crush injuries can leave devitalized tissue inside, near, or beneath the wound. This damaged tissue may impede wound healing, serve as a medium for pathogens, and may be either inaccessible or too extensive for safe debridement. Prophylactic use of antibiotics is often considered in these cases.

High-pressure injection injuries, such as those caused by paint sprayers, pressure washers, or ruptured hydraulic lines, are at very high risk for infection and can cause damage far from the laceration or point of injection (Fig. 2). Skin flora may be carried remotely into the deep tissues and between planes of tissue and the injected medium may also cause direct injury. These wounds require surgical consultation and should have a very low threshold for operative exploration.

Box 3
High-risk wounds

Highly contaminated wounds

Crush injuries that have extensive devitalized tissue

Wounds that have been open for a prolonged time (>8 hours) that may need primary closure

Animal bites or marine injuries

Injuries through the soles of shoes

Sites with poor vascular supply

High-pressure injection injuries

Involvement of vulnerable sites (eg, bone, joint, or cartilage)

Because it is known that wounds that are nearing or have surpassed the so-called golden period of 19-hours have a lesser chance of healing it is also appropriate to consider providing antibiotic prophylaxis when choosing to close these wounds.

Wounds that involve vulnerable sites such as joints, bones, cartilage, and tendon or tendon sheaths are susceptible to serious infections. Greater precautions are taken with these injuries because infections involving these areas can lead to severe illness, amputations, multiple surgeries, disabilities, and other severe complications. Often, these injuries require debridement and washout in the operating suite with immediate initiation of parenteral antibiotics.

Patients with the previously described factors for wound infection or poor healing may be considered for prophylactic antibiotics as well. Whether because of poor vascular flow at an injured site or injury in an immunocompromised host, the inability to adequately fight off infection increases risk for complications.

Patients who need to proceed to the operating room for an emergent surgical intervention receive prophylactic antibiotics before the procedure based on the degree of anticipated contamination. Traumatic wounds are generally considered to be clean, clean-contaminated, contaminated from a foreign body, or grossly contaminated.[14]

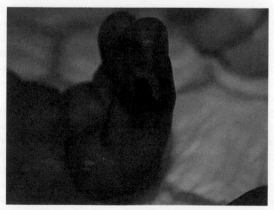

Fig. 2. High-pressure injection injury. (*Data from* Urso-Baiarda F, Stanley PR. The 'Butter Test' to guide effective tissue cleansing after high-pressure injection injury. J Plast Reconstr Aesthet Surg 2010;63(11):e792–5.)

In any procedure deemed anything except a clean procedure, it is generally accepted that prophylactic antibiotics should be initiated.

SELECTING AN AGENT

The antibiotic selected for prophylaxis should provide coverage of the pathogens that are most likely to colonize that wound, based on location and mechanism of injury.[15] Other factors should be considered, such as compliance, resistance, potential adverse reactions, and cost. Medication regimens with more frequent doses and longer duration of therapy may have poorer compliance rates. Some geographic areas have a higher resistance to what would otherwise be considered first-line agents. Selection of therapy may have to be adjusted and the facility antibiogram or infectious disease service should be consulted in these situations.

Staphylococcus aureus and streptococci species are the most common organisms found in soft tissue wound infections. Although they can be pathologic at times, these species are largely found on normal skin flora. When there is a break in the epidermis, these pathogens can colonize wounds and increase the risk for infection. First-generation cephalosporins and penicillinase-resistant B-lactams (eg, dicloxacillin) are effective against *S aureus* and many streptococci, therefore they are the most commonly used agents for prophylactic antibiotic coverage. As methicillin-resistant *S aureus* (MRSA) becomes more prevalent in the community, other medications should be considered.[16] Clindamycin, trimethoprim-sulfamethoxazole, tetracycline (eg, doxycycline or minocycline), and linezolid are effective outpatient treatments that cover MRSA.

Penetration injuries through a shoe may be inoculated with pseudomonas. In this case, B-lactam agents are not sufficient coverage. A fluoroquinolone such as ciprofloxacin is the antibiotic of choice.[17] Mammalian bites, which are discussed in further details later, may require amoxicillin-clavulanate for coverage of *Pasteurella* or *Eikenella* species. Injuries occurring with marine exposure have possibility of infection with *Vibrio vulnificus*, which may be treated with fluoroquinolones or a third-generation cephalosporin plus a tetracycline.

TETANUS PROPHYLAXIS

For every presentation of a recent injury or wound, tetanus vaccination status should be inquired. *Clostridium tetani* is a spore-forming toxin that causes symptoms of uncontrolled muscle spasm and lockjaw. This bacterium is commonly found in soil and feces and may be inoculated into a wound by a thorn, wood, metal, or other material. It affects the nervous system by disrupting the inhibitory neurotransmitter release that affects motor neurons, causing unopposed muscle contractions and rigidity. This condition can ultimately interfere with the respiratory muscles and myocardium and lead to asphyxia or sudden cardiac death. Tetanus is easily preventable with vaccinations but has a high mortality once infection has occurred.[18]

The Centers for Disease Control and Prevention (CDC) recommend children to receive tetanus (diphtheria, tetanus, acellular pertussis) vaccinations at months 2, 4, 6, between 15 and 18 months, and lastly at 4 to 6 years of age. Boosters (tetanus, diphtheria and pertussis [Tdap]) are recommended after the age of 10 years and again every 10 years. Patients presenting with a wound that is simple and clean should be offered a Tdap booster if they have not had a tetanus vaccination within the last 10 years. For contaminated wounds or any wounds not considered simple and clean, the patient should receive a booster within 5 years. For patients with contaminated wounds and of unknown vaccination status or who have received less than 3 tetanus vaccinations, the addition of tetanus immune globin is recommended.

EVALUATION AND MANAGEMENT OF ANIMAL BITES

Statistics for animal bites may be underreported because of some patients not seeking medical attention or reporting. Dog bites account for most animal bites, followed by cats and small rodents. Common concerns for many patients are infection, need for rabies vaccine, and cosmetic outcome. Each of these is addressed separately. Mammalian bites often present as puncture wounds and sometimes tearing, depending on the aggressiveness of the animal.

Initial management of bites is similar to that of any wound. Good hemostasis must be achieved, followed by adequate irrigation. Because of the potential harm from agents such as alcohol or hydrogen peroxide, water is the irrigate of choice. A mild soap may be used if desired. All bites should be considered contaminated; thus, the use of prophylactic antibiotics is often considered. Although the supporting evidence is lacking, it is commonly accepted to use antibiotics in high-risk cases, if the injury is from certain types of animals, or if there is an increased suspicion for a specific pathogen.[19] Large wounds; crush or deep penetrating injuries; and wounds on the hands, feet, or over a joint may also benefit from prophylactic antibiotics. The use of radiographic studies is recommended if there is suspicion of foreign bodies, vascular injury, or underlying fracture.

Although now very rare in the United States, a common concern of patients presenting with dog bite is rabies exposure. The drastically reduced risk of rabies in the United States has been caused by successful animal control programs. More than 90% of rabies exposures are caused by wildlife such as bats and carnivores.[20] Rabies virus is transmitted through saliva and nervous system tissue. When infection is suspected, initiation of treatment with human rabies immunoglobulin followed by a full course of rabies vaccine should be initiated (Table 1). The animal in question should be quarantined for observation of aggressive behavior. If this is not possible, postexposure prophylaxis may be initiated depending on suspicion of the animal. Statistics vary based on geographic locations. Patients may have received preexposure vaccinations because of their risk of exposure, such as those who work with rabid animals or who are traveling. These patients do not require rabies immune globulin with their rabies vaccine (see Table 1).

The practice for wound closure in bite wounds is widely variable. In general, bite wounds are considered contaminated and often do not undergo primary closure. Larger gaping wounds are often considered for loose approximation, in which a few sutures are placed to help the healing process and improve scaring, but this is not as cosmetically appealing as a traditional primary closure. There are insufficient studies addressing the infection rate occurring in bite wounds receiving primary closure versus those left open.[21] One study involved 168 patients with dog bite

Table 1 Rabies vaccine schedule		
Vaccination Status	**Doses**	**Schedule**
Preexposure	3 doses	Days 0, 7, 21–28
Post-exposure		
Never vaccinated[a]	4 doses	Days 0, 3, 7, 14
Completed vaccinations[b]	2 doses	Days 0 and 3

[a] Rabies immune globulin given on day 0.
[b] No rabies immune globulin indicated.

lacerations who were randomized into 2 groups: one that received primary closure and one in which the wounds were left open. Both groups received the same prophylactic antibiotics, and the investigators concluded that there was no significant difference in infection rates and that improved cosmesis was achieved with primary closure.[22] Although most clinicians leave bite wounds open, wounds considered for primary closure are dependent on time of injury to presentation, location, and type of animal. The time frame by which the wound should be closed is debatable, just as in other wounds, but many investigators suggest that it should be within 8 hours of injury. Injuries located on the face are well vascularized and typically heal well with good irrigation and primary closure. However, other locations, such as hands and joints, are at higher risk for infection.[23] Few studies have been done on dog bites showing lower infection rates compared with other animal bites.

Other animal bites, such as cat bites, have a higher risk of infection. Cat bites may not seem as damaging as dog bites, but these wounds are often more difficult to clean out. Studies show that infection rates can range from 20% to 80%.[24] Thus, prophylactic antibiotics are strongly considered and primary wound closure is often deferred.

Human bites tend to have higher rates of infection and often evaluation and treatment are not sought until the infection is well established. Thus, experts recommend antibiotics to be initiated on initial presentation of any human bite wound regardless of location. Antibiotics should be designed to cover *Eikenella corrodens* as well as other common bacterial flora, such as *S aureus* and oral anaerobes.[25] As mentioned earlier, hand wounds tend to have a higher infection rate but human bites involving the hand pose a significant risk. These hand wounds often occur with a closed fist to an open mouth, causing a laceration from teeth over the metacarpophalangeal joint. To novice practitioners, this may seem like a minor injury. However, because the soft tissue is thin and there is close proximity of the wound to tendons, bone, and joint capsule, inoculation of bacteria can easily cause infection.[26] These injuries usually require orthopedic consultation, intravenous antibiotics (eg, ampicillin/sulbactam), and possibly a thorough washout in the operating room.[27]

THERMAL BURNS

Thermal burns are classified by size of the area burned, described as percentage of total body surface area (TBSA) involved, and by depth of tissue involved, which is described as superficial to full thickness. Percentage of TBSA can be determined using either the rule of 9s or a Lund-Browder chart (Fig. 3). Very small TBSA burns may be best measured by using the patients palm to estimate 1%.

The rule of 9s allots 9% TBSA for an adult's head, 9% for each upper extremity, 18% for the anterior torso, 18% for the posterior torso, 18% for each leg, and 1% for the perineum and genitalia. The rule of 9s is not accurate for infants and children because of the disproportionately large head and smaller lower extremities. Use of this rule in infants may lead to over-resuscitation with intravenous fluids. Instead, the rule is modified for infants and children and termed the rule of 5s (Table 2),[9] or the appropriately sized diagram is chosen from the Lund-Browder formula[9] (Table 3).

CLASSIFYING DEPTH OF BURNS

Burn injuries are classified based on the depth of tissue injury. These injuries can be broken down into 5 categories: superficial, superficial partial thickness, deep partial thickness, full thickness, and fourth degree (Fig. 4). Classifying burn injuries helps to determine appropriate wound care in outpatient management or need for surgical intervention.

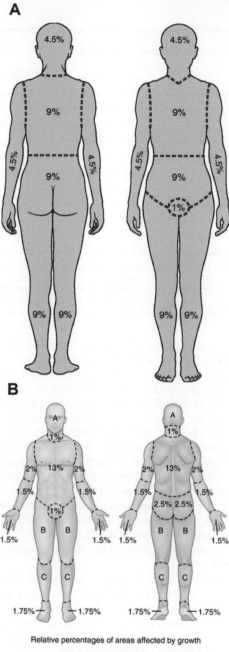

Fig. 3. (*A*) Rule of 9s and (*B*) Lund-Browder chart. (*From* Integumentary system. In: Buck CJ, editor. The next step, advanced medical coding. 2011 edition. Philadelphia: Saunders; 2011; and *Courtesy of* Rosen's Emergency Medicine, 2010.)

Table 2
Rule of 9s (adults) and rule of 5s (children and infants)

Area of Burn	Percentage		
	Adult	Child	Infant
Head and neck	9	15	20
Arm			
Right	9	10	10
Left	9	10	10
Torso			
Anterior	18	20	20
Posterior	18	20	20
Leg			
Right	18	15	10
Left	18	15	10
Genitalia and perineum	1		
Total	100	100	100

From Stone CK, Humphries RL. Current emergency diagnosis & treatment. In: Stone CK, Humphries RL, editors. Current emergency diagnosis & treatment. New York: McGraw-Hill; 2003. p. 580–1.

Superficial burns are erythematous and painful. Commonly seen in sunburns, these involve only the outermost layer of skin (the epidermis). These burns typically blanch, do not form blisters, and heal within 3 to 6 days and without scarring.

Partial thickness injuries are divided into 2 categories: superficial and deep. Superficial partial-thickness burns include the epidermis and upper portions of the dermis. They commonly present as erythematous, moist, and painful areas with blisters, although the hair may still be present. If the blister is unroofed, the underlying skin is erythematous but blanches with pressure. Burns in this category may take 1 to 3 weeks to heal and usually do not scar. Deep partial-thickness burns extend deeper into the dermal layer, affecting hair follicles and glands. These blisters are unroofed easily and underlying skin may be pale with patches of redness, have a weeping or waxy appearance, and may or may not blanch with pressure. These burns are painful to pressure only and take much longer (3–9 weeks) to heal. These injuries are often difficult to differentiate from full-thickness burns and are at risk for scarring or problems with function if involving hands or joints, therefore appropriate follow-up and wound care are necessary.

Full-thickness burns involve all layers of the dermis and often include the subcutaneous tissue destroying glands, hair follicles, and nerve endings. These burns may be gray or a pale color, have a leathery texture, are generally painless, and do not develop blisters. The skin does not blanch and is not sensitive to pressure. These burns can develop eschar tissue, putting patients at risk for scarring, contracture, and functional disability without surgical intervention.

Fourth-degree burns extend through the skin and involve underlying muscle or bone.

TREATMENT OF BURNS

Treatment of burns is based on size, severity, location, patient age, and comorbidities. As with other traumatic wounds, factors that diminish healing capacity, such as

Table 3
Lund-Browder chart

Area	Birth to 1 y	1–4 y	5–9 y	10–14 y	Adult
Head	19	17	13	11	9
Neck	2	2	2	2	2
Torso					
Anterior	13	13	13	13	13
Posterior	13	13	13	13	13
Upper Arm					
Anterior	2	2	2	2	2
Posterior	2	2	2	2	2
Forearm					
Anterior	1.5	1.5	1.5	1.5	1.5
Posterior	1.5	1.5	1.5	1.5	1.5
Hand					
Dorsum	1.25	1.25	1.25	1.25	1.25
Palm	1.25	1.25	1.25	1.25	1.25
Upper Leg					
Anterior	2.75	3.25	4	4.25	4.5
Posterior	2.75	3.25	4	4.25	4.5
Lower Leg					
Anterior	2.5	2.5	2.5	3	3.25
Posterior	2.5	2.5	2.5	3	3.25
Foot					
Dorsum	1.75	1.75	1.75	1.75	1.75
Sole	1.75	1.75	1.75	1.75	1.75
Right buttock	2.5	2.5	2.5	2.5	2.5
Left buttock	2.5	2.5	2.5	2.5	2.5
Genitalia	1	1	1	1	1

nutritional status, body habitus, and immune compromised states, must all be considered when treating patients with burns.

If the burn involves the airway or compromises respiration, these issues must be addressed immediately. Patients with deep burns covering more than 15% TBSA require fluid resuscitation, usually with lactated Ringer to reduce the risk of hyperchloremia from normal saline. There are various formulas for initiating fluid resuscitation, although Parkland formula is the most widely used, followed by the modified Brooke formula. Regardless of initial formula choice, maintenance of hydration status to clinical response, such as a urine output of 0.5 mL/kg/h, is most important. Mortality increases when urine output is minimal. Fluid losses related to larger area burns may also lead to shock or electrolyte disturbances. Hypoxemia or carbon monoxide poisoning could be a result of the environment in which the burn occurred. These issues should be monitored along with cardiac activity. In all but the most minor burns, jewelry such as rings and bracelets should be removed early because ensuing edema can cause them to become constrictive.

Once the ABCs (airway, breathing, circulation) have been evaluated and attended to, the first step in treating any acute burn is cooling the affected area. Cooling not only provides comfort but may help to limit the depth of the burn. Cooling can be done with a towel-wrapped ice pack, or cool saline–soaked gauze. Running cool

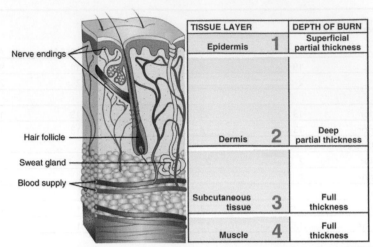

TISSUE LAYER		DEPTH OF BURN
Epidermis	1	Superficial partial thickness
Dermis	2	Deep partial thickness
Subcutaneous tissue	3	Full thickness
Muscle	4	Full thickness

Fig. 4. Burn depths. (*From* Mahan LK, Escott-Stump S. Krause's food and nutrition therapy. 12th edition. St Louis (MO): Saunders; 2008.)

water or soaking may also be used but should be limited to just a few minutes to avoid macerating the skin.

Cleaning of most burns can be done with mild soap and water. As discussed earlier, the use of disinfectants may impede the healing process and should only be used if the burn is otherwise heavily contaminated. Antibiotics should be preserved for infected burns. Tetanus vaccination status needs to be up to date.

Ruptured blisters or sloughing skin should be debrided because they can harbor bacteria and lead to infection. The treatment of intact blisters is controversial, with some clinicians advocating for immediate removal, whereas others argue for blisters being left intact.[28] Those arguing for the removal of blisters do so from the stance that blister fluid may chemically inhibit the healing process and be a medium for bacterial growth. Others think that this is a sterile space that provides and natural barrier for the burn, decreasing both pain and risk of infection. Part of the normal healing process is resorption of the fluid and contraction of the blister. If blisters are large, cover joints, impede physical examination, or are lasting longer than 1 week, they should be removed.

Superficial and small-area, partial-thickness burns do not always require dressings; however, aloe vera, a nonscented lotion, or bacitracin may be used to provide comfort. If a dressing is desired for protection, these items can also help keep it from adhering to the skin. Larger-area, partial thickness, superficial burns can be covered with a variety of dressings but can usually be adequately treated with an antibiotic ointment and petroleum jelly gauze or other nonadhesive dressing. Deep partial-thickness and full-thickness burns should be assessed by a burn specialist and can temporarily be dressed as discussed earlier or with a specialty dressing such as a product containing hydrocolloid or silver.

Areas of burn that are of particular concern are hands, feet, face, eyes, ears, and perineum, and any circumferential burn.[9] Burns such as these, and any partial-thickness burn that crosses a joint, should have a lower threshold for specialist involvement. Circumferential full-thickness burns also pose a special risk around limbs, chest, and abdomen because eschar tissue can form, causing restriction of deeper tissues to swell. In the chest and abdomen, eschar tissue may restrict a

---

Box 4
American Burn Association guidelines on burn center referral

- Partial-thickness burns greater than 10% TBSA
- Involvement of face, hands, feet, genitalia, peritoneum, and major joints
- Third-degree burns
- Electrical or chemical burns
- Inhalation injury
- Comorbidities that may complicate recovery or affect mortality
- Burn injuries with concomitant trauma (eg, fracture) in which burn poses the greatest risk of morbidity or mortality
- If hospital does not have qualified personnel or equipment for the care of burned children
- Burn injury in patients who require special social, emotional, or rehabilitative intervention

---

patient's ability to breathe. In limbs, it may act as a tourniquet and cut off circulation to the distal limb. These circumstances may require an escharotomy, a high-risk procedure in which burn specialists should be consulted. Burns to these areas and all burns greater than 10% TBSA, or any full-thickness burn, are best treated at a burn center. Contact and consultation should be made early in the emergency department course of stay and transfer should be arranged as soon as the patient is stabilized[29] (Box 4).

Whether treating traumatic lacerations or burns, understanding the factors that affect patient healing is key to providing good patient care. Type, location, and tissue type involvement are only a portion of what physician assistants must consider in managing wounds. Patient comorbidities, socioeconomic factors, and access to care must also be kept in mind. Taking all of the elements discussed in this article into account when determining the best methods for wound care/repair and specialist involvement are the only way to ensure the best chances of success for these patients.

REFERENCES

1. Waseem M, Lakdawala V, Patel R, et al. Is there a relationship between wound infections and laceration closure times? Int J Emerg Med 2012;5(1):32.
2. Berk W, Osbourne D, Taylor D. Evaluation of the 'Golden Period' for wound repair: 204 cases from a third world emergency department. Ann Emerg Med 1988; 17(5):496–500.
3. Pfaff JA, Moore GP. Reducing risk in emergency department wound management. Emerg Med Clin North Am 2007;25(1):189–201.
4. Levine MR, Gorman SM, Young CF, et al. Clinical characteristics and management of wound foreign bodies in the ED. Am J Emerg Med 2008;26(8):918–22.
5. Hess CT. Checklist for factors affecting wound healing. Adv Skin Wound Care 2011;24(4):192.
6. Stevenson TR, Thacker JG, Rodeheaver GT, et al. Cleansing the traumatic wound by high pressure syringe irrigation. JACEP 1976;5(1):17–21.
7. Kaysinger KK, Nicholson NC, Ramp WK, et al. Toxic effects of wound irrigation solutions on cultured tibiae and osteoblasts. J Orthop Trauma 1995;9(4):303–11.
8. Owens BD. Comparison of irrigation solutions and devices in a contaminated musculoskeletal wound survival model. J Bone Joint Surg Am 2009;91(1):92.

9. Stone CK, Humphries RL. Current emergency diagnosis & treatment. In: Stone CK, Humphries RL, editors. Current emergency diagnosis & treatment. New York: McGraw-Hill; 2003. p. 580–1.
10. Wheeler CB. Side effects of high pressure irrigation. J Trauma 1977;17(3):256.
11. Ethicon wound closure manual. Somerville (NJ): Ethicon; 1994.
12. Ortho-McNeil Pharmaceuticals, Janssen-Cilag. A brief history of wound healing. Yardley (PA): Oxford Clinical Communications; 1998.
13. Blumm RM, Hollander JE, Singer AJ. Skin and soft tissue injuries and infections: a practical evidence based guide. People's Medical Publishing House (PMPH) USA; 2010.
14. Surgical site infection: pathogenesis and prevention. Available at: http://www.medscape.org/viewarticle/448981_4. Accessed August 2, 2016.
15. National Nosocomial Infections Surveillance (NNIS) System report, data summary from October 1986 April 1998, issued June 1998. Am J Infect Control 1998;26(5):522–33.
16. Baddour MM. MRSA (methicillin resistant *Staphylococcus aureus*) infections and treatment. New York: Nova Science; 2010.
17. Barth R. Plantar puncture wounds. Emergency management of infectious diseases. p. 147–50. http://dx.doi.org/10.1017/cbo9780511547454.029.
18. Tetanus prevention after a disaster. Tetanus prevention|health and safety prevention. Available at: http://www.emergency.cdc.gov/disasters/disease/tetanus.asp. Accessed August 2, 2016.
19. Abrahamian FM, Goldstein EJC. Microbiology of animal bite wound infections. Clin Microbiol Rev 2011;24(2):231–46.
20. Centers for Disease Control and Prevention. Rabies in the U.S. 2011. Available at: http://www.cdc.gov/rabies/location/usa/index.html. Accessed August 2, 2016.
21. Chen E, Horing S, Shepherd SM, et al. Primary closure of mammalian bites. Acad Emerg Med 2000;7(2):157–61.
22. Cheng H-T, Hsu Y-C, Wu C-I. Does primary closure for dog bite wounds increase the incidence of wound infection? A meta-analysis of randomized controlled trials. J Plast Reconstr Aesthet Surg 2014;67(10):1448–50.
23. Myers JP. Bite wound infections. Curr Infect Dis Rep 2003;5(5):416–25.
24. Kennedy SA, Stoll LE, Lauder AS. Human and other mammalian bite injuries of the hand. J Am Acad Orthop Surg 2015;23(1):47–57.
25. Patil P, Panchabhai T, Galwankar S. Managing human bites. J Emerg Trauma Shock 2009;2(3):186.
26. Godoy D, Bonadeo G, Peralta H. Fight bite injuries. Internet J Emerg Med 2003;1(2). http://dx.doi.org/10.5580/1cd.
27. Shewring DJ, Trickett RW, Subramanian KN, et al. The management of clenched fist 'fight bite' injuries of the hand. J Hand Surg Eur Vol 2015;40(8):819–24.
28. Herndon DN. Total burn care. In: Total burn care. Edinburgh (United Kingdom): Saunders Elsevier; 2007. p. 71.
29. Guidelines for the operation of burn centers. Available at: http://www.ameriburn.org/chapter14.pdf. Accessed August 2, 2016.

Deadly Drug Ingestions

 CrossMark

Ann R. Verhoeven, MMSc, PA-C[a],*, Carson R. Harris, MD, DABAM[b]

KEYWORDS

- Acute poisoning management • Emergency department • Toxidrome
- One pill can kill • Overdose

KEY POINTS

- Organized rapid recognition and management is important in patients with a toxic ingestion.
- Toxidrome recognition is an important tool to aid in the identification and ongoing management of potentially lethal drug poisonings.
- Knowledge about prevalence and preparation for skilled management of harmful and potentially fatal ingestions, intentional and unintentional, is important for emergency medicine physician assistants.

INITIAL MANAGEMENT

The initial approach to the clinical evaluation of patients known or suspected to be presenting with toxic ingestion is to focus on the principles of emergent stabilization.[1–3] Adhering to an algorithmic approach to evaluation and management of critically ill patients while considering administering a specific antidote is recommended (Fig. 1).[4] The assessment of airway patency, followed rapidly by the determination of adequate ventilation, are the first vital components. If the airway is determined to be inadequate despite optimal positioning and supplemental oxygen, intubation should be considered as well as the key antidotes (naloxone, hypertonic dextrose). Evaluation of circulatory compromise and intervention should be performed next, with the immediate treatment of dysrhythmia and hemodynamic instability as indicated. Intravenous (IV) access, laboratory draw, and frequently IV fluid administration should be done at this time. Obtaining a 12-lead electrocardiogram (ECG) can aid in identifying a specific toxicity for which an antidote can be given (calcium, glucagon, Fab, sodium bicarbonate). Continuous

Disclosure: The authors have no relevant financial relationships to disclose.
[a] Emergency Medicine Physician Assistant Residency Program, Emergency Medicine Department, Regions Hospital, 640 Jackson Street, MS 11102F, Saint Paul, MN 55101, USA;
[b] Department of Emergency Medicine, Minnesota Poison Control System, Valhalla Place Addiction and Mental Health Services, University of Minnesota Medical School, 800 Great Oaks Lane, Eagan, MN 55123, USA
* Corresponding author.
E-mail address: ann.r.verhoeven@healthpartners.com

Physician Assist Clin 2 (2017) 449–463
http://dx.doi.org/10.1016/j.cpha.2017.02.008
2405-7991/17/© 2017 Elsevier Inc. All rights reserved.
physicianassistant.theclinics.com

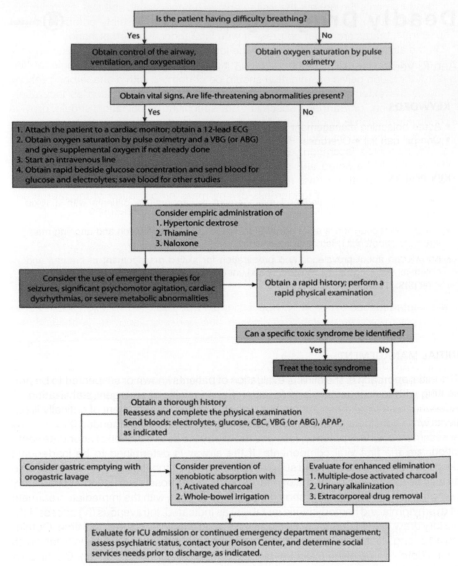

Fig. 1. Basic guide to the management of poisoned patients. A more detailed description of the steps in management is provided in the text. This algorithm is only a guide to management, which must consider the patient's clinical status. APAP, acetaminophen; ABG, arterial blood gas; CBC, complete blood count; ECG, electrocardiogram; ICU, intensive care unit; VBG, venous blood gas. (*From* Hoffman RS, Howland M, Lewin NA, et al. Principles of managing the acutely poisoned or overdosed patient. In: Hoffman RS, Howland M, Lewin NA, et al, editors. Goldfrank's toxicologic emergencies, 10th edition. New York: McGraw-Hill; 2015; with permission. Available at: http://accessemergencymedicinemhmedical.com/content.aspx?bookid=1163&sectionid=65089354. Accessed September 15, 2016.)

cardiac monitoring, pulse oximetry, and end-tidal CO_2 are important tools in the initial evaluation and ongoing management of poisoned patients.

Continue the algorithmic approach by assessing for disability or alteration of mental status. In the patients presenting comatose or stuporous, consider whether an antidote is indicated (hypertonic dextrose, naloxone, thiamine, or flumazenil) (Table 1). When seizures are identified, if hypoglycemia is excluded, an anticonvulsant, typically a benzodiazepine, should be given. When seizures are thought to be caused by isoniazid, consider the need for an antidote (pyridoxine). For organophosphate or carbamate insecticide poisoning, pralidoxime and atropine are used as antidotes. In the case of severe agitation, assess for hypoglycemia, hypoxia, and metabolic disturbance while treating with a sedative. Most commonly a benzodiazepine is indicated. Consider the need for intubation and paralysis in treating benzodiazepine-unresponsive patients. For dyskinesia or rigidity, again, benzodiazepines are indicated. Another critically important complication from a toxic ingestion is hyperthermia, which can cause seizures, agitation, and muscular rigidity. Rapid external cooling, control of shivering, and, for unresponsive patients, intubation and neuromuscular paralysis are appropriate.

Exposure of the patient may give important clues to the cause of the toxic exposure and its complications. Skin findings may include track marks, cyanosis, diaphoresis, urticaria, or edema. Evaluate for signs of trauma or systemic infection, and consider rhabdomyolysis with a history of prolonged immobilization or severe agitation.

DIAGNOSIS OF DEADLY DRUGS

Identification of the constellation of signs, symptoms, laboratory findings, and ECG changes that define a specific toxicologic syndrome, or toxidrome, may narrow the differential diagnosis to a specific class of deadly drugs (or poisons) and guide subsequent management.[5]

Obtaining reliable historical information about the drug ingestion is often difficult. It is important to question the patient, close contacts, and emergency medical service

Table 1 Common antidotes	
Toxin/Drug	Antidote
Carbon monoxide	Oxygen
Opioids	Naloxone
Acetaminophen	N-acetylcysteine
Organophosphates	Atropine, pralidoxime
Cyclic antidepressant–sodium channel antagonists	Sodium bicarbonate
Lead, arsenic, mercury	Dimercaptosuccinic acid (succimer)
Ethylene glycol, methanol	Ethanol, 4-methypyrizole (fomepizole)
Digoxin, cardiac glycosides	Digoxin-specific Fab
Insulin	Glucose/dextrose
Anticholinergic drugs	Physostigmine
Cyanide	Cyanide antidote kit (sodium nitrite, sodium thiosulfate), hydroxocobalamin
Isoniazid, hydrazines	Pyridoxine
β-Adrenergic antagonist	Glucagon, high-dose insulin/euglycemia
Calcium channel blocker	Calcium chloride, high-dose insulin/euglycemia

Adapted from Harris CR, Stellpflug SJ. Suspected intoxication and overdose. In: McKean SC, Ross JJ, Dressler DD, et al, editors. Principles and practice of hospital medicine. China: McGraw-Hill Medical; 2012. p. 699; with permission.

providers where applicable for as much information regarding the ingestion as possible. A useful mnemonic in obtaining the relevant historical information regarding drug ingestions is Tox MATTERS (Box 1).[6] This information assists in estimating the potential lethality of the drug poisoning.

PHYSICAL EXAMINATION TOXIDROMES

Although many of the toxidromes have overlapping features and many ingestions involve multiple substances, identification of signs and symptoms consistent with a specific toxidrome can indicate a specific drug/toxin class.[5,7] The physical examination toxidromes discussed in this article include anticholinergics, cholinergics, opioids, sympathomimetics, and sedative hypnotics/alcohol (Table 2).[8] In addition, looking for signs and symptoms of serotonin and neuroleptic malignant syndrome are important when selective serotonin reuptake inhibitors (SSRIs) and neuroleptic medications are involved.

Anticholinergic Toxidrome

Anticholinergic drugs act by inhibiting muscarinic receptors and toxic symptoms are a result primarily of antagonism of the parasympathetic nervous system.[5] Common anticholinergic pharmaceutical agents include antihistamines, antipsychotics, antispasmodics, tricyclic antidepressants (TCAs), and mydriatics. The signs of anticholinergic toxicity have been long described in the following mnemonic: hot as a hare, red as a beet, dry as a bone, blind as a bat, mad as a hatter, and tachy as polyester suit, which corresponds with hyperthermia, flushing, anhidrosis, mydriasis, delirium, and tachycardia, respectively.[5,7,9] The central nervous system (CNS) effects of this class of drugs may lead to severe agitation, hallucinations, choreoathetosis, seizures, and coma.[7] Significant tachycardia and hypertension can occur. Suppression of sweat glands, innervated by the sympathetic nervous system but modulated by muscarinic receptors, can result in life-threatening hyperthermia. Treatment involves aggressive external cooling measures, judicious use of benzodiazepine, and IV crystalloids. The antidote, physostigmine, is recommended in patients presenting with a pure anticholinergic overdose and the absence of TCA toxicity.[7,9] The contraindication of physostigmine in TCA overdose is based on a case report of 2 patients with asystolic arrests following lethal ingestions of a TCA and receiving physostigmine,[10] but this contraindication has been perpetuated in the medical texts.

Box 1
Key points in the toxicology history of ingestions

The toxicology history mnemonic MATTERS:

Medications or substances ingested

Amount ingested/concentration

Time the medication was Taken

Emesis and presence of pill fragments

Reasons for ingestion

Signs and symptoms

Adapted from Harris CR, Stellpflug SJ. Suspected intoxication and overdose. In: McKean SC, Ross JJ, Dressler DD, et al, editors. Principles and practice of hospital medicine. China: McGraw-Hill Medical; 2012. p. 697; with permission.

Table 2
Characteristics of common toxidromes

	Mental Status	Vital Signs	Pupils	Skin
Anticholinergic	Increased	Increased	Enlarged	Dry
Cholinergic	Increased/decreased	Bradycardia	Small	Wet
Opioid	Decreased	Decreased	Small	—
Sympathomimetic	Increased	Increased	Enlarged	Wet
Sedative Hypnotic	Decreased	Decreased	Small	—
Serotonin	Increased/decreased	Increased/decreased	Enlarged	Wet

Adapted from Harris CR, Stellpflug SJ. Suspected intoxication and overdose. In: McKean SC, Ross JJ, Dressler DD, et al, editors. Principles and practice of hospital medicine. China: McGraw-Hill Medical; 2012. p. 697; with permission.

Cholinergic Toxidrome

The agents considered classically to cause the cholinergic toxidrome are organophosphates and carbamate insecticides, and toxic exposures are most commonly secondary to agricultural worker exposure. Cholinergic agents activate muscarinic acetylcholine receptors, but many cholinergic agents also act on other receptors (eg, sympathetic stimulation) causing variable clinical presentations.[5] Mnemonics used to describe the cholinergic toxidrome include DUMBBELS (defecation, urination, miosis, bronchorrhea, bronchoconstriction, emesis, lacrimation, and salivation) and SLUDGE (salivation, lacrimation, urination, defecation, gastrointestinal dysfunction, and emesis).[5,11] The respiratory system effects are considered the major factor leading to death; however, the patients are at risk for significant dehydration, seizures, as well as flaccid paralysis that can lead to nonconvulsive status epilepticus.[5] In addition to supportive treatment, atropine is the antidote given for cholinergic poisoning, and in severe cases multiple doses are required to reach the desired clinical effect. Pralidoxime chloride in addition to atropine is recommended for patients poisoned with organophosphates.[5,11] There is still some controversy in the effectiveness of pralidoxime in organophosphate poisoning.[12] High-quality critical care management is extremely important in yielding the best outcome.

Opioid Toxidrome

According to the National Center for Health Statistics, 40% of drug-poisoning deaths involved opioid analgesics in 2014 (18,893 deaths).[1] Opioids include naturally derived narcotics (eg, codeine and morphine), synthetic compounds (eg, methadone, tramadol, and fentanyl), and semisynthetic compounds (eg, heroin, hydromorphone, oxycodone, and hydrocodone). Opioids exert their clinical effects by binding to 3 major classes of opioid receptors: mu, kappa, and delta (or OP3, OP2, and OP1 respectively).[5] The opioid toxidrome consists of bradycardia, hypotension, bradypnea, hypothermia, CNS depression, miosis, and decreased peristalsis. CNS and respiratory depression can lead to anoxic brain injury, aspiration pneumonia, and rhabdomyolysis.[5] Treatment with the opioid antagonist naloxone reverses the opioid toxicity and can be used for diagnostic purposes. The goal of therapy is partial reversal to ensure airway protection but not full reversal and fulminant opioid withdrawal.[7] Because of the short half-life of naloxone (30 to 60 minutes), redosing is often necessary and a continuous infusion may be needed in ingestions of longer-acting opioids (eg, methadone). Short-acting opioid overdose requires at least 2 hours of observation before discharge from the ED in the care of a responsible adult. If repeat dosing of naloxone is required, that is an indication that the patient needs an extended period of observation or admission. Fentanyl is estimated to be 80 to 100 times more potent than morphine and 40 to 50 times more potent than pure heroin.[13] There is a current "epidemic" of prescription opioid abuse and overdose deaths, as well as a resurgence of heroin use among opioid addicts.[14] The number of heroin-related deaths in the United States increased 244% between 2007 (2402) and 2013 (8257).[15] One of the suspected reasons is that there have been incidences of heroin adulterated with fentanyl.[15]

Sympathomimetic Toxidrome

Illicit drug use of stimulants causes the largest percentage of toxicity in the sympathomimetic drug category (eg, cocaine, methamphetamine, 3,4-methylenedioxymethamphetamine). Stimulant street drugs are among the top 5 categories of substances associated with the most fatalities in the AAPCC 2014 annual report of the NPDS.[2] The sympathomimetics exert their effects by activation of a combination of α and β receptors, resulting in an excessive fight-or-flight reaction.[7] The signs include tachycardia, hypertension, tachypnea, hyperthermia, agitation, mydriasis, and diaphoresis. In severe cases, cardiac dysrhythmias, hypertensive crises, rhabdomyolysis, seizures, cardiovascular injury, and cerebrovascular injury (ischemic or hemorrhagic) may occur.[16,17] Sympathetic stimulation results in many of the same signs as the anticholinergic syndrome, such as tachycardia, hypertension, agitation, and hyperthermia. The key finding that differentiates the syndromes is that sympathetic stimulation results in diaphoresis, as opposed to dry skin in anticholinergic toxicity. The recommended treatment includes use of benzodiazepines in incremental boluses titrated to effect; IV crystalloid hydration; and, with hyperthermia, aggressive external cooling measures. Further control of hypertension should be achieved using α-adrenergic receptor antagonists (eg, phentolamine), nitrites, or nitroprusside. β-Blockers are contraindicated because β_2-receptor blockade theoretically leads to unopposed α_1-adrenergic receptor stimulation.[16,17] Antipsychotics as second-line agents for the control of agitation should be used with caution because they lower the seizure threshold, can induce hypotension and dysrhythmias, and impair heat dissipation.[17]

Hyperthermic Toxidromes

Hyperthermia has been found to be an independent risk factor of poor outcomes.[7] The finding of hyperthermia in a patient who is known to be taking an SSRI or neuroleptic should prompt consideration of these medications contributing to or causing the toxic syndrome. In addition to hyperthermia, patients with serotonin syndrome may present with alterations in mental status, autonomic nervous system disturbances, muscle rigidity, hyperreflexia, and clonus.[5] Neuroleptic malignant syndrome (NMS) is clinically similar, with signs including hyperthermia, muscle rigidity, autonomic instability, and mental status changes.[5,18] Hyperthermia syndromes lead to a severe imbalance of the autonomic nervous system accompanied by rhabdomyolysis, disseminated intravascular coagulopathy, and eventually multiorgan failure.[19] A diagnostic aid to distinguish between the two syndromes of serotonin syndrome and NMS, in addition to history, is an increased serum creatine kinase level. This finding is more consistent with NMS. Treatment recommendations are the same: discontinuance of the inciting drug, supportive care, aggressive external cooling measures, and benzodiazepines. Drug antagonists may be considered: cyproheptadine for serotonin syndrome, and bromocriptine, amantadine, and dantrolene have been used in NMS.[5,20] In treatment-unresponsive cases, endotracheal intubation and paralysis should be considered.[21]

Sedative Hypnotic Toxidrome

As a class, the sedative hypnotics are defined by their agonism at gamma-aminobutyric acid A receptors in the CNS.[7] Ethanol is the most available and highly used substance resulting in this toxidrome. The 2 major pharmaceutical categories are barbiturates and benzodiazepines. The signs of sedative hypnotic toxicity include hypotension, bradycardia, bradypnea, mild confusion to complete obtundation, and hypothermia. The hypothermia may be a direct result of the drug in the case of barbiturates, or from environmental exposure.[7] Treatment recommendations include aggressive supportive care, particularly with respect to respiratory failure. Flumazenil, a benzodiazepine antagonist, can be considered with caution in known benzodiazepine toxicity, because there is risk for seizures resistant to standard therapy, particularly in chronic benzodiazepine-dependent patients.[7] Abrupt discontinuation of long-term benzodiazepine use precipitates a potentially lethal withdrawal syndrome.[22] Deaths from ingestion of benzodiazepine alone are rare; however, combinations with alcohol or other coingestants are responsible for a large proportion of deaths, especially when coingested with opioids.[2,7] Sedative hypnotics are in the category found to have the highest increase of human exposures in the 2014 AAPCC NPDS report.[2]

LABORATORY TESTING CONSIDERATIONS

The metabolic profile tests that are most useful in the initial evaluation of most cases of suspected toxic drug ingestion include a basic metabolic panel and an acetaminophen level for potentially suicidal patients. A basic metabolic panel allows for the evaluation of glucose, electrolytes, acid/base balance, anion gap, and renal function, all of which are important in guiding further evaluation and treatment decisions.

Subsequent metabolic tests may be considered on a case-by-case basis, including osmolality, venous or arterial blood gas, lactate level, hepatic function panel, complete blood count (CBC), pregnancy test (in women of childbearing age), thyroid-stimulating hormone (TSH) level, total creatine kinase (CK), and urine myoglobin level (Box 2). Crystals in a urinalysis may indicate ethylene glycol ingestion. Specific drug levels, as indicated by the patient's history and initial metabolic test results, should be obtained, with consideration of acetaminophen, salicylate, carbon monoxide, cyanide, and volatile alcohol screening.

Indiscriminate use of urine drug screening (UDS) rarely provides clinically useful information.[4] Interpretation of routine UDS results is plagued by many confounders, including delayed drug metabolism, false-positive results caused by cross reactivity, false-negative results, and the possibility that not all drugs within a class will be detected.[5] Many investigators have shown that UDS test results rarely affect management decisions.[5,8,23]

Box 2
Laboratory testing in suspected toxic drug ingestion

Initial evaluation: basic metabolic profile, acetaminophen level

Targeted evaluation: osmolality, venous/arterial blood gas, lactate, hepatic function panel, CBC, pregnancy test, TSH, total CK, urine myoglobin, urinalysis, salicylate, carbon monoxide, cyanide, volatile alcohol screen, suspected specific drug level.

Toxins Inducing Osmolar Gap

The osmolar gap may be increased in the presence of low-molecular-weight substances, such as ethanol, other alcohols, and glycols, any of which can contribute to the measured, but not the calculated, osmolality.[24] The lack of an established normal range is problematic with regard to using the osmolar gap as a screening tool in the evaluation of potentially toxic alcohol-poisoned patients.[5] If clinical suspicion is high for toxic alcohol ingestion, even in the setting of a normal osmolar gap, presumptive treatment measures should be considered, including fomepizole or ethanol infusion and consideration of hemodialysis.

Toxins Inducing Anion Gap Metabolic Acidosis

Obtaining a basic metabolic panel in all poisoned patients is generally recommended and evaluation of the cause of an increased anion gap is important for successful treatment.[6] The normal anion gap is 8 to 16 mEq/L and accounts for the unmeasured anions (eg, phosphate, sulfate, and anionic proteins). Anion gap = $Na^+ - (Cl^- + HCO3^-)$.

An increased anion gap suggests metabolic acidosis. Toxin as well as nontoxin causes of metabolic acidosis are organized in the popular mnemonic CATMUDPILES (Box 3).[25] Many symptomatic poisoned patients have an initial mild metabolic acidosis on presentation secondary to increase of serum lactate level.[5] If the anion gap metabolic acidosis worsens despite adequate supportive care, either toxins that form acidic metabolites (eg, ethylene glycol, methanol, or ibuprofen) or toxins that cause lactic acidosis by interfering with aerobic energy production (eg, cyanide or iron) should be considered.[5,25]

ELECTROCARDIOGRAPHIC TOXIC EFFECTS
QT Prolongation

Drugs that block the cardiac potassium efflux channels result in QT interval prolongation and may lead to ventricular tachycardia, most often the polymorphic ventricular

---

Box 3
Potential causes of anion gap metabolic acidosis

Mnemonic: CATMUDPILES

- CO, CN
- Alcoholic ketoacidosis and starvation ketoacidosis
- Toluene
- Metformin, methanol
- Uremia
- DKA
- Pyroglutamic acidosis, paracetamol, phenformin, propylene glycol
- Iron, isoniazid
- Lactic acidosis
- Ethylene glycol
- Salicylates

Abbreviations: CN, cyanide; CO, carbon monoxide; DKA, diabetic ketoacidosis.
  Data from Fernando J. Anion Gap. In: Life in the Fast Lane 2015. Available at: http://lifeinthefastlane.com/ccc/anion-gap/. Accessed June 26, 2016.

tachycardia known as torsades de pointes. The QT interval is corrected for heart rate influence by a formula calculation (corrected QT = $QT/\sqrt{RR}$). An interval of greater that 500 milliseconds is concerning for potential arrhythmia. Drugs associated with QT prolongation are numerous and include antihistamines; antipsychotics; class IA, IC, and III antiarrhythmics; and fluoroquinolones. Consider other causes of QT prolongation, such as hypokalemia, hypomagnesemia, hypothermia, myocardial ischemia, neurologic catastrophes, and hypothyroidism.[5,26]

QRS Prolongation

Drugs that induce cardiac sodium channel blockade prolong the QRS interval and toxicity may lead to profoundly slowed intraventricular conduction and eventual asystole.[5,27] Myocardial Na^+ channel–blocking drugs comprise a diverse group of pharmaceutical agents, including TCAs, and many produce additional effects involving the anticholinergic, opioid, or sympathomimetic syndromes.[5] Na^+ channel–blocking drugs may respond to treatment with hypertonic saline or sodium bicarbonate.[5]

Bradycardia

The cardiovascular drug classes causing bradycardia include calcium channel blockers (CCB) and β-adrenergic receptor blockers. Toxicity of CCBs and β-blockers is variable; however, in addition to bradydysrhythmias, marked hypotension can occur, and the potential for lethality exists, particularly if ingested by pediatric patients.[27] Sustained-release preparations prolong the toxicity. Treatment of a toxic ingestion of CCBs begins with IV calcium ion infusion, which increases the extracellular ionized calcium concentration, competitively binding calcium receptors. Toxicity from CCBs and β-blockers may be treated with IV fluid resuscitation, atropine, glucagon, and vasopressors, and cardiac pacing may be indicated. The early use of high-dose insulin therapy with glucose supplementation should be instituted and may prevent the need for vasopressors and pacing.[28–33] Fat emulsion therapy and extracorporeal life support may be considered in patients who fail to respond to all pharmaceutical interventions.[28]

ONE PILL CAN KILL

Deadly drug ingestions from a single dose are a special consideration for the pediatric patient population. Although it may take more than 1 pill or 1 dose, it is important to be familiar with the medications and substances that are potentially lethal when ingested by a child. A list of medications or substances that are potentially lethal for toddlers in 1 dose, compiled from a review of the literature, is shown in Box 4.[34–39] In 2014, slightly less than half of all exposure cases managed by poison control centers involved children younger than 6 years. However, as in previous years, the number of fatalities was small (34 cases).[2] The first ranked substances associated with fatalities of children less than or equal to 5 year old were fumes/gases/vapors (7), analgesics (6), household cleaning substances (3), antihistamines (2), cardiovascular drugs (1), and 6 other substances (1 each).[2]

DECONTAMINATION
Gastrointestinal Decontamination

The role of gastrointestinal (GI) decontamination is highly controversial and assessment should be based on the type of ingestion, estimated quantity and size of pill or tablet, time since ingestion, concurrent ingestions, ancillary medical conditions, and

---

Box 4
Medications or substances with lethal potential for toddlers in 1 dose

- Sulfonylureas: oral hypoglycemic
- Calcium channel blockers
- Cyclic antidepressants
- Opiates
- Clonidine
- Antimalarials: chloroquine/quinine derivatives
- Antiarrhythmics: flecainide
- Antipsychotics: clozapine, olanzapine, chlorpromazine, thioridazine
- Toxic alcohols
- Camphor
- Methyl salicylate
- Imidazoline decongestants
- Diphenoxylate/atropine
- β-Blockers
- Theophylline
- Podophyllin

---

age and size of the patient.[4] Evidence now points away from the routine use of GI decontamination of most patients presenting to the ED with an oral pharmaceutical overdose.[4] Syrup of ipecac–induced emesis is no longer recommended for use in the emergency department.[8,40,41]

Gastric lavage

There is no evidence in the medical literature for routine use of gastric lavage.[42] Studies have shown that, after a delay of 60 minutes or more, little of the ingested dose is removed[24] and the procedure may be associated with serious complications. It has been performed for ingestions of large amounts of drugs poorly absorbed by activated charcoal and large amounts of sustained-release or enteric-coated medications. Experienced providers should only perform gastric lavage when the airway is protected and no caustic material is involved. There is weak evidence of benefit of gastric lavage and it generally does not offer any more advantage compared with activated charcoal.[8]

Activated charcoal

There are no well-designed studies showing the effectiveness of activated charcoal (AC) in poisoned patients[42]; however, AC continues to be recognized as an effective method for reducing the systemic absorption of many drugs and may be considered if the patient has ingested a potentially toxic amount of poison.[24,40,43] AC is highly effective in adsorbing most toxins when given in a ratio of 10 to 1 (charcoal to toxin). The use of a 1-hour time frame from drug ingestion to AC administration should be used as a guide rather than an absolute time limit, because there may be delayed gastric emptying and prolonged absorption.[40] Contraindications for the use of AC include an ingestion in which AC is known not to adsorb a clinically meaningful amount of the toxin, concern for high aspiration potential in a patient who is not intubated, or caustic ingestions.[24,40]

Multiple-dose AC (MDAC) administration serves 2 purposes: (1) to prevent ongoing absorption of a drug that persists in the GI tract (modified-release preparation) and (2) to enhance elimination in the postabsorptive phase by disrupting either enterohepatic recirculation or enteroenteric recirculation.[40] According to the 1999 position statement from the American Academy of Clinical Toxicology (AACT) and the European Association of Poisons Centres and Clinical Toxicologists (EAPCCT), MDAC should be considered only if the patient has ingested a potentially life-threatening amount of carbamazepine, dapsone, phenobarbital, quinine, or theophylline.[40,44] Volunteer studies have shown increased elimination of amitriptyline, digoxin, phenytoin, salicylates, and sotalol with MDAC treatment; however, there is insufficient research to support a recommendation for use of MDAC in these overdoses.[44] MDAC should not be used in the presence of intestinal obstruction.

Whole-bowel irrigation

Although no clear evidence-based studies have been done to recommend it, whole-bowel irrigation (WBI) has been performed in certain circumstances. WBI is achieved through the use of oral or nasogastric administration of large amounts of an osmotically balanced polyethylene glycol electrolyte lavage solution. The indications for which WBI has been considered include large ingestions of drugs poorly absorbed by AC (eg, iron, lithium, or potassium), situations in which other methods of decontamination are unlikely to be either safe or beneficial, large ingestions of sustained-release or enteric-coated pharmaceuticals, and removal of drug-filled packets.[24,40,45] WBI is contraindicated in patients with bowel obstruction, perforation, or ileus, and in patients with hemodynamic instability or compromised unprotected airways.[45]

Enhanced Elimination

Enhanced elimination involves interventions taken to attempt to eliminate drugs already absorbed from the GI tract. Available techniques of enhanced elimination include manipulation of urinary pH (ion trapping), hemodialysis, and hemoperfusion, with the alkalinization of the urine used the most frequently.[46] Their use is limited to circumstances of critical intoxication with deterioration despite maximal support, impaired route of elimination, ingestion of a known lethal dose of a toxin, and underlying medical problems that increase the hazard.[24]

Alkalinization of the urine can be used to enhance the elimination of weak acids and should be considered as first-line treatment of patients with moderately severe salicylate poisoning who do not meet criteria for hemodialysis.[46] Drugs with low molecular weight, water solubility, and low protein-binding properties, such as lithium, ethylene glycol, methanol, salicylates, and valproic acid, can be treated with hemodialysis. Hemoperfusion should be considered for theophylline, phenobarbital, and carbamazepine overdoses.[47]

DISPOSITION

Early consultation with a clinical toxicologist is recommended for discussion of complicated patient presentations and for controversial management decisions. Providers can speak directly with a physician at a regional poison control center (1-800-222-1222) when immediate feedback is crucial (Box 5). It is advisable to observe the patient for at least 6 to 8 hours before disposition in all potentially serious toxic ingestions.[24] Repeated evaluation is essential for identifying new or developing toxic syndromes, for early identification of deteriorating condition, as well as or development

Box 5
Toxicology resources

Poison Center Hotline: 1-800-222-1222

Textbooks
- Hoffman RS, et al, editors. Goldfrank's toxicologic emergencies, 10th edition
- Brent J, et al, editors. Critical care toxicology: diagnosis and management of the critically poisoned patient
- Olson K, et al, editors. Poisonings and drug overdose, 6th edition
- Nelson LS, et al, editors. Handbook of poisonous and injurious plants

Online resources
- www.erowid.org (Erowid)
- www.acmt.net (American College of Medical Toxicology)
- www.clintox.org (AACT)
- www.aapcc.org (American Association of Poison Control Centers)
- www.thepoisonreview.com (The Poison Review)

From Harris CR, Stellpflug SJ. Suspected intoxication and overdose. In: McKean SC, Ross JJ, Dressler DD, et al, editors. Principles and practice of hospital medicine. China: McGraw-Hill Medical; 2012. p. 700; with permission.

of a withdrawal syndrome.[4,8] Consider repeat serum levels. An extended observation may be required in sustained-release or enteric-coated medications. Intensive care admission is appropriate for patients with hemodynamic instability and those with the potential to deteriorate. In addition, all patients with intentional poisoning should have a psychosocial evaluation, and the possibility that the ingestion was not accidental should be considered with a toxic ingestion involving a child.

SUMMARY

The number of drug-induced deaths surpassed the number of motor vehicle collision deaths as the number 1 cause of injury-related death in the United States in 2008, and although the number of motor vehicle collision deaths has declined, the number of drug-induced deaths continues to increase. According to the 2015 National Drug Threat Assessment, more than 120 people die each day as a result of drug overdose.[15] Emergency medicine physician assistants frequently encounter poisoned patients and must be well informed about the clinical presentation and the critical management principles of patients with potentially lethal drug ingestion. An algorithmic approach using critical care management principles is useful in the initial management of these patients. Rapid initiation of supportive care and, in some circumstances, immediate antidote administration should be performed. Toxidrome recognition is important, in addition to a thorough history, laboratory testing, and ECG testing, in identifying undifferentiated drug ingestions and assisting with more specific management.

REFERENCES

1. CDC/National Center for Health Statistics (/nchs/indes.htm). Page last updated: April 5, 2016. Available at: http://www.cdc.gov/nchs/data/factsheets/factsheet_drug_poisoning.htm. Accessed June 26, 2016.
2. Mowry JB, Spyker DA, Brooks DE, et al. 2014 annual report of the American Association of Poison Control Centers' National Poison Data System (NPDS): 32nd annual report. Clin Toxicol (Phila) 2015;53(10):962–1147.

3. Albert M, McCaig LF, Uddin S. Emergency department visits for drug poisoning: United States, 2008-2011. NCHS data brief, no. 196. Hyattsville (MD): National Center for Health Statistics; 2015.

4. Hoffman RS, Howland M, Lewin NA, et al. Principles of managing the acutely poisoned or overdosed patient. In: Hoffman RS, Howland M, Lewin NA, Nelson LS, Goldfrank LR, editors. Goldfrank's toxicologic emergencies, 10th edition. New York: McGraw-Hill; 2015. Available at: http://accessemergencymedicinemhmedical.com/content.aspx?bookid=1163&sectionid=65089354. Accessed March 16, 2017.

5. Holstege CP, Borek HA. Toxidromes. Crit Care Clin 2012;28:479–98.

6. Harris CR. Common ingestions and exposures you might see. In: Harris CR, editor. The toxicology handbook for clinicians. Philadelphia: Mosby Elsevier; 2006. p. 1–3.

7. Meehan TJ, Bryant SM, Aks SE. Drugs of abuse: the highs and lows of altered mental states in the emergency department. Emerg Med Clin North Am 2010; 28:663–82.

8. Harris CR, Stellpflug SJ. Suspected intoxication and overdose. In: McKean SC, Ross JJ, Dressler DD, et al, editors. Principles and practice of hospital medicine. China: McGraw-Hill Medical; 2012. p. 696–701.

9. Holger JS. Antihistamines and anticholinergics. In: Harris CR, editor. The toxicology handbook for clinicians. Philadelphia: Mosby Elsevier; 2006. p. 50–3.

10. Suchard JR. Assessing physostigmine's contraindication in cyclic antidepressant ingestions. J Emerg Med 2003;25(2):185–91.

11. DeLisle C. Organophosphate pesticides. In: Harris CR, editor. The toxicology handbook for clinicians. Philadelphia: Mosby Elsevier; 2006. p. 54–60.

12. Eddleston M, Eyer P, Worek F, et al. Pralidoxime in acute organophosphorus insecticide poisoning—a randomized controlled trial. PLoS Med 2009;6(6): e1000104.

13. Fentanyl: Incapacitating agent. In: National Institute for Occupational Safety and Health (NIOSH) (/niosh) Education and Information Division. 2014. Available at: http://www.cdc.gov/niosh/ershdb/EmergencyResponseCard_29750022.html. Accessed September 19, 2016.

14. Kanouse AB, Compton P. The epidemic of prescription opioid abuse, the subsequent rising prevalence of heroin use, and the federal response. J Pain Palliat Care Pharmacother 2015;29(2):102–14.

15. 2015 National drug threat assessment summary. DEA Strategic Intelligence Section. October 2015. DEA-DCT-DIR-008–16. Available at: https://www.dea.gov/resource-center/statistics.shtml. Accessed September 19, 2016.

16. Schep LJ, Slaughter RJ, Beasley DM. The clinical toxicology of metamfetamine. Clin Toxicol 2010;48:675–94.

17. Greene SL, Kerr F, Braitberg G. Review article: amphetamines and related drugs of abuse. Emerg Med Australas 2008;20:391–402.

18. Perry PJ, Wilborn CA. Serotonin syndrome vs. neuroleptic malignant syndrome: a contrast of causes, diagnoses, and management. Ann Clin Psychiatry 2012; 24(2):155–62.

19. Grander W. Malignant hyperthermia syndrome in the intensive care unit: differential diagnosis and acute measures. Med Klin Intensivmed Notfmed 2016;111(5): 407–16.

20. Ebadi M, Pfeiffer RF, Murrin LC. Pathogenesis and treatment of neuroleptic malignant syndrome. Gen Pharmacol 1990;21(4):367–86.

21. Vassallo SU, Delaney KA. Thermoregulatory principles. In: Hoffman RS, Howland M, Lewin NA, et al, editors. Goldfrank's toxicologic emergencies, 10th edition. New York: McGraw-Hill; 2015. Available at: http://accessemergencymedicine.mhmedical.com/content.aspx?bookid=1163&sectionid=65092584. Accessed March 16, 2017.

22. Holger JS. Benzodiazepines. In: Harris CR, editor. The toxicology handbook for clinicians. Philadelphia: Mosby Elsevier; 2006. p. 37–8.

23. Kellermann AL, Fihn SD, LoGerfo JP, et al. Impact of drug screening in suspected overdose. Ann Emerg Med 1987;16(11):1206–16.

24. Olson KR. Emergency evaluation and treatment. In: Olson KR, Anderson IB, Benowitz, et al, editors. Poisoning and drug overdose. 5th edition. USA: Lange Medical Books/McGraw-Hill; 2007. p. 1–67.

25. Fernando J. Anion gap. In: Life in the fast lane 2015. Available at: http://lifeinthefastlane.com/ccc/anion-gap/. Accessed June 26, 2016.

26. Priori SG, Cantu F, Schwartz PJ. The long QT syndrome: new diagnostic and therapeutic approach in the era of molecular biology. Schweiz Med Wochenschr 1996;126(41):1727–31.

27. Kolecki PF, Curry SC. Poisoning by sodium channel blocking agents. Crit Care Clin 1997;13(4):829–48.

28. Gordon B. Cardiovascular drugs. In: Harris CR, editor. The toxicology handbook for clinicians. Philadelphia: Mosby Elsevier; 2006. p. 61–75.

29. Jang DH, DeRoos J. Calcium channel blockers. In: Hoffman RS, Howland M, Lewin NA, et al, editors. Goldfrank's toxicologic emergencies, 10th edition. New York: McGraw-Hill; 2015. Available at: http://accessemergencymedicine mhmedical.com/content.aspx?bookid=1163&sectionid=65096376. Accessed March 16, 2017.

30. Brubacher JR. β-Adrenergic antagonists. In: Hoffman RS, Howland M, Lewin NA, et al, editors. Goldfrank's toxicologic emergencies, 10th edition. New York: McGraw-Hill; 2015. Available at: http://accessemergencymedicinemhmedical.com/content.aspx?bookid=1163&sectionid=65096471. Accessed March 16, 2017.

31. Holger JS, Stellpflug SJ, Cole JB, et al. High-dose insulin: a consecutive case series in toxin-induced cardiogenic shock. Clin Toxicol 2011;49(7):653–8.

32. Engebretsen KM, Kaczmarek KM, Morgan J, et al. High-dose insulin therapy in beta-blocker and calcium channel-blocker poisoning. Clin Toxicol 2011;49(4):277–83.

33. St-Onge M, Dubé PA, Gosselin S, et al. Treatment for calcium channel blocker poisoning: a systematic review. Clin Toxicol 2014;52(9):926–44.

34. Bar-Oz B, Levichek Z, Koren G. Medications that can be fatal for a toddler with one tablet or teaspoonful: a 2004 update. Paediatr Drugs 2004;6(2):123–6.

35. Henry K, Harris C. Deadly ingestions. Pediatr Clin North Am 2006;53:293–315.

36. Wong DC, Curtis LA. Are 1 or 2 dangerous? Clozapine and olanzapine exposure in toddlers. J Emerg Med 2004;27(3):273–7.

37. White CC, De Baltz G. One pill can kill: pediatric poisonings caused by one dose of adult medication. JEMS 2015;56–9.

38. Dobson JV, Webb SA. Life-threatening pediatric poisonings. J S C Med Assoc 2004;100:327–32.

39. Ranniger C, Roche C. Are one or two dangerous? Calcium channel blocker exposure in toddlers. J Emerg Med 2007;33(2):145–54.

40. Hoegberg LCG, Gude AB. Techniques used to prevent gastrointestinal absorption. In: Hoffman RS, Howland M, Lewin NA, et al, editors. Goldfrank's toxicologic emergencies, 10th edition. New York: McGraw-Hill; 2015. Available at: http://accessemergencymedicinemhmedical.com/content.aspx?bookid=1163&sectionid=65089810. Accessed March 16, 2017.

41. Höjer J, Troutman WG, Hoppu K, et al. Position paper update: ipecac syrup for gastrointestinal decontamination. Clin Toxicol 2014;51:134–9.
42. Benson BE, Hoppu K, Tourman WB, et al. Position paper update: gastric lavage for gastrointestinal decontamination. Clin Toxicol 2013;51:140–6.
43. Vale JA, Krenzelok EP, Barceloux GD. Position paper: single-dose activated charcoal. Clin Toxicol 2005;43:61–87.
44. Vale JA, Krenzelok EP, Barceloux GD. Position statement and practice guidelines on the use of multi-dose activated charcoal in the treatment of acute poisoning. Clin Toxicol 1999;37(6):731–51.
45. Thanacoody R, Caravati EM, Troutman WG, et al. Position paper update: whole bowel irrigation for gastrointestinal decontamination of overdose patients. Clin Toxicol (Phila) 2015;53(1):5–12.
46. Proudfoot AT, Krenzelok EP, Vale JA. Position paper on urine alkalinization. Clin Toxicol 2004;42(1):1–26.
47. Goldfarb DS, Ghannoum M. Principles and techniques applied to enhance elimination. In: Hoffman RS, Howland M, Lewin NA, et al, editors. Goldfrank's toxicologic emergencies, 10th edition. New York: McGraw-Hill; 2015. Available at: http://accessemergencymedicinemhmedical.com/content.aspx?bookid=1163& sectionid=65090072. Accessed March 16, 2017.

Asymptomatic Hypertension in the Emergency Department

Jed Grant, MPAS, PA-C[a],*, Karimeh Borghei, MSN, FNP-C, PA-C[b]

KEYWORDS

- Asymptomatic hypertension • Hypertensive urgency • Hypertensive emergency
- Hypertension in the ED • ED workup hypertension • ED treatment hypertension

KEY POINTS

- Data are limited, and there is a paucity of evidence on which to base treatment of asymptomatic patients with elevated blood pressure.
- A recheck of the blood pressure at 90 minutes following triage often shows improvement and helps guide the emergency department evaluation and follow-up decisions.
- The routine ordering of diagnostic studies to screen for end-organ damage in asymptomatic patients is not beneficial.
- Consider a basic metabolic panel and discharge with prescription for antihypertensive medication for African American patients, indigent patients, and those with unreliable or poor follow-up.
- Acute treatment is not indicated and possibly harmful. If you must treat, give patients a dose of the antihypertensive medication that is already prescribed by their primary care provider or one you will prescribe at discharge.

INTRODUCTION

Approximately 30% of Americans have hypertension, and about 5% of emergency department (ED) patients will have a blood pressure (BP) that is elevated. Of those with elevated BP on initial presentation to the ED, about 40% will have a BP high enough to be associated with end-organ damage.[1,2] Although pain and the stress of visiting the ED may contribute to an elevated BP at presentation, one study showed that 75% of those presenting with uncontrolled hypertension were noncompliant with medications.[3] Another showed that on recheck of the BP at 90 minutes most patients

[a] PA Program, University of the Pacific, 3200 Fifth Avenue, Sacramento, CA 95817, USA; [b] UC Davis CTSC Clinical Research Center, 2221 Stockton Boulevard, Suite D, Sacramento, CA 95817, USA
* Corresponding author.
E-mail address: jgrant@pacific.edu

Physician Assist Clin 2 (2017) 465–472
http://dx.doi.org/10.1016/j.cpha.2017.02.009
2405-7991/17/© 2017 Elsevier Inc. All rights reserved.
physicianassistant.theclinics.com

returned to their baseline BP; therefore, a repeat BP at 90 minutes is an important component in the evaluation of these patients.[4,5]

The real question is what to do with those patients who have no symptoms but may have occult end-organ damage. Data in establishing guidelines for evaluation and treatment of patients with asymptomatic hypertension in the ED setting are limited because of lack of large outcome studies to help determine the validity of such guidelines. The American College of Emergency Physicians has a policy regarding this issue that was updated in 2013; however, there is a paucity of evidence on which to base guidance.[4] This article focuses on the evaluation and treatment of asymptomatic hypertensive patients.

DEFINITIONS

The definition of hypertension is based on the Eighth Joint National Committee's guidelines as published in 2014.[6] These guidelines are for adults 18 years and older with hypertension and is focused on the primary care setting. The definition of hypertension is further delineated in the general population and in populations with diabetes or chronic kidney disease. In individuals less than 60 years of age in the general population, hypertension is defined as a systolic BP of 140 mm Hg or greater and/or a diastolic BP of 90 mm Hg or greater.[6] In individuals who are aged 60 years or older in the general population, hypertension is defined as a systolic BP of 150 mm Hg or greater and/or a diastolic BP of 90 mm Hg or greater. In the population with diabetes and no chronic kidney disease (CKD), hypertension is defined as a systolic BP of 140 mm Hg or greater and/or a diastolic BP of 90 mm Hg or greater in all adults.[6] In the population with CKD, regardless of the presence of diabetes, hypertension is defined as systolic BP of 140 mm Hg or greater and/or a diastolic BP of 90 mm Hg or greater in all adults (Table 1).

CLASSIFICATIONS OF HYPERTENSION

Hypertension is most commonly primary (essential) but may be due to secondary causes on occasion. In 90% to 95% of individuals with hypertension, no cause can be identified.[7] There are current implications that genetics may play a role in the development of high BP, such as hypertension being more prevalent in some families and in African Americans. Primary or essential hypertension can also be caused by increased sodium consumption, excessive alcohol use, obesity, sedentary lifestyle, use of tobacco and nicotine products, polycythemia, aggressiveness, and poor stress coping skills.[7]

In approximately 5% of all individuals a root cause for hypertension is found. Secondary hypertension should be considered in individuals with sudden onset of

Table 1 Definition of hypertension			
Classification	Age (y)	Systolic BP	Diastolic BP
General population	18–59	≥140	≥90
General population	≥60	≥150	≥90
Diabetes present and no CKD	≥18	≥140	≥90
CKD present with or without diabetes	≥18	≥140	≥90

Adapted from JNC 8 hypertension guideline algorithm 2014.

hypertension, in individuals less than 30 years of age without a family history of hypertension, and in patients with suddenly uncontrolled BP that had previously been well controlled.

Medication-related causes of secondary hypertension include the use of oral contraceptives, hormone therapies as used in infertility and transgender treatments, sympathomimetics, decongestants, nonsteroidal antiinflammatory drugs, appetite suppressants, antidepressants, corticosteroids, anabolic steroids, cyclosporine, and erythropoietin. Hypertension is also caused by excessive consumption of caffeine, excessive ingestion of black licorice, and use of illicit drugs, such as cocaine and methamphetamines.[7]

Systemic causes of secondary hypertension include acute kidney disease and CKD, renal artery stenosis, hyperthyroidism, hypothyroidism, primary hyperaldosteronism, Cushing syndrome, coarctation of the aorta, pheochromocytoma, and obstructive sleep apnea.[7]

Hypertension in the ED is most commonly situationally transient, acutely elevated, chronic hypertension.[5] In this setting, hypertension can further be classified as hypertensive emergency or hypertensive urgency.

Chronic Hypertension

In the ED, hypertension may be caused by pain due to a traumatic injury, a procedure or illness, and by anxiety secondary to the setting. In all of these situations the elevated BP is situational and transient, usually returning to the patients' baseline within 90 minutes. Only about 6% of patients with BP that remains elevated 90 minutes after arrival will have a normal BP outside the ED and likely have underlying chronic hypertension.[4,5,8] Although these patients are most appropriately managed in the primary care setting, this may be a valuable opportunity for the ED provider to start therapy for those patients who have poor follow-up or are at increased risk of end-organ damage.[2]

Hypertensive Emergency

Hypertensive emergency is classified as systolic BP of 180 mm Hg or greater or a diastolic BP of 110 mm Hg or greater associated with acute end-organ damage. There is poor correlation between the BP numbers and presence of end-organ damage, so how high is too high for asymptomatic patients? There is some discordance in the literature, but generally asymptomatic patients may be discharged safely with a prescription for antihypertensive medication and a BP as high as 180/110 mm Hg.[4,9,10]

Signs and Symptoms

Hypertension in itself does not cause any symptoms but over time may have a profound effect on the brain, eyes, heart, and kidneys. An appropriate history and physical examination focused on the end organs most affected by hypertension should be performed. Interestingly, one study found that emergency providers are not particularly adept at recognizing hypertension until it reaches the range associated with hypertensive urgency, and then only 36% of patients with BP greater than 180/100 mm Hg had fundoscopy performed in the ED.[5] Acute changes in vision may be reported due to retinal hemorrhages, though the more concerning finding on funduscopic examination would be papilledema indicating elevated intracranial pressure.

Concerning signs and symptoms of hypertension related to brain injury include altered mental status, confusion, irritability, headache, and focal neurologic findings, all of which may be suggestive of intracranial hemorrhage.[7,9] Any change in the baseline level of neurologic function combined with a markedly elevated BP suggests ongoing insult to the brain.

Hypertension is the second most common cause of end-stage renal disease. African American patients and those with coexisting diabetes are at increased risk for progression to renal failure associated with hypertension. Symptoms of azotemia may be absent and when present may be vague depending on whether the cause of renal insult is prerenal, intrarenal, or postrenal. Symptoms may include hematuria, edema, pericardial friction rub caused by uremic pericarditis, abdominal bruit, palpable kidney, or asterixis (flapping tremor) in the setting of hypertensive nephropathy.[7,9] Asterixis and pericarditis are indications for emergency dialysis.

Aortic dissection occurs when the intima and media dissect in the aorta. It may occur in the setting of profound hypertension and classically presents dramatically with a sudden onset of a tearing pain radiating to the intrascapular area. BP differential may exist in the upper extremities or between the upper and lower extremities depending on the location and severity of the tear. Any chest pain radiating to the back in the setting of markedly elevated BP should prompt concern for dissection.

Acute coronary syndrome and pulmonary edema may occur in the setting of markedly elevated BP. Chest pain, shortness of breath, dizziness or syncope, and rales on auscultation of the lungs are commonly associated with these diagnoses and should spur prompt intervention from the clinician.

Preeclampsia/eclampsia is associated with hypertension in pregnant patients. In healthy patients, BP should decrease during early gestation and gradually return to normal by full term. Hypertension with proteinuria and edema occur in preeclampsia, whereas the onset of seizure heralds eclampsia.

Asymptomatic hypertension only occurs in stable patients without signs or symptoms of end-organ damage. Presence of end-organ damage as evidenced by history, physical examination, or diagnostic studies is an indication for further evaluation and treatment in the ED; however, the focus here is on asymptomatic patients with hypertension.

Diagnostic Evaluation

Although a proper history and physical examination are required, multiple studies have shown that routine ordering of diagnostic studies to screen for end-organ damage in asymptomatic patients is not beneficial.[1,11] Complete blood count, chest radiograph, computed tomography of the brain or chest, electrocardiogram (ECG), and urinalysis (UA) were all found to be of no benefit in the evaluation of asymptomatic hypertensive patients and should not be routinely ordered.[1,4,11]

A basic metabolic panel (BMP) or serum creatinine may be ordered for African American patients because they are at risk for accelerated end-organ damage particularly in the setting of comorbid diabetes mellitus.[2,3] Likewise, indigent patients or those with poor access to care may have either a creatinine alone or BMP performed because those patients with long-standing untreated hypertension are most likely to have occult hypertensive nephropathy.[2,3,9]

Patients with BPs greater than 180/110 mm Hg may also have a serum creatinine or BMP in the ED. A benefit of obtaining the BMP rather than just the serum creatinine is that the additional information provided is helpful in determining which medications are safe to prescribe on discharge and may reveal comorbidities with significant prognostic value. Obtain a pregnancy test on hypertensive female patients before prescribing an angiotensin-converting enzyme inhibitor (ACEI) or angiotensin receptor blocker (ARB).

Table 2
Oral agents for hypertensive urgencies

Medication Name	Drug Class	Dosage	Onset of Action (min)	Duration (h)	Contraindications
Captopril	ACEI	12–25 mg PO	15–30	4–6	Renal artery stenosis, pregnancy
Clonidine (for rebound hypertension only)	Central α2-agonist	0.1–0.2 mg PO	30–60	6–8	CHF, second- or third-degree AV block
Furosemide	Loop diuretic	20–80 mg PO	30–60	6–8	Anuria
Labetalol	α₁-β adrenergic blocker	200–400 mg PO, repeat every 2–3 h	30–120	6–12	Asthma, COPD, bradycardia, heart block, heart failure
Lisinopril	ACEI	2.5–40.0 mg PO	60	24	Aliskiren, renal artery stenosis, pregnancy
Losartan	ARB	50 mg PO	60	12–24	Second and third trimesters of pregnancy
Nifedipine ER (for preeclampsia only)	Ca++ channel blocker	10 mg PO, may repeat every 30–60 min	10–15	3–6	Angina, acute hypertension

Abbreviations: AV, atrioventricular; CHF, congestive heart failure; COPD, chronic obstructive pulmonary disease; ER, extended release.

Indications for Initiation of Antihypertensive Medications in the Emergency Department

It may ultimately take several months and multiple treatment modalities to get the BP to goal. The goal of initiating antihypertensive medications for patients with asymptomatic hypertension in an ED setting is not to treat the numbers and bring the BP to goal but to begin the process of treatment to reduce end-organ damage in those patients at most risk.[2,4,8,9] There is no difference in outcomes for those patients with hypertensive urgency admitted or treated as an outpatient.[10] Likewise there are no studies associating hypertensive urgency with acute risk of end-organ injury, and most patients with hypertensive urgency have uncontrolled hypertension 6 months later.[10] Caution should be taken when considering lowering BP acutely, such as when requested by law enforcement to lower BP for medical clearance for incarceration. Chronically elevated asymptomatic BP should not be lowered to a normal goal during a brief ED visit because there is a paradoxically increased risk of damage to end organs, particularly to the brain.[4,8,9]

One dose of patients' usual prescribed antihypertensive for those patients with chronic hypertension may be given in the ED if the BP is greater than or equal to 180/110 mm Hg. Although caution is advised, for antihypertensive-naïve patients with a markedly elevated BP medications listed in Table 2 may be used, with treatment choice depending on patient race, comorbidities, and socioeconomic factors. After initiating medications, ideal follow-up by a primary care provider should be within 1 week.[9] It is appropriate to prescribe 30 days of medication; however, refills and medications for more than 30 days are not recommended because of the need for close follow-up.

SUMMARY

Asymptomatic hypertension is chronically uncontrolled hypertension that has a very low risk of causing acute end-organ damage.[10] As with other chronic problems, it is best treated over the long-term by the primary care provider. No serious hypertensive-related adverse events occurred when delaying medical intervention until follow-up out to 6 months, though placing patients on antihypertensive therapy at discharge may protect from further end-organ damage.[2,4,9–11]

Although there is limited evidence on which to base guidelines for treatment in the ED, the current recommendation is that routine screening for acute target organ injury is not required in this population unless patients are African American, have poor follow-up, or

Table 3
Current guidelines for evaluation and treatment of asymptomatic hypertension in the emergency department

BP (mm Hg)	Demographic	Order	Follow-up
≥140/90 but ≤180/110	Good follow-up available	Consider DC Rx	1 mo with PCP
≥140/90 but ≤180/110	AA, indigent, poor access to care	Serum Cr or BMP DC with Rx	1 mo with PCP
≥180/110	All	Recheck BP at 90 min If >180/110 then: serum Cr or BMP Consider acute Tx DC Rx	1 wk to 1 mo with PCP

Abbreviations: AA, African American; DC, discharge; PCP, primary care provider; Rx, outpatient prescription, Serum Cr, serum creatinine; TX, treatment.

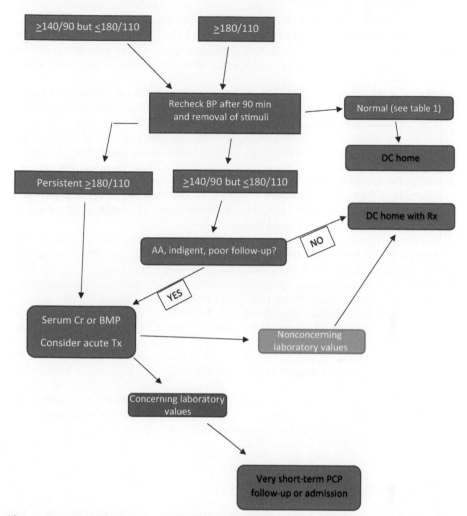

Fig. 1. Current guidelines for evaluation and treatment of asymptomatic hypertension in the ED. AA, African American; Cr, creatinine; DC, discharge; PCP, primary care provider; Rx, outpatient prescription; Tx, treatment.

have limited access to care.[1–3] For those patients, and for patients with a BP greater than or equal to 180/110 mm Hg that does not normalize after 90 minutes of observation, serum creatinine or BMP may be appropriate to order to evaluate for occult kidney dysfunction and to determine patient disposition[2,4] (**Table 3**). Routine screening of UA, chest radiograph, and an ECG were shown to be of no benefit in all populations studied and should not be routinely performed.[1] Most of these patients are safe to discharge with follow-up with their primary care provider within 1 week (**Fig. 1**).

REFERENCES

1. Karras DJ, Kruus LK, Cienki JJ, et al. Utility of routine testing for patients with asymptomatic severe blood pressure elevation in the emergency department. Ann Emerg Med 2008;51:231–9.

2. Brody A, Rahman T, Reed B, et al. Safety and efficacy of antihypertensive prescription at emergency department discharge. Acad Emerg Med 2015;22:632–5.

3. Nishijima DK, Paladino L, Sinert R. Routine testing in patients with asymptomatic elevated blood pressure in the emergency department. Am J Emerg Med 2010; 28:235–42.

4. Wolf SJ, Lo B, Shih RD, et al. Clinical policy: critical issues in the evaluation and management of adult patients in the emergency department with asymptomatic elevated blood pressure. Ann Emerg Med 2013;62:59–68.

5. Tilman K, DeLashaw M, Lowe S, et al. Recognizing asymptomatic elevated blood pressure in emergency department patients: how good (bad) are we? Am J Emerg Med 2007;25:313–7.

6. James PA, Oparil S, Carter BL, et al. 2014 evidence-based guideline for the management of high blood pressure in adults: report from the panel members appointed to the Eighth Joint National Committee (JNC 8). JAMA 2014. http://dx.doi.org/10.1001/jama.2013.284427.

7. Sutters M. Systemic hypertension. In: Papadakis MA, McPhee SJ, Rabow MW, editors. Current medical diagnosis and treatment 2016, vol. 11, 55th edition. New York: McGraw Hill; 2016. p. 435–67.

8. Lawson L, Robelli S. Best evidence on management of asymptomatic hypertension in emergency department patients. J Emerg Nurs 2011;37:174–8.

9. Baumann BM. Systemic hypertension. In: Tintinalli JE, editor. Emergency medicine: a comprehensive study guide, vol. 57, 8th edition. New York: McGraw Hill; 2016. p. 399–408.

10. Patel KK, Young L, Howell EH, et al. Characteristics and outcomes of patients presenting with hypertensive urgency in the office setting. JAMA Intern Med 2016;176(7):981–8.

11. Karras DJ, Kruus LK, Cienki JJ, et al. Evaluation and treatment of patients with severely elevated blood pressure in academic emergency departments: a multi-center study. Ann Emerg Med 2006;43:230–6.

Orthopedic Pearls and Pitfalls

Jonathan D. Monti, DSc, PA-C*, Aaron Cronin, DSc, PA-C

KEYWORDS

- Orthopedic emergencies • Compartment syndrome • Septic arthritis • Fractures
- Dislocations

KEY POINTS

- Orthopedic emergencies generate a significant number of visits to emergency departments and are a common source of malpractice claims.
- Prompt identification of orthopedic injuries and illnesses requiring urgent intervention and referral is a key factor in executing proper management.
- Septic arthritis is a crucial diagnostic consideration in the setting of acute joint pain due to potential for rapid joint destruction, resultant permanent function loss, and associated systemic illness.
- Known or suspected compartment syndrome requires urgent orthopedic consultation to prevent permanent tissue damage and/or muscle contracture.

INTRODUCTION

Orthopedic-related injuries and illnesses are commonplace in the emergency department (ED). Orthopedic injuries (especially undiagnosed/missed fractures) are a leading cause of ED malpractice claims and dollars paid.[1–3] Although many orthopedic injuries and illnesses are effectively treated by ED staff without orthopedic specialty consultation, prompt and accurate recognition of conditions requiring specialty intervention remains a vital emergency clinician skill. This article's intent is to provide emergency clinicians a cognitive framework of how to best approach the evaluation of potential orthopedic emergencies and to briefly review several critical orthopedic emergencies encountered in the ED. As a result, it is the authors' intent to assist their colleagues in avoiding pitfalls when diagnosing and managing these high-risk emergencies.

Disclosure Statement: The authors have nothing to disclose.
The views expressed are those of the authors and do not reflect the official policy or position of the US Army Medical Department, Department of the Army, Department of Defense or the U.S. Government.
Department of Emergency Medicine, US Army/Baylor EMPA Residency Program, Madigan Army Medical Center, 9040A Jackson Avenue, Tacoma, WA 98431, USA
* Corresponding author.
E-mail address: jonathan.d.monti.mil@mail.mil

EVALUATION CONSIDERATIONS
History

As with all emergency cases, a detailed patient history regarding the orthopedic complaint is crucial in achieving an accurate diagnosis. Specifically, ED clinicians must elicit a precise mechanism of injury (whenever possible). The mechanism of injury provides the clinician essential injury severity clues as well as clues for potential underlying or associated injuries.

A general medical history remains imperative as well as a thorough review of systems. Clinicians should specifically inquire of systemic symptoms such as fever in the setting of potential infectious orthopedic emergencies as well as function of affected anatomic regions. Functional assessment questions include signs and symptoms related to range of motion (ROM), resistance/strength, ambulation, weight-bearing, and associated neurologic dysfunction. The patient's past medical history is completed with a baseline functional status, previous injuries/surgeries/therapies and vaccinations, and pertinent family, social, and travel history. The review of systems includes comorbidity inquires, to include coagulopathies, autoimmune disorders, and immunecomprised states.

Physical Examination

A thorough physical examination includes, but is not limited to, the following components.

Inspection
Inspection includes observing for antalgic gait and the presence of the patient's reluctance or compensation in using the affected limb/area. The affected area is completely exposed and inspected for gross deformities, overlying skin lesions, ecchymosis, and overall skin integrity. Visual comparison to the contralateral side, when possible, is recommended.

Neurovascular function
Vascular status is assessed early by palpating correlating vessels and capillary refill. Neurologic evaluation includes associated, bilateral sensory and motor function, to include 2-point discrimination, deep tendon reflexes, and strength.

Palpation
Palpation is performed systematically, with the clinician specifically noting areas of induration, edema, crepitus, bony step-off, skin temperature if concern for infection or vascular compromise, and areas of maximal tenderness. The area of concern/maximal pain is best palpated last to avoid the patient limiting further examination.

Range of motion
The clinician and patient range the joints both proximal and distal to the affected area. Acutely diminished ROM or pain with axial load should increase clinical suspicion of acute bony/orthopedic injury. High-yield functional tests specific to the injured anatomic region may be appropriate.

CONSULTATION CONSIDERATIONS

Urgent orthopedic consultation in the ED is generally indicated in the following circumstances.

Open Fracture

An open fracture is defined as a fracture with overlying soft tissue injury. Open fractures are associated with increased risk of osteomyelitis, a major complication that may result in chronic pain, permanent disability, and requisite prolonged therapies, including prescriptions, multiple surgeries, and/or amputation. Thus, urgent and meticulous intervention is required, including updating tetanus vaccination, copious irrigation, debridement, and early antibiotic administration. The Gustilo-Anderson Classification system, outlined in Table 1, is a widely used prognostic tool used to grade open fractures and guide management based on size of wound, extent of soft tissue involvement, type of fracture, and wound contamination.[4] This classification system, in conjunction with local antibiograms, can guide prophylactic antibiotic regimens. A first-generation cephalosporin is often chosen for type I and type II fractures. A third-generation cephalosporin, aminoglycoside, or penicillin/beta-lactam combination should be considered for larger or significantly contaminated (type III) fractures.[5–7]

Irreducible Fracture/Dislocation

Occasionally the emergency clinician is unable to reduce displaced fractures/dislocations despite adequate anesthesia/analgesia. Technique may not be the only reason for irreducibility. At times, deep sedation may be required. Open reduction in the operating room may be necessary if reduction cannot be achieved in the ED.

Neurovascular Compromise

Closed reductions in the ED often result in acute restoration of neurovascular function. Postreduction, consultative evaluation of nerve/vessel integrity may still be warranted from an orthopedic specialist.

Compartment Syndrome

Compartment syndrome can lead to irreversible muscle and nerve damage within 6 to 8 hours after injury, resulting in devastating permanent sequelae. Early orthopedic consultation is recommended in known or suspected cases of compartment syndrome.

Need for Surgical Intervention

Although operative intervention is often required for orthopedic injuries and illnesses, it may be appropriately delayed in certain circumstances. Telephonic consultation, at a

Table 1 Gustilo-Anderson classification of open fractures	
Type I	Wound <1 cm, minimal soft tissue damage and contamination
Type II	Wound >1 cm but <10 cm without extensive soft tissue damage, flap, or avulsion
Type IIIA	Open segmental fracture, wound >10 cm with extensive soft tissue damage but adequate soft tissue coverage of periosteum
Type IIIB	Wound >10 cm with extensive soft tissue damage, significant contamination, inadequate soft tissue to cover periosteum
Type IIIC	Any open fracture with accompanying vascular injury requiring repair

Data from Gustilo RB, Anderson JT. Prevention of infection in the treatment of one thousand and twenty-five open fractures of long bones: retrospective and prospective analyses. J Bone Joint Surg Am 1976;58:453–8.

minimum, is recommended to discuss the most appropriate timeline for any injury or illness requiring operative intervention.

CRITICAL UPPER EXTREMITY ORTHOPEDIC EMERGENCIES
Sternoclavicular Dislocation

Sternoclavicular dislocations (SCDs), most of which are anterior, account for less than 1% of all joint dislocations.[8] These injuries are most often the result of a significant anterior thrust of the shoulder joint or direct force to the anterior chest. Most commonly, motor vehicle collisions (MVCs), athletics, and falls are the inciting mechanisms.[9] Posterior SCDs are rare due to the posterior sternoclavicular joint's strength, but may be associated with life-threatening injuries.[10,11] Patients with posterior SCD may complain of dysphagia, dyspnea, or unilateral arm edema because of esophageal compression, pneumothorax, tracheal compression/rupture, or compression/laceration of great vessels, making accurate diagnosis crucial.

Immediate bedside ultrasound (US) should be performed if pneumothorax is suspected, and US has been reported to be useful in the detection of posterior SCD.[12] By comparison, routine radiographs have a low sensitivity for detecting SCD. Special serendipity view may be useful; however, CT is the imaging modality of choice, particularly in posterior SCDs due to risk of associated life-threatening injuries to adjacent non-bony structures[13] (Fig. 1). Orthopedic consultation is required for posterior SCD for closed or open reduction.

Posterior Shoulder Dislocations

Posterior shoulder dislocations (PSDs) are comparatively infrequent versus anterior dislocations, but up to 60% to 70% of posterior dislocations may be missed during initial evaluation.[14,15] Most commonly the result of high energy trauma, seizures, or electrocution, 90% of PSDs are subacromial.[16] Standard anteroposterior (AP) radiographic evaluation may miss in up to 50% of PSDs.[17] As such, Y-scapular view and axillary views are imperative if PSD is suspected (Fig. 2). PSDs are commonly associated with humeral fractures (reverse Hill-Sachs lesions), lesser tuberosity fractures, posterior glenoid rim fractures, and rotator cuff tears in 20% of cases.[14,18]

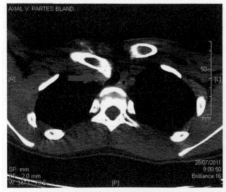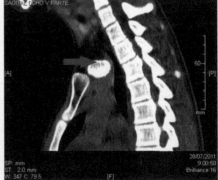

Fig. 1. CT imaging revealing compression of trachea secondary to posterior SCD (*arrows*). (*Reprinted from* Rodríguez Suárez PM, Hussein Serhal M, Freixinet Gilart JL. Tracheal compression secondary to posterior sternoclavicular dislocation. Arch Bronconeumol 2014;50:306; with permission from Elsevier.)

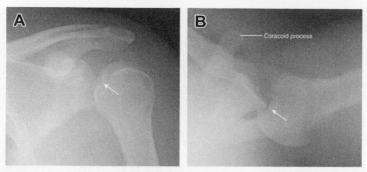

Fig. 2. Radiographs of PSD, not immediately recognized on AP view (*A*), with arrow annotating the subtle finding of internal rotation of humeral head, which may be the only finding on AP view. Axillary view (*B*) of the same patient reveals obvious PSD, with arrow pointing to humeral head impacted onto posterior glenoid rim. (*Reprinted from* Andrews JR, Wilk KE, Reinold MM. The athlete's shoulder. 2nd edition. Philadelphia: Churchill Livingstone; 2008; with permission from Elsevier.)

Orthopedic consultation should be pursued before reduction attempts. Although closed reduction, accomplished with axial traction on an adducted shoulder, is often successful, severe pain and muscle spasms are common; therefore, sedation and analgesia are often required. Indications for open reduction of PSD include significant displacement of lesser tuberosity, articular surface involvement of greater than 25%, and chronic dislocations.[15]

Elbow Fracture/Dislocation: The "Terrible Triad"

Although the elbow is a relatively stable joint, it is the second most commonly dislocated large joint.[19] Ninety percent of elbow dislocations are posterolateral.[20] Elbow dislocations are associated with neurovascular complications in up to 21% of cases, making early assessment of neurovascular status the clinician's first priority.[19] Ulnar nerve entrapment and subsequent compromise, characterized by paresthesias or loss of sensation in ulnar nerve distribution, or inability to hold a piece of paper between the fourth and fifth fingers, is the most common of these complications, but brachial artery injury may also occur.[19]

The "terrible triad" consists of an elbow dislocation associated with fractures of the radial head and coronoid process (Fig. 3). These injuries result in gross elbow joint instability and are associated with significant stiffness and resultant long-term disability. If spontaneous reduction has not already occurred, expeditious closed reduction is required in conjunction with an orthopedic surgeon's consultation. ROM-testing should be avoided when radial head and coronoid fractures are present, because this can exacerbate the injury. Suspected vascular injuries require further evaluation with arteriography in the ED. Immobilization with a posterior splint with the elbow flexed at 90° is recommended with prompt orthopedic consultation for definitive management, commonly requiring operative fixation.

Scaphoid Fractures

The scaphoid is the most commonly fractured carpal bone, often secondary to falling onto an outstretched hand or forced dorsiflexion of the wrist.[21] Anatomic snuff box tenderness remains the key diagnostic examination finding. Snuffbox tenderness in the setting of normal wrist radiographs clue the clinician to the possibility of occult

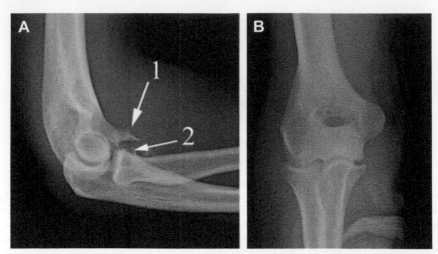

Fig. 3. Lateral (A) and AP (B) radiographs of an elbow revealing fractures of coronoid process (arrow 1) and radial head (arrow 2). (Reprinted from Chen NC, Ring D. Terrible triad injuries of the elbow. J Hand Surg 2015;40:2300; with permission from Elsevier.)

fracture. Up to 25% of acute wrist injuries with negative initial radiographs are associated with occult scaphoid fracture.[22]

MRI yields 97.7% sensitivity, and computed tomography (CT) yields 83% sensitivity in detecting scaphoid fractures. However, these modalities are costly and may not be readily available to ED clinicians.[23] In such ED environments, management for suspected (based on presence of snuffbox tenderness and negative initial radiograph) and actual scaphoid fractures consists of thumb spica cast/splint immobilization and outpatient hand surgeon referral. Repeat radiographs obtained in 7 to 10 days are necessary for those patients whose initial radiographs are negative and who can tolerate immobilization.

Malunion or nonunion occurs in up to 15% of scaphoid fractures, and avascular necrosis occurs in 20% of all scaphoid fractures and 80% of proximal scaphoid fractures, because the scaphoid's vascular supply originates from the distal portion of the bone. These complication rates highlight the importance of early immobilization, accurate diagnosis, and appropriate consultation.[21]

CRITICAL LOWER EXTREMITY ORTHOPEDIC EMERGENCIES
Hip Fracture Radiographic Considerations

Delayed or misdiagnosis of hip fractures is associated with increased mortality, increased hospitalization, and dramatically decreased functionality.[23] Although plain radiographs are sufficient to identify most fracture/dislocations, occult hip fractures occur in 10% of patients with initially negative radiographs.[24] Occult fracture is suspected in any patient complaining of axial load-/weight-bearing pain despite normal radiographs.[25] Even CT, although widely available, may miss up to 2% of fractures.[25] Thus, MRI remains the diagnostic study of choice to exclude occult hip fracture in equivocal cases of suspected hip fracture.[24,25]

Knee Dislocation

Knee dislocations are potentially limb threatening, because they are commonly associated with severe vascular injury.[26] They are most commonly the result of MVCs, falls, or sports-related injuries.[27] Most knee dislocations result in an obvious deformity; however, significant edema may result in a less obvious deformity. The knee will be grossly unstable due to ligamentous disruption. Peroneal nerve function should be evaluated by assessing strength when asking the patient to actively dorsiflex the foot/toes of the ipsilateral limb against resistance, because up to one-third of knee dislocations result in peroneal nerve injury.[27] Reduction may occur spontaneously before ED arrival, causing clinicians to disregard the potential for vascular injury.

All patients with known or suspected knee dislocation should undergo ankle-brachial index (ABI) evaluations for potential popliteal artery injury. ABI score greater than 0.9 has a negative predictive value of nearly 100% for ruling out popliteal artery injury.[28] Recent literature suggests that CT angiography for evaluation of popliteal artery injury is unnecessary when a distal pulse is palpable and ABI greater than 0.9.[28,29] Vascular surgery consultation is indicated for suspicion or known popliteal artery injury. Otherwise, ED management includes closed reduction with longitudinal traction and orthopedic consultation for knee instability and need for operative repair.

Maisonneuve Fracture

This unstable injury consists of (1) a deltoid ligament tear or medial malleolar fracture, (2) disruption of the tibiofibular ligament/interosseous membrane, and (3) proximal fibular fracture. A Maisonneuve fracture is a devastating soft tissue injury to the ankle that may have subtle findings on ankle radiographs. The proximal fibula is often not examined and therefore not imaged, and the bones of the ankle may not exhibit significant radiographic findings.

Standard ankle radiographs may reveal subtle mortise or distal tibiofibular syndesmosis widening (Fig. 4). The astute ED clinician should, therefore, always palpate the proximal fibula for tenderness in the setting of any ankle injury and order radiographs of the lower leg if tenderness is present (Fig. 5). Along with bimalleolar and trimalleolar ankle fractures, a Maisonneuve fracture requires ED orthopedic consultation secondary to acute and chronic ankle instability requiring operative repair.[30]

Lisfranc Injury

The Lisfranc (tarsometatarsal) joint complex includes the articulation of the proximal first, second, and third metatarsals with the cuneiform bones, and fourth and fifth metatarsals with the cuboid. It significantly contributes to overall midfoot stability. Injuries to this complex can range from stable sprains to fracture dislocations. Up to 20% of Lisfranc injuries may be misdiagnosed, making them a common source of ED malpractice claims.[31] They are associated with a high incidence of chronic pain and functional disability.[32] Mechanism of injury is typically high energy, most commonly a fall or MVC, or a rotational force when the foot is in a plantarflexed position.[33] Patients typically present with midfoot pain, with examination revealing midfoot tenderness, swelling, and possible dorsal foot ecchymosis and instability with midfoot stress. Pain with passive toe ROM may suggest an acute compartment syndrome (ACS).

Radiographic evaluation of midfoot injuries initially consists of AP, lateral, and oblique images (Fig. 6). Weight-bearing views, if tolerated, are also recommended, because this stresses the midfoot and may prevent 10% of missed Lisfranc diagnoses.[31] CT can be useful if the patient cannot tolerate stress radiographs, and CT has been shown to be more sensitive in diagnosing Lisfranc injuries.[34] Patients with known or suspected Lisfranc injuries are placed in a posterior splint, made non-weight-bearing, and provided with close orthopedic or podiatry follow-up. Compartment syndrome of the foot can occur and, if suspected, requires emergent

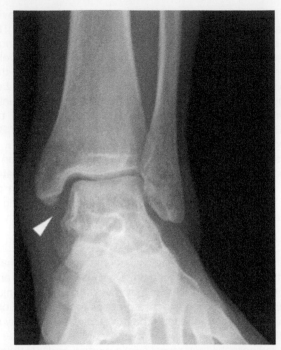

Fig. 4. AP radiographs of Maisonneuve fracture of an ankle with subtle finding of widening of tibiotalar joint medially (*arrowhead*). (*Reprinted from* Taweel NR, Raikin SM, Karanjia HN, et al. The proximal fibula should be examined in all patients with ankle injury: a case series of missed maisonneuve fractures. J Emerg Med 2013;44:e252; with permission from Elsevier.)

consultation/intervention. Many Lisfranc injuries require operative intervention for reduction/fixation.[35]

COMPARTMENT SYNDROME

ACS affects 200,000 people annually. ACS manifests when increased pressure within a limited space ultimately compromises the space's tissue circulation and function.[36] Compartment syndrome, if left untreated, leads to contracture deformities, paralysis, or amputation. Maintaining a high index of suspicion is therefore critical to the timely diagnosis and management of ACS.

ACS is most commonly the result of traumatic fractures to the extremities (75%),[37,38] but can occur after both minor trauma and atraumatic settings. Causes of ACS are listed in Box 1. The lower leg and forearm are most commonly affected[36]; however, other locations affected can include hand, foot, thigh buttocks, abdomen, and ocular orbit.

Clinical Features

The classic clinical findings of ACS are described as "The 5 'P's" (Box 2). The earliest and most common finding in ACS is pain out of proportion to apparent injury. The pain of compartment syndrome is commonly described as a deep, unrelenting ache. Presence of paresthesias suggests nerve ischemia and usually occurs within 30 minutes to 2 hours. Pain with passive stretching is the most sensitive sign of compartment

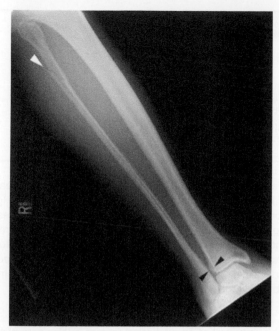

Fig. 5. AP radiographs of tibia/fibula in a patient with maisonneuve fracture revealing subtle widening of syndesmosis (*black arrowheads*) and proximal fibular fracture (*white arrowhead*). (*Reprinted from* Taweel NR, Raikin SM, Karanjia HN, et al. The proximal fibula should be examined in all patients with ankle injury: a case series of missed maisonneuve fractures. J Emerg Med 2013;44:e253; with permission from Elsevier.)

syndrome.[39] Other classic findings typically associated with ACS (pallor, pulselessness, paralysis) are insensitive and often very late findings.[40]

Diagnosis

Direct measurement of compartment pressures is the most important adjunct in diagnosis of ACS. Typical methods of measurement include a Stryker handheld manometer or simple needle manometer. Normal compartment pressures are less than

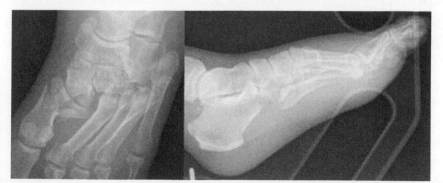

Fig. 6. AP and lateral foot radiographs revealing Lisfranc injury of midfoot. (*Reprinted from* Demirkale I, Tecimel O, Celik I, et al. The effect of the Tscherne injury pattern on the outcome of operatively treated Lisfranc fracture dislocations. Foot Ankle Surg 2013;19:190; with permission from Elsevier.)

Box 1
Common causes of acute compartment syndrome

Traumatic fracture

Crush injury

Burns

Constriction (ie, casts/bandages)

Prolonged immobilization and compression

Vascular injury

---

10 mm Hg. Capillary blood flow compromise begins at pressures greater than 20 mm Hg, and ischemic necrosis occurs at pressures greater than 30 mm Hg.[41–44] Because diastolic blood pressure correlates with tissue perfusion pressures, experts now recommend using a "delta pressure" (diastolic blood pressure – compartment pressure) as a threshold for diagnosing ACS. A delta pressure of 20 to 30 mm Hg or less warrants orthopedic intervention.[45–47] Serial pressures over the course of 6 hours are recommended if a clinical suspicion for ACS exists, as a single compartment pressure cannot reliably exclude ACS.

Management

Adequate analgesia, removal of exacerbating factors such as cast/dressings, and a neutral position of the affected area are recommended. The mainstay of ACS treatment is immediate fasciotomy. Affected compartment tissues will tolerate ischemia for up to 4 hours; after 8 hours damage becomes irreversible, thus increasing morbidity.[48] If concern for muscle ischemia exists, the patient should undergo evaluation for rhabdomyolysis, consisting of urine myoglobin, renal function, and serum creatine phosphokinase levels.

SEPTIC ARTHRITIS

Septic arthritis remains the most important diagnostic consideration in ED patients presenting with acute joint pain, due to the potential for both rapid joint destruction and sepsis. Septic arthritis affects 2 to 10 persons per 100,000 annually in the United States and is more prevalent in children and older adults.[49] Risk factors are listed in **Box 3**.

Clinical Presentation

Patients with bacterial arthritis most commonly present acutely with a single swollen and painful joint. Polyarthropathies occur in 20% of bacterial cases, most commonly

---

Box 2
Classic clinical findings of acute compartment syndrome

Pain

Paresthesias

Pallor[a]

Pulselessness[a]

Paralysis[a]

   [a] Late finding.

Box 3
Risk factors for septic arthritis
Age greater than 80
Recent joint surgery
Diabetes/immunocompromised states
Alcoholism
Intravenous (IV) drug use
Skin infection
Rheumatoid or other chronic arthritis
Previous corticosteroid injection
History/presence of prosthetic joint
Adapted from Margaretten ME, Kohlwes J, Moore D, et al. Does this adult patient have septic arthritis? JAMA 2007;297:1478.

in patients with rheumatoid arthritis or other systemic connective tissue disease.[50,51] Larger joints are more commonly affected; the knee is involved in greater than 50% of cases,[52] but smaller axial joints such as the sternoclavicular joint and pubic symphysis can be involved. Most patients present with fever, although less frequently in the elderly and immunocompromised.[50] Gonococcal arthritis, the most common cause of bacterial arthritis in sexually active young adults, may present with a prodromal phase consisting of a migratory arthritis and/or tenosynovitis.[53,54] Given the variability of septic joint patient presentations, particularly across certain at-risk populations, history and physical examination are considered unreliable in excluding the diagnosis of septic arthritis.

Diagnosis

Laboratory tests commonly drawn in septic arthritis evaluation include complete blood count, erythrocyte sedimentation rate, and C-reactive protein. However, no serum markers values have been determined to reliably rule in or out this condition.[50,55] Radiographs are also unreliable in diagnosing acute septic arthritis, because bony changes/destruction occur late in the disease process and the presence of effusion cannot accurately distinguish cause.

The diagnostic gold standard for septic arthritis is a positive synovial fluid culture. Arthrocentesis is performed for any patient wherein septic arthritis is clinically suspected. Overlying skin at the needle penetration point must be free of cellulitis/lesions, and caution is used in the setting of coagulopathy. Final culture results may take days, however. As such, the ED clinician relies on synovial fluid analysis in determining initial management and disposition.

Synovial fluid analysis should include culture (aerobic and anaerobic), Gram stain, white blood cell count, cell differential, synovial lactate, and evaluation for crystals. Synovial glucose and protein levels are not helpful in diagnosing septic arthritis.[55] Synovial fluid findings typical of bacterial arthritis compared with normal joint and inflammatory arthritis are shown in **Table 2**.

Management

The mainstay of septic arthritis treatment is prompt administration of appropriate parenteral antibiotics and orthopedic consultation for possible joint irrigation.

Table 2
Synovial fluid characteristics

	Normal	Inflammatory	Septic
Appearance/viscosity	Clear/yellow/high	Yellow/white/low	Cloudy/purulent/variable
White blood cells (mm^3)	<200	2000–100,000	15,000–100,000
Cell differential	<25% PMNs	>50% PMNs	>75% PMNs
Synovial lactate	<5.6 mmol/L	<5.6 mmol/L	>5.6 mmol/L
Synovial LDH	<250 U/L	<250 U/L	>250 U/L
Gram stain	Negative	Negative	Positive in 70% of septic joints
Culture	Negative	Negative	Positive

Abbreviations: LDH, lactate dehydrogenase; PMN, polymorphonuclear leukocytes.
Adapted from Genes N, Chisolm-Straker M. Monoarticular arthritis update: current evidence for diagnosis and treatment in emergency department. Emerg Med Pract 2012,14:5–7; and Sholter DE, Russell AS. Synovial fluid analysis. In: Post TW, editor. UpToDate. Waltham (MA): UpToDate. Accessed July 15, 2016.

Appropriate initial antibiotic therapy is based on likely causative agent, gram-stain results, and immune status (Table 3). *Staphylococcus* remains the most common bacteria implicated in adults with septic arthritis.[56] Gonococcal arthritis is much less likely to cause joint destruction and therefore rarely requires joint irrigation.[57]

PEDIATRIC ORTHOPEDIC CONSIDERATIONS

Pediatric bone anatomy is unique because, until puberty, the bones are undergoing growth at open physes. Physeal injuries potentially affect future growth; thus, they remain a primary consideration when managing pediatric fractures. Salter and Harris developed a classification system based on fracture appearance (Fig. 7) and each fracture type's potential to affect growth.

Type I fractures, if not significantly displaced, may be radiographically undetectable but have a low incidence of growth disturbance.[58] Type II fractures account for 75% of all physeal fractures.[19] They, along with type III fractures, generally have a positive prognosis. However, type III intra-articular fractures require open reduction to ensure

Table 3
Empiric antibiotic therapy for suspected septic arthritis

Gram Stain Results	Antibiotic	Alternative Antibiotic
(+) Gram-positive cocci	Vancomycin 15 mg/kg IV	Imipenem 500 mg IV
(+) Gram-negative bacilli	Ceftriaxone 2 g IV	Ciprofloxacin 400 mg IV
Negative Gram stain with clinical & synovial fluid findings consistent with septic joint	Immunocompetent: Vancomycin 15 mg/kg IV Immunocompromised/IV drug users: vancomycin 15 mg/kg IV Plus Third-generation cephalosporin	Imipenem 500 mg IV

Data from Burton JH, Fortuna TJ. Joints and bursae. In: Tintinalli JE, editor. Emergency medicine: a comprehensive study guide. 8th edition. New York: McGraw Hill, Inc; 2016. p. 1933; Goldenberg DL, Sexton DJ, Septic Arthritis in Adults. In: UpToDate, Post TW (Ed), UpToDate, Waltham, MA.

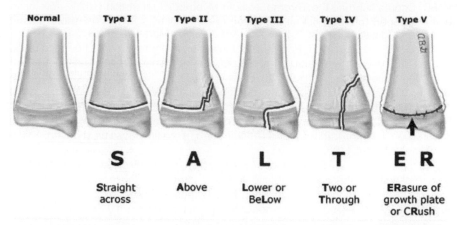

Fig. 7. Salter-Harris classification of physeal fractures. The growth plate is shown in green. The mnemonic refers to the fracture line and its relationship to the growth plate. The metaphysis is the bone above the growth plate, and the epiphysis is the bone below. Type I fractures disrupt the physis. Type II fractures involve a break from the growth plate up into the metaphysis, with the periosteum usually remaining intact. Type III fractures are intraarticular fractures through the epiphysis that expand across the physis. Type IV fractures cross the epiphysis, physis, and metaphysis. Type V fractures are compression injuries to the physis. (*Reproduced from* Beutler A, Stephens MB. General principles of fracture management: bone healing and fracture description. In: Post TW, editor. UpToDate. Waltham (MA): UpToDate. For more information, visit www.uptodate.com; with permission.)

proper articular surface alignment. Type IV fractures account for 10% of physeal fracture and are at significant risk of growth disturbance, requiring precise realignment.[19] Therefore, open reduction and fixation is often required. Type V fractures, although also frequently radiographically undetectable, is typically secondary to a significant mechanism. These require close orthopedic monitoring for anticipated growth arrest.

SUMMARY

Orthopedic-related injuries and illnesses are common but challenging encounters due to the wide range of acuity with which they can present to the ED. Likewise, management of orthopedic injuries and illness can range from expectant to life- or limb-saving intervention. Key for ED clinicians who manage orthopedic emergencies is their ability to recognize the need for urgent intervention, appropriately use diagnostic modalities and adjuncts, and coordinate timely consultation and/or referral for care.

REFERENCES

1. Kachalia A, Gandhi TK, Puopolo AL, et al. Missed and delayed diagnoses in the emergency department: a study of closed malpractice claims from 4 liability insurers. Ann Emerg Med 2007;49(2):196–205.

2. American College of Emergency Physicians Medical-Legal Committee. Summary of Malpractice Claim Data & Trends from Three Sources. An Information Paper 2013. Available at: https://www.acep.org/summary-of-malpractice-claim-data—trends-from-three-sources. Accessed October 13, 2016.

3. Karcz A, Korn R, Burke MC, et al. Malpractice claims against emergency physicians in Massachusetts: 1975-1993. Am J Emerg Med 1996;14(4):341–5.
4. Gustilo RB, Anderson JT. Prevention of infection in the treatment of one thousand and twenty-five open fractures of long bones: retrospective and prospective analyses. J Bone Joint Surg Am 1976;58:453–8.
5. Wilkins J, Patzakis M. Choice and duration of antibiotics in open fractures. Orthop Clin North Am 1991;22:433.
6. Russell GV Jr, King C, May CG, et al. Once daily high-dose gentamicin to prevent infection in open fractures of the tibial shaft: a preliminary investigation. South Med J 2001;94:1185.
7. Patzakis MJ, Bains RS, Lee J, et al. Prospective, randomized, double-blind study comparing single-agent antibiotic therapy, ciprofloxacin, to combination antibiotic therapy in open fracture wounds. J Orthop Trauma 2000;14:529.
8. Ferrera PC, Wheeling HM. Sternoclavicular joint injuries. Am J Emerg Med 2000; 18(1):58–61.
9. Wirth MA, Rockwood CA Jr. Acute and chronic traumatic injuries of the sternoclavicular joint. J Am Acad Orthop Surg 1996;4(5):268–78.
10. Sewell MD, Al-Hadithy N, Le Leu A, et al. Instability of the sternoclavicular joint: current concepts in classification, treatment and outcomes. Bone Joint J 2013;95:721.
11. Glass ER, Thompson JD, Cole PA, et al. Treatment of sternoclavicular joint dislocations: a systematic review of 251 dislocations in 24 case series. J Trauma 2011; 70:1294.
12. Blakeley CJ, Harrison HL, Siow S, et al. The use of bedside ultrasound to diagnose posterior sterno-clavicular dislocation. Emerg Med J 2011;28(6):542.
13. Groh GI, Wirth MA. Management of traumatic sternoclavicular joint injuries. J Am Acad Orthop Surg 2011;19(1):1–7.
14. Kowalsky MS, Levine WN. Traumatic posterior glenohumeral dislocation: classification, pathoanatomy, diagnosis, and treatment. Orthop Clin North Am 2008; 39(4):519–33.
15. Cicak N. Posterior dislocation of the shoulder. J Bone Joint Surg Br 2004;86(3): 324–32.
16. Elberger ST, Brody G. Bilateral posterior shoulder dislocations. Am J Emerg Med 1995;13(3):331–2.
17. Gor DM. The trough line sign. Radiology 2002;224(2):485–6.
18. Saupe N, White LM, Bleakney R, et al. Acute traumatic shoulder dislocation: MR findings. Radiology 2008;24(1):185–93.
19. Simon R, Sherman S. Emergency orthopedics. 6th edition. New York: McGraw-Hill; 2011. p. 298.
20. Hobgood ER, Khan SO, Field LD. Acute dislocations of the adult elbow. Hand Clin 2008;24:1.
21. Abraham MK, Scott S. The emergent evaluation and treatment of hand and wrist injuries. Emerg Med Clin North Am 2010;28(4):789–809.
22. Carpenter CR, Pines JM, Schuur JD, et al. Adult scaphoid fracture. Acad Emerg Med 2014;21(2):101–21.
23. Belmont PJ Jr, Garcia EJ, Romano D, et al. Risk factors for complications and in-hospital mortality following hip fractures: a study using the National Trauma Data Bank. Arch Orthop Trauma Surg 2014;134(5):597–604.
24. Cannon J, Silvestri S, Munro M. Imaging choices in occult hip fracture. J Emerg Med 2009;37(2):144–52.
25. Hossain M, Barwick C, Sinha AK, et al. Is magnetic resonance imaging (MRI) necessary to exclude occult hip fracture? Injury 2007;38:1204.

26. Green NE, Allen BL. Vascular injuries associated with dislocation of the knee. J Bone Joint Surg Am 1977;59(2):236–9.

27. Brautigan B, Johnson DL. The epidemiology of knee dislocations. Clin Sports Med 2000;19(3):387–97.

28. Mills WJ, Barei DP, McNair P. The value of the ankle-brachial index for diagnosing arterial injury after knee dislocation: a prospective study. J Trauma 2004;56(6): 1261–5.

29. Abou-Sayed H, Berger DL. Blunt lower-extremity trauma and popliteal artery injuries: revisiting the case for selective arteriography. Arch Surg 2002;137(5): 585–9.

30. Valderrabano V, Wiewiorski M, Frigg A, et al. Chronic ankle instability. Unfallchirurg 2007;110(8):691–9 [in German].

31. Gupta RT, Wadhwa RP, Learch TJ, et al. Lisfranc injury: imaging findings for this important but often-missed diagnosis. Curr Probl Diagn Radiol 2008;37(3): 115–26.

32. Philbin T, Rosenberg G, Sferra JJ. Complications of missed or untreated Lisfranc injuries. Foot Ankle Clin 2003;8(1):61–71.

33. Thompson MC, Mormino MA. Injury to the tarsometatarsal joint complex. J Am Acad Orthop Surg 2003;11(4):260–7.

34. Haapamaki V, Kiuru M, Koskinen S. Lisfranc fracture-dislocation in patients with multiple trauma: diagnosis with multidetector computed tomography. Foot Ankle Int 2004;25(9):614–9.

35. Meyer SA, Callaghan JJ, Albright JP, et al. Midfoot sprains in collegiate football players. Am J Sports Med 1994;22(3):392–401.

36. Konstantakos EK, Dalstrom DJ, Nelles ME, et al. Diagnosis and management of extremity compartment syndromes: an orthopaedic perspective. Am Surg 2007; 73(12):1199–209.

37. Elliott KG, Johnstone AJ. Diagnosing acute compartment syndrome. J Bone Joint Surg Br 2003;85:625.

38. Köstler W, Strohm PC, Südkamp NP. Acute compartment syndrome of the limb. Injury 2005;36:992.

39. Yamaguchi S, Viegas SF. Causes of upper extremity compartment syndrome. Hand Clin 1998;14(3):365–70.

40. Newton EJ, Love J. Acute complications of extremity trauma. Emerg Med Clin North Am 2007;25:751.

41. Klenerman L. The evolution of the compartment syndrome since 1948 as recorded in the JBJS (B). J Bone Joint Surg Br 2007;89:1280.

42. Reneman RS, Slaaf DW, Lindbom L, et al. Muscle blood flow disturbances produced by simultaneously elevated venous and total muscle tissue pressure. Microvasc Res 1980;20:307.

43. Wiederhielm CA, Weston BV. Microvascular, lymphatic, and tissue pressures in the unanesthetized mammal. Am J Physiol 1973;225:992.

44. Dahn I, Lassen NA, Westling H. Blood flow in human muscles during external pressure or venous stasis. Clin Sci 1967;32:467.

45. McQueen MM, Court-Brown CM. Compartment monitoring in tibial fractures. The pressure threshold for decompression. J Bone Joint Surg Br 1996;78:99.

46. White TO, Howell GE, Will EM, et al. Elevated intramuscular compartment pressures do not influence outcome after tibial fracture. J Trauma 2003;55:1133.

47. Ovre S, Hvaal K, Holm I, et al. Compartment pressure in nailed tibial fractures. A threshold of 30 mmHg for decompression gives 29% fasciotomies. Arch Orthop Trauma Surg 1998;118:29.

48. Whitesides TE, Heckman MM. Acute compartment syndrome: update on diagnosis and treatment. J Am Acad Orthop Surg 1996;4(4):209–18.
49. Dubost JJ, Soubrier M, De Champs C, et al. No changes in the distribution of organisms responsible for septic arthritis over a 20 year period. Ann Rheum Dis 2002;61(3):267–9.
50. Margaretten ME, Kohlwes J, Moore D, et al. Does this adult patient have septic arthritis? JAMA 2007;297:1478.
51. Mikhail IS, Alarcón GS. Nongonococcal bacterial arthritis. Rheum Dis Clin North Am 1993;19:311.
52. Goldenberg DL. Septic arthritis and other infections of rheumatologic significance. Rheum Dis Clin North Am 1991;17:149.
53. Rice PA. Gonococcal arthritis (disseminated gonococcal infection). Infect Dis Clin North Am 2005;19:853.
54. Belkacem A, Caumes E, Ouanich J, et al. Changing patterns of disseminated gonococcal infection in France: cross-sectional data 2009–2011. Sex Transm Infect 2013;89:613.
55. Carpenter CR, Schuur JD, Everett WW, et al. Evidence-based diagnostics: adult septic arthritis. Acad Emerg Med 2011;18(8):781–96.
56. Frazee BW, Fee C, Lambert L. How common is MRSA in adult septic arthritis? Ann Emerg Med 2009;54(5):695–700.
57. Garcia-DeTorre I, Nava-Zavala A. Gonococcal and nongonococcal arthritis. Rheum Dis Clin North Am 2009;35:63.
58. Black KJ, Duffy C, Hopkins-Mann C, et al. Musculoskeletal disorders in children. In: Tintinalli JE, editor. Emergency medicine: a comprehensive study guide. 8th edition. New York: McGraw Hill, Inc; 2016. p. 915–34.

Antibiotic Stewardship
Choosing Wisely

Joshua F. Knox, MA, PA-C, Mary Jo P. Wiemiller, MS, PA-C*

KEYWORDS

- Antibiotic stewardship • Antibiotic resistance • Sepsis

KEY POINTS

- Most cases of acute otitis media resolve without complications. A period of observation before antibiotic therapy may be beneficial for many patients with acute otitis media.
- Most cases of acute pharyngitis are viral in cause.
- Antibiotics have not demonstrated any consistent benefit in the symptoms or natural history of acute bronchitis.
- Indications for antibiotic therapy in acute rhinobacterial sinusitis include (1) persistent signs or symptoms for ≥10 days without evidence of improvement, (2) severe symptoms or signs of fever and purulent nasal discharge or facial pain lasting 3 to 4 consecutive days at the beginning of the illness, or (3) worsening symptoms or signs following an upper respiratory infection that was initially improving.

INTRODUCTION

Emergency department (ED) providers routinely prescribe antibiotics to treat common and life-threatening infections. Whenever antibiotics are used, biologic pressure is placed on bacteria, promoting resistance. Excessive antibiotic use facilitates the emergence, persistence, and transmission of antibiotic-resistant bacteria and increases health care costs.[1–3] Contemporary research demonstrates that antibiotics are frequently overprescribed in ambulatory settings, including the ED.[4] In addition to the development of resistance, adverse reactions from antibiotics, particularly in children, are a very common reason for seeking emergency care.[5,6] Responsible antibiotic use, known as *antimicrobial stewardship*, includes the appropriate use of antimicrobials to improve patient outcomes, reduce microbial resistance, and decrease the spread of multidrug-resistant infections.

Disclosure: There are no financial or commercial disclosures or additional funding sources for either author.
Physician Assistant Studies, Marquette University, 1700 W Wells Street, Milwaukee, WI 53233, USA
* Corresponding author.
E-mail address: maryjo.wiemiller@marquette.edu

Physician Assist Clin 2 (2017) 489–501
http://dx.doi.org/10.1016/j.cpha.2017.02.011
2405-7991/17/© 2017 Elsevier Inc. All rights reserved.

According to the Centers for Disease Control and Prevention (CDC) and the World Health Organization, antibiotic resistance is at crisis levels.[7,8] Antibiotic-resistant infections affect 2 million people per year and are associated with approximately 23,000 deaths per year in the United States.[7] The loss of antibiotic efficacy due to resistance makes treatment of common and serious infections more complicated, costly, and in some cases, impossible.

In response to this crisis, the CDC has launched a comprehensive hospital-based program to support antibiotic stewardship, improve patient care, and diminish resistance.[9] Furthermore, a practical guideline, the *Antibiotic Stewardship Playbook*, was recently developed by a team of experts to reduce antibiotic misuse and overuse.[10] The Centers for Medicare and Medicaid Services and the Joint Commission are both taking steps toward mandated antibiotic stewardship programs in acute care hospitals.[11,12] This article discusses appropriate initial antibiotic choices and treatment indications for acute otitis media (AOM), pharyngitis, sinusitis, acute bronchitis, and sepsis.

ACUTE OTITIS MEDIA
Diagnosis

AOM is the most common infection requiring medical therapy for children less than 5 years old. The American Academy of Pediatrics (AAP) has recently published updated guidelines for the diagnosis and management of AOM in children.[13] The diagnosis of AOM should be made in children when there is moderate or severe bulging of the tympanic membrane (TM) or new onset otorrhea without otitis externa. The diagnosis of AOM should additionally be made for children with mild bulging of the TM and recent onset of ear pain or pronounced TM erythema. The peak incidence of AOM is in children between 3 and 18 months of age. *Streptococcus pneumoniae* is the most common bacteria responsible for AOM in children and adults, followed by *Haemophilus influenzae*.

Antibiotic Therapy Versus Observation

Antibiotic treatment of AOM provides statistically significant benefits over placebo in reducing pain at 2 to 3 days, decreasing tympanic membrane perforations and contralateral AOM episodes. However, these benefits come at the expense of increased adverse events from pharmacologic treatment, including rash, diarrhea, or vomiting. Furthermore, most cases of AOM in developed nations resolve spontaneously without complications.[14] Several recent ED studies suggest that a period of observation with follow-up, or a wait-and-see prescription for antibiotics, instead of immediate antibiotic administration reduces antibiotic usage without an increase in complications.[15–17]

The AAP currently recommends that antibiotics for AOM be prescribed for the following:

- Children older than 6 months who have severe signs or symptoms of AOM.
- Children 6 to 23 months with bilateral AOM.

For all other children, clinicians may either prescribe antibiotics or offer an observation period after jointly deciding this with caregivers when close follow-up can be assured.[13]

Amoxicillin (80–90 mg/kg/d) is recommended for most children as first-line therapy for AOM. If a child has taken amoxicillin in the last 30 days, has concurrent conjunctivitis, or has a history of unresponsiveness to amoxicillin, then amoxicillin-clavulanate

(90 mg/kg/d amoxicillin and 6.4 mg/kg/d clavulanate) is recommended. This recommendation applies to both therapies at AOM diagnosis or after the period of observation. For children who have failed an initial 2 to 3 days of antibiotic therapy, either amoxicillin-clavulanate or ceftriaxone (50 mg/kg intramuscularly or intravenously for 3 days) is recommended.[13]

Duration of Therapy

Although there is some uncertainty in the optimal duration of AOM antibiotic therapy for children, several studies suggest a 10-day course of antibiotics is preferred over shorter durations for children under 2 and for any child with severe symptoms.[18–22] For children with mild to moderate symptoms, a 7-day course is recommended for children aged 2 to 5 years and a 5- to 7-day course for children aged 6 or older.[13]

PHARYNGITIS
Epidemiology and Diagnosis

Pharyngitis is defined as infection or inflammation of the pharynx or tonsils. Most cases of pharyngitis are viral in origin. Group A streptococcus (GAS) is the only common bacterial cause of pharyngitis, representing approximately 10% of adult sore throats and 24% to 37% in children.[23,24] The highest incidence of GAS pharyngitis is found in children and adolescents from 5 to 15 years old in the winter and early spring months. Although antibiotics modestly shorten the duration of the illness, they are given predominantly for the prevention of acute rheumatic fever. Acute rheumatic fever, however, has been on the decline in the United States over the last several decades.[25]

Sore throat is a commonly encountered complaint in the ED, representing 2.3% of adult ED visits.[26] Despite the low incidence of GAS in adults, recent studies demonstrate that more than 50% of adult ED visits receive antibiotic therapy for sore throat, often times with second-line or nonrecommended therapies.[26] Similar patterns of overprescribing and inappropriate antimicrobial coverage have been found in children who are treated in ambulatory settings for pharyngitis.[27]

The Infectious Diseases Society of America (IDSA) guidelines recommend that patients with sore throat be tested for GAS to distinguish between GAS and viral pharyngitis.[28] Testing by a rapid antigen detection test (RADT) and culture is recommended. If the RADT is negative, a throat culture should be obtained in children and adolescents. Throat culture is not necessary in adults due to the low incidence of GAS. Current guidelines recommend selective testing based on clinical symptoms and signs to avoid identifying GAS carriers rather than acute GAS infections. Testing for GAS is not recommended for the following individuals: (1) persons with sore throat and associated symptoms such as cough, rhinorrhea, or oral ulcers that more strongly suggest a viral cause; (2) children less than 3 years, due to the rarity of acute rheumatic fever in this age group; and (3) asymptomatic household contacts of patients with GAS pharyngitis.[28] Clinicians should consider the possibility of chronic GAS carriage or colonization in the setting of frequent recurrent episodes of RADT positive pharyngitis.

Antibiotic Therapy

IDSA recommends oral penicillin or amoxicillin for 10 days as first-line therapy for adults and children without a penicillin allergy. The recommendation for penicillin is based on efficacy, narrow spectrum of activity, minimal cost, and low frequency of side effects.[28] Penicillin courses less than 10 days in length are inferior to 10-day courses for bacterial cure rates.[29] First-generation cephalosporins are appropriate therapy in patients who have a non-type I penicillin hypersensitivity. Cephalosporins have clinical and bacterial cure rates slightly superior to penicillins in double-blinded clinical trials.[29] Clindamycin and the macrolide antibiotics are also appropriate therapy for penicillin allergic patients. However, clinicians should consider the increasing rates of macrolide resistance and treatment failures in the United States before prescribing them.[30] Table 1 lists the full IDSA recommendations on drug, dose, and duration.[28]

ACUTE BRONCHITIS

Acute bronchitis is defined as inflammation of the bronchi, clinically manifests as cough with or without phlegm production, and can last for up to 3 weeks.[31] Acute bronchitis should be distinguished from chronic bronchitis present in patients with chronic obstructive pulmonary disease. Those patients have cough and sputum production on most days of the month for at least 3 months of the year during 2 consecutive years.

Viruses are responsible for 90% to 95% of acute bronchitis.[31] The 3 most common bacterial causes for acute bronchitis are *Mycoplasma pneumonia*, *Chlamydia pneumonia*, and *Bordetella pertussis*.[32] Treatment of *M pneumonia* and *C pneumonia* rarely results in clinically significant improvement in the setting of acute bronchitis. The possibility of *B pertussis*, the organism responsible for whooping cough, should be considered in settings of outbreaks, cough lasting greater than 2 weeks, and middle age or older adults with partially senescent immunity.[33] Classical inspiratory whooping and post-tussive emesis are relatively rare findings in adults with pertussis.[34] Children and adults with confirmed or probable pertussis should receive a macrolide antibiotic and be isolated for 5 days from the start of treatment.[31]

Table 1
Antibiotic regimens recommended for group A streptococcal pharyngitis

Drug, Route	Dose or Dosage	Duration or Quantity	Recommendation Strength, Quality
Without penicillin allergy			
Penicillin V, oral	Child: 250 mg twice daily or 3 times daily. Adults: 250 mg 4 times daily or 500 mg twice daily	10 d	Strong, high
Amoxicillin, oral	50 mg/kg once daily (max: 1000 mg) or 25 mg/kg (max: 500 mg) twice daily	10 d	Strong, high
Benzathine, penicillin G intramuscularly	<27 kg 600,000 U >27 kg 1,200,000 U	1 dose	Strong, high
With penicillin allergy			
Cephalexin oral	20 mg/kg/dose twice daily (max 500 mg/dose)	10 d	Strong, high
Cefadroxil, oral	30 mg/kg once daily (max: 1 g)	10 d	Strong, high
Clindamycin, oral	7 mg/kg/dose 3 times daily (max 300 mg/dose)	10 d	Strong, moderate
Azithromycin, oral	12 mg/kg once daily (max 500 mg)	5 d	Strong, moderate
Clarithromycin, oral	7.5 mg/kg twice daily (max 250 mg/dose)	10 d	Strong, moderate

Diagnosis

Patients with acute bronchitis present with a cough lasting more than 5 days that may be associated with sputum production. It is a frequently encountered diagnosis in the ED among both children and adults.[35] For most patients, the diagnosis is based upon the history and physical examination alone. Further testing is usually not needed. Viral cultures, serologic testing, or sputum analyses should not be routinely performed because the causative organism is rarely identified in clinical practice.[31] The diagnosis of acute bronchitis should be made when there is no clinical or radiographic evidence of pneumonia, and the common cold, asthma exacerbation, or exacerbation of chronic obstructive pulmonary disease have been excluded.[31] Consequently, the evaluation of the patient with suspected acute bronchitis should focus on exclusion of severe illnesses, such as pneumonia and influenza. Purulent sputum is present in 50% of patients with acute bronchitis and is not indicative of a bacterial cause. Physical examination may reveal rhonchi or wheezing due to bronchospasm. Fever is a rare finding in acute bronchitis. When influenza is present in the community, the presence of both cough and fever within 2 days of symptom onset is a strong predictor of influenza, and testing should be considered. When abnormal vital signs are present or there are rales or other signs of consolidation on physical exam, a chest radiograph should be ordered to exclude pneumonia.

Treatment

Because viruses are the usual causative agent in acute bronchitis, antibiotics have not demonstrated any consistent benefit in the symptoms or natural history of acute bronchitis.[36] In a recent meta-analysis of treatment trials for acute bronchitis, there was no difference in subjects described as being clinically improved between the antibiotic and placebo groups at follow-up and a significant trend toward increased adverse events in the antibiotic group.[37] Despite this evidence, approximately 70% to 80% of patients receive antibiotics for acute bronchitis, and the percentage is even higher in ED settings.[36,38,39] The national goal since 2005 has been no routine antibiotic prescriptions for acute bronchitis.[39]

Symptomatic therapy for acute bronchitis may include nonsteroidal anti-inflammatory medications, acetaminophen, cough suppressants, or inhaled β2-agonists. The American College of Chest Physicians guidelines weakly recommend central cough suppressants, such as codeine and dextromethorphan for short-term symptomatic relief of coughing in patients of all ages with acute bronchitis. There is no evidence to support the use of β2-agonists in children with acute cough who do not have evidence of airflow restriction. In select adult patients with acute bronchitis and wheezing accompanying a cough, treatment with β2-agonist bronchodilators appears to shorten the cough duration.[40] Orally inhaled anticholinergic agents have not been studied for acute bronchitis and therefore are not recommended based on the evidence.[40] Nonsteroidal anti-inflammatories or acetaminophen may be helpful in symptomatically treating constitutional symptoms including mild pain.

SINUSITIS
Epidemiology and Diagnosis

Rhinosinusitis is the symptomatic inflammation of the paranasal sinuses and nasal cavity.[41] It is classified as acute if lasting less than 4 weeks and chronic if lasting more than 12 weeks. Furthermore, acute rhinosinusitis can be subdivided into acute bacterial rhinosinusitis (ABRS) or viral rhinosinusitis. The distinction becomes important because guidelines for both children and adults recommend differentiating the entities before initiating antibiotics for ABRS because approximately 90% of acute rhinosinusitis cases start as a viral infection.[41,42] The IDSA recommends making the diagnosis of ABRS in children or adults when there are any of the following present: (1) persistent signs or symptoms of acute rhinosinusitis for ≥10 days without evidence of improvement, (2) severe symptoms or signs of fever and purulent nasal discharge or facial pain lasting 3 to 4 consecutive days at the beginning of the illness, or (3) worsening symptoms or signs following an upper respiratory infection that was initially improving.[42] The American Academy of Otolaryngology clinical practice guidelines are similar, with an emphasis on purulent nasal discharge and/or facial pain/pressure for 10 days or worsening of signs/symptoms within 10 days of onset.[41] Routine imaging is not recommended in uncomplicated acute rhinosinusitis.[41]

Approximately 12% of adults reported being diagnosed with rhinosinusitis in a recent national survey.[43] Rhinosinusitis is the most common outpatient diagnosis that generates an antibiotic prescription among adults.[44] In fact, antibiotics are prescribed in more than 80% of visits for rhinosinusitis.[45]

Therapy

Initial management of ABRS can include watchful waiting for uncomplicated cases for which reliable follow-up is available or antibiotics.[41] For adults, initial therapy with either amoxicillin or amoxicillin-clavulanate is the recommended first-line therapy for 5 to 7 days[41,42] (Table 2). The IDSA recommends amoxicillin-clavulanate as first-line therapy rather than amoxicillin alone but acknowledges that the data supporting this recommendation are weak.[42] For children, amoxicillin-clavulanate is the recommended first-line therapy for 10 to 14 days[42] (Table 3).

Although recommended in the guidelines as second-line therapy for children and adults, the US Food and Drug Administration recently advised against the use of respiratory fluoroquinolones for patients with uncomplicated acute sinusitis and acute bronchitis who have other treatment options.[46] Macrolides and trimethoprim/sulfamethoxazole are also not recommended for ABRS.[42] Clinicians may recommend analgesics, nasal steroids, or saline irrigation for symptomatic relief of ABRS.[41,42]

SEPSIS
Definition

In 2016, the Third International Consensus redefined sepsis. Sepsis is defined as life-threatening organ dysfunction caused by a dysregulated host response to infection and is clinically characterized by an acute change of 2 or more points in the Sequential Organ Failure Assessment (SOFA) score. SOFA scores of 2 can predict 10% mortality or more in the hospitalized patient.[47] Table 4 lists SOFA scoring. Septic shock is a subset of sepsis in which underlying circulatory and cellular/metabolic abnormalities are profound enough to substantially increase mortality.

Sepsis had historically been defined as a patient with 2 or more criteria of the systemic inflammatory response syndrome (SIRS criteria) with a documented or suspected source of infection. The SIRS criteria include a temperature greater than 100.4°F or less than 96.8°F, heart rate greater than 90 beats/min, respiratory rate greater than 20 breaths/min or $Paco_2$ less than 32 mm Hg, and white blood cell count greater than 12,000 cells/mm^3 or less than 4000 cells/mm^3 or greater than 10 immature cells (bands).[47] Because of the severity of the disease, the third international consensus task force thought health care providers required improved clinical tools and diagnostics to earlier identify and properly treat sepsis.[47]

Table 2
Antimicrobial regimens for acute bacterial rhinosinusitis in children

Indication	First Line (Daily Dose)	Second Line (Daily Dose)
Initial empirical therapy	• Amoxicillin-clavulanate (45 mg/kg/d PO bid)	• Amoxicillin-clavulanate (90 mg/kg/d PO bid)
β-Lactam allergy		
Type 1 hypersensitivity		• Levofloxacin (10–20 mg/kg/d PO every 12–24 h)
Non-type 1 hypersensitivity		• Clindamycin[a] (30–40 mg/kg/d PO tid) plus Cefixime (8 mg/kg/d PO bid) or Cefpodoxime (10 mg/kg/d PO bid)
Risk for antibiotic resistance or failed initial therapy		• Amoxicillin-clavulanate (90 mg/kg/d PO bid) • Clindamycin[a] (30–40 mg/kg/d PO tid) plus Cefixime (8 mg/kg/d PO bid) or Cefpodoxime (10 mg/kg/d PO bid) • Levofloxacin (10–20 mg/kg/d PO every 12–24 h)
Severe infection requiring hospitalization		• Ampicillin/sulbactam (200–400 mg/kg/d IV every 6 h) • Ceftriaxone (50 mg/kg/d IV every 12 h) • Cefotaxime (100–200 mg/kg/d IV every 6 h) • Levofloxacin (10–20 mg/kg/d IV every 12–24 h)

Abbreviations: bid, twice daily; IV, intravenously; PO, orally; qd, daily; tid, 3 times a day.
[a] Resistance to clindamycin (~31%) is found frequently among S pneumoniae serotype 19A isolates in different regions of the United States.
From Chow AW, Benninger MS, Brook I, et al; Infectious Diseases Society of America. IDSA clinical practice guideline for acute bacterial rhinosinusitis in children and adults. Clin Infect Dis 2012;54(8):e24; with permission of Oxford University Press.

Diagnosis and Antibiotic Therapy

When patients present to the ED, it is crucial that health care providers properly diagnose sepsis. One frequent tool that is gaining use is the quick SOFA score, or qSOFA. Patients have a positive qSOFA score if they have 2 or more of the following criteria: respiratory rate greater than 22 breaths/min; systolic blood pressure less than 100 mm Hg; altered mental status. A positive qSOFA score supports identification of patients with suspicion of an infection and an increased risk of hospitalized death.[48]

Once sepsis is diagnosed, appropriate antibiotic therapy selection is one of the most critical factors to decrease mortality and optimize patient outcomes. Initial empiric therapy should be directed against the resident flora of the primary suspected infectious organ. Blood cultures should be obtained on all patients to appropriately direct therapy that is pathogen specific. Any site that is infected can lead to sepsis. Sites include but are not limited to, in the most prevalent order: respiratory tract, urinary tract, abdominal cavity, and skin and soft tissue. Pneumonia is the most common infectious source of sepsis in the United States.[49] Undiagnosed or untreated sepsis can progress to septic shock.

Per the 2012 Surviving Sepsis Campaign (SSC) Guidelines, patients with "severe sepsis" or septic shock have little margin for error in the choice of therapy. Therefore,

Table 3
Antimicrobial regimens for acute bacterial rhinosinusitis in adults

Indication	First Line (Daily Dose)	Second Line (Daily Dose)
Initial empirical therapy	• Amoxicillin-clavulanate (500 mg/125 mg PO tid, or 875 mg/125 mg PO bid)	• Amoxicillin-clavulanate (2000 mg/125 mg PO bid) • Doxycycline (100 mg PO bid or 200 mg PO qd)
β-Lactam allergy		• Doxycycline (100 mg PO bid or 200 mg PO qd) • Levofloxacin (500 mg PO qd) • Moxifloxacin (400 mg PO qd)
Risk tor antibiotic resistance or failed initial therapy		• Amoxicillin-clavulanate (2000 mg/125 mg PO bid) • Levofloxacin (500 mg PO qd) • Moxifloxacin (400 mg PO qd)
Severe infection requiring hospitalization		• Ampicillin-sulbactam (1.5–3 g IV every 6 h) • Levofloxacin (500 mg PO or IV qd) • Moxifloxacin (400 mg PO or IV qd) • Ceftriaxone (1–2 g IV every 12–24 h) • Cefotaxime (2 g IV every 4–6 h)

From Chow AW, Benninger MS, Brook I, et al; Infectious Diseases Society of America. IDSA clinical practice guideline for acute bacterial rhinosinusitis in children and adults. Clin Infect Dis 2012;54(8):e23; with permission of Oxford University Press.

the initial selection of antimicrobial therapy should be broad enough to cover all likely pathogens. Antibiotic choices should be guided by local prevalence patterns of bacterial pathogens, susceptibility data, and recent antimicrobial exposure. Substantial evidence demonstrates that failure to initiate appropriate therapy (ie, therapy with activity against the pathogen that is subsequently identified as the causative agent) correlates with increased morbidity and mortality in patients with severe sepsis or septic shock.[49] Narrowing the spectrum of antimicrobial once the pathogen is identified via Gram stain and one or more cultures leads to the shortest duration of therapy and the best outcomes. There are isolated instances in which combination therapies are recommended, such as infection with multidrug-resistant *Acinetobacter* and *Pseudomonas* species.[49] Treatment length should be 7 to 10 days per the guidelines, although patient factors may influence the total length of therapy. It is important that clinicians continue to monitor treatment and improvements.

Recommendations from the 2012 SSC state "initial broad-spectrum coverage in the emergency setting should include an antipseudomonal penicillin (or antipseudomonal cephalosporin) plus an aminoglycoside (or fluoroquinolone) plus vancomycin. In the case of selecting only an antipseudomonal cephalosporin, metronidazole should be added to the regimen for suspected anaerobic coverage. An alternate option would include an antipseudomonal carbapenem plus an aminoglycoside (or fluoroquinolone) plus vancomycin."[50]

In the ED, broad-spectrum antibiotics selected to cover the suspected infectious organ or process is a key step to complying with early goal-directed therapy. Equally as important is early identification and source control of any specific anatomic diagnosis of infection. Examples include necrotizing soft tissue infection, pyelonephritis, peritonitis, cholangitis, and intestinal infarction. Rapid identification and early source removal are optimal to improving patient outcomes.

Table 4
Sequential (sepsis-related) organ failure assessment score

Score System	0	1	2	3	4
Respiration					
PaO$_2$/FiO$_2$ mm Hg (kPa)	>400 (53.3)	≤400 (53.3)	<300 (40)	<200 (26.7) with respiratory support	<100 (13.3) with respiratory support
Coagulation					
Platelets × 10^3/uL	≥150	<150	<100	<50	<20
Liver					
Bilirubin, mg/dL (umol/L)	<1.2 (20)	1.2–1.9 (20–32)	2.0–5.9 (33–101)	6.0–11.9 (102–204)	>12 (204)
Cardiovascular	Mean Arterial Pressure >70 mm Hg	Mean Arterial Pressure <70 mm Hg	Dopamine (<5) or Dobutamine (any dose)	Dopamine (5.1–15) or Epinephrine (<0.1) or Norepinephrine <0.1)	Dopamine >15, Epinephrine (>0.1) or Norepinephrine (>0.1)
CNS					
Glascow Coma Scale	15	13–14	10–12	6–9	<6
Renal					
Creatinine (mg/dL)	<1.2 (110)	1.2–1.9 (110–170)	2–3.4 (171–299)	3.5–4.9 (300–440)	>5 (440)
Urine output (mL/day)	—	—	—	<500	<200

Abbreviation: CNS, central nervous system.

SUMMARY

Improving future ED antibiotic prescribing for common infections will require complementary strategies of educating clinicians about appropriate prescribing patterns and educating patients and families about the role of antibiotics in medical care. The implementation of hospital-based antibiotic stewardship programs has been shown to aid not only in improving appropriate use of antibiotics but also in the correct selection and dosing of optimal agents specific to each cause.[51] Antibiotic stewardship programs have the potential to reduce adverse drug-related events, reduce antimicrobial resistance rates, and improve patient outcomes.

REFERENCES

1. Gaynes R. The impact of antimicrobial use on the emergence of antimicrobial-resistant bacteria in hospitals. Infect Dis Clin North Am 1997;11:757–65.
2. Hicks LA, Chien YW, Taylor TH, et al. Outpatient antibiotic prescribing and non-susceptible Streptococcus pneumoniae in the United States, 1996–2003. Clin Infect Dis 2011;53:631–9.
3. Suda KJ, Hicks LA, Roberts RM, et al. A national evaluation of antibiotic expenditures by healthcare setting in the United States, 2009. J Antimicrob Chemother 2013;68(3):715–8.
4. Fleming-Dutra KE, Hersh AL, Shapiro DJ, et al. Prevalence of inappropriate antibiotic prescriptions among US ambulatory care visits, 2010-2011. JAMA 2016; 315(17):1864–73.
5. Shehab N, Patel PR, Srinivasan A, et al. Emergency department visits for antibiotic-associated adverse events. Clin Infect Dis 2008;47(6):735–43.
6. Bourgeois FT, Mandl KD, Valim C, et al. Pediatric adverse drug events in the outpatient setting: an 11-year national analysis. Pediatrics 2009;124(4):e744–50.
7. Centers for Disease Control and Prevention. Antibiotic Resistance Threats in the United States. 2013. Available at: http://www.cdc.gov/drugresistance/pdf/ar-threats-2013-508.pdf. Accessed June 1, 2016.
8. World Health Organization. Global action plan on antimicrobial resistance. 2015. Available at: http://apps.who.int/iris/bitstream/10665/193736/1/9789241509763_eng.pdf?ua=1. Accessed June 30, 2016.
9. Centers for Disease Control and Prevention. Core elements of hospital antibiotic stewardship programs. Atlanta (GA): US Department of Health and Human Services, CDC; 2014. Available at: http://www.cdc.gov/getsmart/healthcare/implementation/core-elements.html. Accessed June 30, 2016.
10. National Quality Forum. Antibiotic Stewardship Action Team. National Quality Partners Playbook: Antibiotic Stewardship in Acute Care. 2016. Available at: http://www.qualityforum.org/Publications/2016/05/Antibiotic_Stewardship_Playbook.aspx. Accessed June 30, 2016.
11. CMS issues proposed rule that prohibits discrimination, reduces hospital-acquired conditions, and promotes antibiotic stewardship in hospitals. Centers for Medicare and Medicaid Services. Available at: https://www.cms.gov/Newsroom/Media ReleaseDatabase/Fact-sheets/2016-Fact-sheets-items/2016-06-13.html. Accessed July 1, 2016.
12. New Antimicrobial Stewardship Standard. The Joint Commission. Available at: https://www.jointcommission.org/assets/1/6/HAP-CAH_Antimicrobial_Prepub.pdf. Accessed July 1, 2016.

13. Lieberthal AS, Carroll AE, Chonmaitree T, et al. The diagnosis and management of acute otitis media. Pediatrics 2013;131(3):e964–99 [Erratum appears in Pediatrics 2014;133(2):346].
14. Venekamp RP, Sanders SL, Glasziou PP, et al. Antibiotics for acute otitis media in children. Cochrane Database Syst Rev 2015;(6):CD000219.
15. Fischer T, Singer AJ, Chale S. Observation option for acute otitis media in the emergency department. Pediatr Emerg Care 2009;25(9):575–8.
16. McCormick DP, Chonmaitree T, Pittman C, et al. Nonsevere acute otitis media: a clinical trial comparing outcomes of watchful waiting versus immediate antibiotic treatment. Pediatrics 2005;115(6):1455–65.
17. Spiro DM, Tay KY, Arnold DH, et al. Wait-and-see prescription for the treatment of acute otitis media: a randomized controlled trial. JAMA 2006;296(10):1235–41.
18. Cohen R, Levy C, Boucherat M, et al. A multicenter, randomized, double-blind trial of 5 versus 10 days of antibiotic therapy for acute otitis media in young children. J Pediatr 1998;133(5):634–9.
19. Pessey JJ, Gehanno P, Thoroddsen E, et al. Short course therapy with cefuroxime axetil for acute otitis media: results of a randomized multicenter comparison with amoxicillin/clavulanate. Pediatr Infect Dis J 1999;18(10):854–9.
20. Cohen R, Levy C, Boucherat M, et al. Five vs. ten days of antibiotic therapy for acute otitis media in young children. Pediatr Infect Dis J 2000;19(5):458–63.
21. Pichichero ME, Marsocci SM, Murphy ML, et al. A prospective observational study of 5-, 7-, and 10-day antibiotic treatment for acute otitis media. Otolaryngol Head Neck Surg 2001;124(4):381–7.
22. Kozyrskyj AL, Klassen TP, Moffatt M, et al. Short-course antibiotics for acute otitis media. Cochrane Database Syst Rev 2010;(9):CD001095.
23. Wessels MR. Clinical practice: streptococcal pharyngitis. N Engl J Med 2011;364(7):648–55.
24. Shaikh N, Leonard E, Martin JM. Prevalence of streptococcal pharyngitis and streptococcal carriage in children: a meta-analysis. Pediatrics 2010;126(3):e557–64.
25. Bhatia S, Tariq A. Characteristics and temporal trends of patients diagnosed with acute rheumatic fever in the United States from 2001-2011. J Am Coll Cardiol 2016;67:1892.
26. Barnett ML, Linder JA. Antibiotic prescribing to adults with sore throat in the United States, 1997–2010. JAMA Intern Med 2014;174:138–40.
27. Dooling KL, Shapiro DJ, Van Beneden C, et al. Overprescribing and inappropriate antibiotic selection for children with pharyngitis in the United States, 1997-2010. JAMA Pediatr 2014;168(11):1073–4.
28. Shulman ST, Bisno AL, Clegg HW, et al. Clinical practice guideline for the diagnosis and management of group A streptococcal pharyngitis: 2012 update by the Infectious Diseases Society of America. Clin Infect Dis 2012;55(10):1279–82 [Erratum appears in Clin Infect Dis 2014;58(10):1496].
29. Casey JR, Pichichero ME. Metaanalysis of short course antibiotic treatment for group a streptococcal tonsillopharyngitis. Pediatr Infect Dis J 2005;24(10):909–17.
30. Logan LK, McAuley JB, Shulman ST. Macrolide treatment failure in streptococcal pharyngitis resulting in acute rheumatic fever. Pediatrics 2012;129:e798–802.
31. Raman SS. Chronic cough due to acute bronchitis: ACCP evidence-based clinical practice guidelines. Chest 2006;129(1 Suppl):95S–103S.
32. MacKay DN. Treatment of acute bronchitis in adults without underlying lung disease. J Gen Intern Med 1996;11(9):557–62.

33. Nennig ME, Shinefield HR, Edwards KM, et al. Prevalence and incidence of adult pertussis in an urban population. JAMA 1996;275(21):1672–4.

34. Cornia PB, Hersh AL, Lipsky BA, et al. Does this coughing adolescent or adult patient have pertussis? JAMA 2010;304(8):890–6.

35. Centers for Disease Control and Prevention. National Hospital Ambulatory Medical Care Survey: 2011 Emergency Department Summary Tables. Available at: http://www.cdc.gov/nchs/data/ahcd/nhamcs_emergency/2011_ed_web_tables.pdf. Accessed July 15, 2016.

36. Kroening-Roche JC, Soroudi A, Castillo EM, et al. Antibiotic and bronchodilator prescribing for acute bronchitis in the emergency department. Emerg Med 2012;43(2):221.

37. Smith SM, Fahey T, Smucny J, et al. Antibiotics for acute bronchitis. Cochrane Database Syst Rev 2014;(3):CD000245.

38. Barnett ML, Linder JA. Antibiotic prescribing for adults with acute bronchitis in the United States, 1996-2010. JAMA 2014;311(19):2020–2.

39. National Committee for Quality Assurance. HEDIS 2015 Measures. Report Cards » Health Plans » State of Health Care Quality » 2015 Table of Contents » Acute Bronchitis. Available at: http://www.ncqa.org/report-cards/health-plans/state-of-health-care-quality/2015-table-of-contents/acute-bronchitis#sthash.Zf7fO9cX.dpufhttp://www.ncqa.org/report-cards/health-plans/state-of-health-care-quality/2015-table-of-contents/acute-bronchitis. Accessed July 10, 2016.

40. Becker LA, Hom J, Villasis-Keever M, et al. Beta2-agonist drugs for treating cough or a clinical diagnosis of acute bronchitis. Cochrane Database Syst Rev 2015;(9):CD001726.

41. Rosenfeld RM, Piccirillo JF, Chandrasekhar SS, et al. Clinical practice guideline (update): adult sinusitis. Otolaryngol Head Neck Surg 2015;152(2 Suppl):S1–39.

42. Chow AW, Benninger MS, Brook I, et al, Infectious Diseases Society of America. IDSA clinical practice guideline for acute bacterial rhinosinusitis in children and adults. Clin Infect Dis 2012;54(8):e72–112.

43. Blackwell DL, Lucas JW, Clarke TC. Summary health statistics for U.S. adults: National Health Interview Survey, 2012. National Center for Health Statistics. Centers for Disease Control and Prevention. Vital Health Stat 10 2014;(260):1–171. Available at: http://www.cdc.gov/nchs/data/series/sr_10/sr10_260.pdf.

44. Smith SS, Evans CT, Tan BK, et al. National burden of antibiotic use for adult rhinosinusitis. J Allergy Clin Immunol 2013;132(5):10.

45. Smith SS, Kern RC, Chandra RK, et al. Variations in antibiotic prescribing of acute rhinosinusitis in United States ambulatory settings. Otolaryngol Head Neck Surg 2013;148(5):852–9.

46. U.S. Food and Drug Administration. FDA Drug Safety Communication: FDA advises restricting fluoroquinolone antibiotic use for certain uncomplicated infections; warns about disabling side effects that can occur together. 2016. Available at: http://www.fda.gov/Drugs/DrugSafety/ucm500143.htm. Accessed July 20, 2016.

47. Singer M, Deutschman CS, Seymour CW, et al. The Third International Consensus Definitions for Sepsis and Septic Shock (Sepsis-3). Caring for the critically ill patient. JAMA 2016;315(8):801–10.

48. Chen YX, Wang JW, Guo SB. Use of CURB-65 and quick Sepsis-related Organ Failure Assessment to predict site of care and mortality in pneumonia patients in the emergency department: a retrospective study. Crit Care 2016;20:167.

49. Dellinger RP, Levy MM, Rhodes A. Surviving Sepsis Campaign: international guidelines for management of severe sepsis and septic shock: 2012. Crit Care Med 2013;41:580–637.
50. Surviving Sepsis Campaign. 2016 guidelines. Available at: www.survivingsepsis.org. Accessed July 30, 2016.
51. Barlam TF, Cosgrove SE, Abbo LM, et al. Implementing an antibiotic stewardship program: guidelines by the Infectious Diseases Society of America and the Society for Healthcare Epidemiology of America. Clin Infect Dis 2016;62:1–27.

Headache Mistakes You Do Not Want to Make

Karen A. Newell, MMSc, PA-C, DFAAPA*

KEYWORDS

- Life-threatening causes of headache • Acute headache • Subarachnoid hemorrhage
- Giant cell arteritis • Temporal arteritis • Cerebral venous sinus thrombosis
- Cerebral venous thrombosis • Meningitis

KEY POINTS

- Subarachnoid hemorrhage (SAH), cerebral venous sinus thrombosis (CVST)/cerebral venous thrombosis (CVT), giant cell arteritis (GCA)/temporal arteritis, and meningitis/encephalitis are all life-threatening causes of headache in adult patients.
- Thunderclap headache (ie, the worse headache of my life) is a sudden, severe unilateral or occipital headache that begins abruptly and peaks within minutes is the classic description used for SAH. The diagnosis can be confirmed by noncontrast head computed tomography (CT) in most cases and is treated largely with supportive measures and neurosurgical intervention for prevention of rebleed.
- Headache is present in about 90% of CVST/CVT cases and is generally described as gradual in onset and increasing in severity over several days; however, in some cases patients have presented with sudden severe headaches mimicking SAH. Specialized imaging, such as MRI or magnetic resonance venography, may be needed to establish the diagnosis of CVST/CVT, as head CT is read as normal in up to 30% of cases.
- The diagnosis of GCA/temporal arteritis is made clinically. Treatment with corticosteroids should NOT be delayed while awaiting biopsy confirmation.
- Meningitis is suspected when patients present with the classic signs and symptoms of fever, nuchal rigidity, headache, and altered mental status.

OBJECTIVES

List the life-threatening causes of acute headache in adults.
Describe the clinical features, diagnosis, and management of subarachnoid hemorrhage (SAH).
Describe the pitfalls in the diagnosis and management of cerebral venous sinus thrombosis (CVST)/cerebral venous thrombosis (CVT).
Discuss pitfalls in the diagnosis of giant cell arteritis (GCA)/temporal arteritis.
Describe the clinical features, diagnosis, and management of meningitis.

Disclosure Statement: The author has nothing to disclose.
PA Program, Emory University School of Medicine, 1648 Pierce Dr NE, Atlanta, GA 30307, USA
* 1462 Clifton Road, Suite 280, Atlanta GA 30322.
E-mail address: knewell@emory.edu

Physician Assist Clin 2 (2017) 503–517
http://dx.doi.org/10.1016/j.cpha.2017.02.012
2405-7991/17/© 2017 Elsevier Inc. All rights reserved.

physicianassistant.theclinics.com

Headache in adult patients is an extremely common complaint in an acute care setting. It represents about 1% to 2% of all emergency medicine visits in the United States every year. Of these visits, fewer than 5% are from life-threatening causes. Given that the cause of headache is very broad, it is vital that the emergency medicine physician assistant be able to recognize and initiate emergent management of the life-threatening causes. Box 1 lists some of the life-threatening causes for acute headache.

History is a critical component in differentiating life-threatening causes of headache. Box 2 lists some of the more common questions to ask when evaluating patients with headache.

Headaches can be categorized into either primary or secondary causes. Primary headache represents about 90% of cases. They are considered benign and are often recurrent. Examples of primary headache include migraine, tension, cluster, or rebound. The remainder of headache cases can be considered secondary, occur abruptly and are severe or rapidly progressive. They are often associated with infection, head injury, tumor, or from vascular issues. Examples of secondary headache include meningitis, SAH, intracranial hemorrhage (ICH), hypertensive crisis, and acute glaucoma. Table 1 lists some of the causes for primary and secondary headache.

Physical examination in patients with headache should include a thorough head and neck examination, focusing on the eyes (including a funduscopic examination), ears, nose, teeth, and throat as well as assessing for cervical stiffness or lymph nodes. Additionally, a thorough neurologic examination should be performed, including attention to the cranial nerves, sensory, motor, and coordination components, as well as an assessment of mental status.

It is important to understand that many structures in the brain lack the ability to sense pain, including the brain parenchyma, the lining of the ventricles, and the choroid plexus. Because of this, clinical presentation can be complicated and difficult to interpret. Intracranial structures that do sense pain include the dural sinuses, the intracranial part of the trigeminal nerve, and the large arteries.

Differentiating acute from chronic causes of headache is crucial so that prompt treatment of life-threatening causes of headache can be initiated. In general, acute forms of headache can be defined as pain or discomfort that starts suddenly and gets worse quickly. Table 2 highlights some of the clinical features of acute headaches associated with a more serious cause.

| Box 1 |
Life-threatening causes of acute headache
SAH
CVST/CVT
GCA/temporal arteritis
Meningitis/encephalitis
Intracranial tumor

SUBARACHNOID HEMORRHAGE

SAH is defined as bleeding into the subarachnoid space, which is located between the pia mater and the arachnoid membranes.

Box 2
Key questions in the assessment of headache

How long have you been having headaches?

What were the headaches like when they first began? Were they intermittent, daily persistent, or progressive from the beginning?

What is the length of time from the start of the headache until its peak intensity?

Are there any warning symptoms (eg, aura)?

Are you aware of any specific triggers (eg, foods, stress, lack of sleep, menstrual cycle)?

Does the headache interfere significantly with normal activity (eg, work, school)?

What aggravates the headache (eg, light, noise, odors)?

What do you do for relief from the headache (eg, rest, move around, take medication)?

What time of day are the headaches most likely to occur? Do they regularly awaken you from sleep?

Does anyone else in the family have headaches?

Adapted from Counihan TJ. Key questions in the assessment of headache, Cecil essentials of medicine. 2016. p. 994. Table 111-4; with permission from Elsevier.

Most bleeds are spontaneous and occur from cerebral aneurysm rupture or arteriovenous malformation (AVM), but SAH can also occur in the case of severe head trauma.

Of the cases that rupture, 80% occur from saccular or berry aneurysms which are found at the bifurcation of major arteries. AVM make up another 10% of cases. The remainder are largely associated with head trauma, although other atraumatic etiologies are possible.

Epidemiology

The incidence is 10 to 15 per 100,000. SAH affects roughly 30,000 patients each year in the United States; mortality is about 50%, with 10% to 15% dying before arrival to the hospital.[1] Interestingly, postmortem cadaveric studies suggest that most cerebral aneurysms never rupture and that many millions of people live their lives never knowing that they even had an aneurysm. Risk factors for SAH are listed in Box 3.

Table 1
Comparison of primary versus secondary causes of headache

Primary Headache	Secondary Headache
Migraine	Posttraumatic
Tension	Vascular: SAH, vasculitis, arterial dissection
Cluster	Nonvascular: pseudotumor cerebri, low CSF pressure, tumor, Chiari
Exertional	malformation
	Infection: meningitis, abscess, sinusitis
	Disordered homeostasis: hypoxia or hypercapnia, hypoglycemia
	Medication: side effect, withdrawal
	Cervicogenic

Abbreviation: CSF, cerebrospinal fluid.
Adapted from Counihan TJ. Primary and secondary headache syndromes, Cecil essentials of medicine. 2016. p. 994. Tables 111-1 and 111-2; with permission from Elsevier.

Table 2	
Clinical features of headaches suggesting a structural brain lesion	
Symptoms	**Signs**
Worst headache of patients' life	Nuchal rigidity
Progressive	Fever
Onset >50 y of age	Papilledema
Worse in the early morning, awakens patients	Pathologic reflexes or reflex asymmetry
Marked exacerbation with straining	Altered state of consciousness
Focal neurologic dysfunction	

Adapted from Counihan TJ. Clinical features of headaches suggesting a structural brain lesion, Cecil essentials of medicine. 2016. p. 999. Table 111-8; with permission from Elsevier.

Clinical Presentation

Thunderclap headache (worse headache of patients' life) is a sudden severe unilateral or occipital headache sometimes associated with loss of consciousness due to acute vessel rupture and meningeal irritation from bleeding. Rupture often occurs suddenly and is quickly followed by meningeal signs, such as nuchal rigidity/stiff neck, photophobia or other visual changes, nausea/vomiting (70%), delirium, dizziness, and seizure but usually presents with NO focal neurologic deficits.

Physical examination should include assessment of blood pressure (BP) for signs of mild to moderate elevation; checking for an increase in temperature; evaluation of pulse, which may reveal tachycardia; and doing a thorough funduscopic examination looking for evidence of papilledema or retinal hemorrhage.

Traditionally, a noncontrast head computed tomography (CT) could establish the diagnosis of SAH in 93% to 98% of cases if it was obtained within 12 hours.[2] The image in **Fig. 1** demonstrates typical findings found in patients with SAH. In the past, when a noncontrast head CT was obtained and was read as negative, a lumbar puncture (LP) was usually obtained looking for blood in the cerebrospinal fluid (CSF) (not as a result of traumatic tap) to confirm any recalcitrant cases so that prompt intervention, such as endovascular coiling/surgical clipping, could prevent the possibility of a rebleed. More recently, because of improvements in imaging techniques, studies indicate that a qualified radiologist can detect SAH with 100% accuracy using a noncontrast head CT if performed within 6 hours.[3–6] Other imaging studies may include CT

Box 3
Risk factors for subarachnoid hemorrhage
Previous ruptured aneurysm (multiple aneurysms in 20%–30% of patients)
Family history (3–7 times increased risk in first-degree relative with SAH)
Hypertension
Smoking
Alcohol abuse
Sympathomimetic drug use (cocaine, methamphetamine and ecstasy [3,4-methylenedioxymethamphetamine])
Females > males
African American > Caucasian
80% occur in patients aged 40 to 65 years

angiography, magnetic resonance angiography with or without contrast, and/or MRI without contrast. Helpful ancillary studies may include serum chemistry panel, complete blood count, prothrombin time (PT), activated partial thromboplastin time (aPTT), blood type/screen, cardiac enzymes, arterial blood gas, chest radiograph, and electrocardiogram (Fig. 1).

Treatment

Treatment is mainly supportive with emergent intubation for declining level of consciousness, oxygenation, intravenous (IV) access, cardiac monitoring, immediate neurosurgical consult, as well as pharmacologic BP control (goal mean arterial pressure <110 mm Hg and systolic BP <160 mm Hg), other measures may include elevating the head of the bed to 30°, mannitol, antiemetics and stool softeners to minimize increases in ICP. The neurosurgeon may consider using neuroprotective agents, such as nimodipine, as well as consideration of operative intervention for clipping the ruptured aneurysm or endovascular coiling. Guidelines for the management of aneurysmal SAH for health care professionals from the American Heart Association/American Stroke Association are useful references for more detailed information on treatment.

Common complications may include rebleeding in 20% of patients within 2 weeks, which can carry a mortality between 50% and 80%.[1] Other complications include cerebral ischemia, seizures, hydrocephalus caused by obstruction of CSF flow, as well as increased ICP. Additionally, there are numerous grading scales, such as the Hunt and Hess, that may be used after SAH to help predict prognosis and mortality.

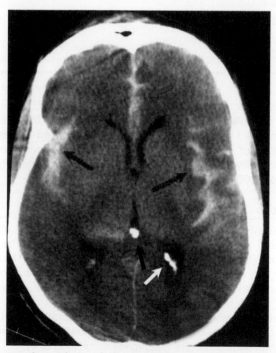

Fig. 1. Non–contrast-enhanced CT of the brain demonstrating an SAH. There is high-attenuation blood in the Sylvian fissures (*blue arrows*) and the interhemispheric fissure (*red arrow*). Do not confuse normal, physiologic calcifications (*white* and *black arrows*) for blood. (*From* http://learningradiology.com/archives2007/COW%20266-Subarachnoid%20hemorrhage/subarachnoidcorrect.html; with permission.)

CEREBRAL VENOUS SINUS THROMBOSIS OR CEREBRAL VENOUS THROMBOSIS

CVST or CVT is a relatively uncommon condition in which a thrombosis or occlusion located in the venous channels in the brain can cause brain herniation from unilateral mass effect. It presents with the complaint of headache and if unrecognized and untreated is associated with a high morbidity and mortality. Risk factors for developing CVST/CVT include hypercoagulable conditions, including those listed in Box 4.

Box 4
Cerebral venous sinus thrombosis/cerebral venous thrombosis risk factors

Patients using oral contraceptives

Pregnancy and postpartum malignancy

Women > men by 3:1

Underlying inflammatory (inflammatory bowel disease) or infectious processes

Protein C deficiency

Protein S deficiency

Antithrombin III deficiency

Antiphospholipid syndrome

Factor V Leiden mutation

Lupus anticoagulant

Prothrombin G20210A gene mutation

May be associated with certain medications

May be associated with sinusitis, trauma, or recent surgery

Epidemiology

The incidence is difficult to determine, but CVT is generally thought to be very rare (estimated incidence <1.5 per 100,000 annually in the United States), although with a high clinical index of suspicion and advancing imaging techniques the reported cases may be increasing. In the United States, the reported incidence during pregnancy was 11.6 per 100,000 deliveries.[7]

Clinical Presentation

Patients may present with a variety of manifestations, including 3 major syndromes. The first is isolated intracranial hypertension headache syndrome that can occur with or without vomiting, papilledema, and/or visual changes. The second is focal syndrome, which may include focal neurologic deficits and/or seizures. The last is encephalopathy syndrome, which can present with multifocal signs, mental status changes, stupor, and/or coma.[8–10]

Headache is present in about 90% of cases and is generally described as gradual in onset and increasing in severity over several days; however, in some cases patients have presented with sudden severe headaches mimicking SAH.

Diagnostic Studies

Head CT is often the first study obtained; but because it can be read as normal in up to 30% of CVT cases, additional studies, such as CT venography, MRI or magnetic resonance venography, may be needed to demonstrate the thrombus or occlusion. Other helpful studies used to distinguish an infectious process, such as meningitis, may include CBC, serum chemistry panel, PT, aPTT, and LP.

Treatment

Treatment should begin as soon as the diagnosis is confirmed and consists of treating the underlying cause, controlling seizures and intracranial hypertension, and initiating antithrombotic therapy. Anticoagulation is the mainstay of acute and subacute treatment of CVT.[11]

Prognosis is generally favorable (80%) if CVT is recognized and promptly treated with subcutaneous low molecular weight heparin (LMWH) or IV heparin, but mortality and permanent disability is high if left unrecognized and untreated. Box 5 lists some of the predictors of poor prognosis.

Box 5
Predictors of poor long-term prognosis

CNS infection

Malignancy

Deep CVT location

Intracranial hemorrhage

Glasgow coma scale of less than 9 on admission

Mental status abnormality

Aged greater than 37 years

Male sex

Abbreviation: CNS, central nervous system.
  Data from Canhao P, Ferro JM, Lindgren AG, et al. Causes and predictors of death in cerebral venous thrombosis. Stroke 2005;36:1720.

GIANT CELL ARTERITIS OR TEMPORAL ARTERITIS/CRANIAL ARTERITIS
Background

GCA is a chronic systemic inflammatory vasculitis affecting medium and large arteries throughout the entire body but most commonly associated with unilateral involvement of the superficial temporal artery. In about half of these patients they will also have or be diagnosed with polymyalgia rheumatica (PR), a disease with painful stiffness affecting the neck, shoulders, and pelvis. For several years, it has been unclear if these conditions were 2 separate entities or part of the same pathophysiologic process but presenting differently. Current thought seems to indicate that there are numerous studies suggesting that GCA consists of several clinical subsets rather than one uniform disease.[12,13] In any case, there seems to be much overlap and similarity between patients with PR and patients with GCA. GCA often affects females more than males (3.7–1.0) and is associated with advancing age (80% of patients are older than 70 years of age). It is rare to encounter in patients less than 50 years of age.

Even though there has been a dramatic advancement of the understanding of the inflammatory cascade, the initial trigger that begins the cascade remains uncertain. Genetic, environmental, and autoimmune factors have all been identified.[14]

Epidemiology

There are 0.5 to 27.0 cases per 100,000 people aged 50 years or older, with the most cases occurring in the northern United States and in those of Scandinavian descent.[15]

Clinical Presentation

GCA presents with the complaint of headache in 60% of cases. Patients may be tender and swollen over the superficial temporal artery. The artery may lack a palpable pulse. The pain is described as worse at night and worse after exposure to cold. It may also be associated with complaints of malaise, fever, weight loss, neck pain, scalp tenderness, sore throat, and jaw claudication/trismus. Visual changes, including blindness (amaurosis fugax), can occur and are associated with ischemia of the optic nerve. Other ocular involvement may include diplopia, ptosis, extraocular muscle weakness, scotomata, or blurry vision.

Diagnostic Studies

Erythrocyte sedimentation rate (ESR) (>100 mm/h) and C-reactive protein (CRP) (>2.45 mg/dL) are often both elevated. Normochromic normocytic anemia may also be present. Leukocyte counts are usually normal or mildly elevated. Diagnosis is confirmed by a temporal artery biopsy; but a negative result on biopsy does not rule out the diagnosis, which may be related to collection of a sample without evidence of the disease because the artery may have skip lesions. Therefore, multiple biopsies and contralateral samples may be needed to confirm the diagnosis. However, the diagnosis should be made clinically. Patients suspected of disease with negative biopsies should also be considered for more specialized imaging of other large vessels to determine and rule out their involvement.

If left untreated, patients with GCA could develop permanent blindness or other serious sequelae, such as transient ischemic attacks (TIAs), cerebral vascular accidents due to vasculitis, or aneurysm of other large arteries, such as the aorta and its branches.

Treatment

Therapy may include corticosteroids (40–60 mg by mouth per day or higher) given for 4 to 6 weeks and then gradually tapered. Patients usually respond quickly to this therapy (within 24–72 hours). Therapy should not be delayed due to awaiting biopsy results and should be initiated promptly, especially in the case of visual changes to avoid permanent impairment or, in rare cases, blindness. Patients with serious visual changes may require higher doses of corticosteroids given intravenously (eg, 1000 mg methylprednisolone each day for several days) to initiate therapy before switching to an oral regimen. Some patients may need corticosteroids for several years. In the case of patients unable to take corticosteroids, cyclosporine, azathioprine, or methotrexate may also be considered.

Additionally, many recommend antiplatelet therapy with low-dose aspirin (81–100 mg/d) to decrease the risk of visual loss, TIAs, or stroke. Because most patients with GCA are older, it is prudent to consider concurrent treatment with a proton pump inhibitor or other gastroprotective medication.

Many challenges are encountered when tapering corticosteroids to include detection of disease recurrence. Using acute-phase reactants, such as ESR and CRP, can be helpful in this process but can be challenging to interpret as elevated levels do not always correlate with disease recurrence. Monitoring serum levels of interleukin 6 and soluble intercellular adhesion molecule-1 may hold promise as additional potential assays to assess active disease.[16,17]

MENINGITIS/ENCEPHALITIS

Meningitis is an inflammation or infection of the meninges that covers the brain and spinal cord (central nervous system). This inflammation has many causes: bacteria, viruses, fungi, parasites, autoimmune diseases, malignancy, and medications. Meningitis can be acute and occur rapidly within several hours to days to chronic developing over several weeks to months. Encephalitis is infection of the brain parenchyma and is associated with earlier and more pronounced altered mental status (AMS). Table 3 shows common bacterial pathogens and other predisposing factors associated with meningitis.

Table 3
Common bacterial pathogens and other predisposing factors associated with meningitis

Predisposing Factor	Bacterial Pathogens
Age	
<1 mo	*Streptococcus agalactiae, Escherichia coli, Listeria monocytogenes*
1–23 mo	*Streptococcus agalactiae, Escherichia coli, Haemophilus influenzae, Streptococcus pneumoniae, Neisseria meningitidis*
2–50 y	*Streptococcus pneumoniae, N meningitidis*
>50 y	*S pneumoniae, N meningitidis, L monocytogenes*, aerobic gram-negative bacilli
Immunocompromised state	*S pneumoniae, N meningitidis, L monocytogenes*, aerobic gram-negative bacilli (including *Pseudomonas aeruginosa*)
Basilar skull fracture	*S pneumoniae; Haemophilus influenzae;* group A, β-hemolytic streptococci
Head trauma; after neurosurgery	*Staphylococcus aureus*, coagulase-negative staphylococci (especially *Staphylococcus epidermidis*), aerobic gram-negative bacilli (including *P aeruginosa*)

Data from Tunkel AR, van de Beek D, Scheld WM. Acute meningitis. In: Bennett JE, Dolin R, Blaser M, editors. Mandell, Douglas, and Bennett's principles and practice of infectious diseases. 8th edition. Philadelphia: Saunders; 2015. p. 853. Table 90–1.

Epidemiology

The cause of bacterial meningitis has changed dramatically over time because of the advent of *Haemophilus influenza* and *Streptococcus pneumonia* vaccines. However, meningitis remains a relatively common diagnosis, with viral causes occurring more often than bacterial.

Clinical Presentation

Clinical presentation may include fever/chills (95%), headache, and complaints of stiff neck, photosensitivity, nausea/vomiting, AMS, and/or seizures. For those patients with complaints of stiff neck, physical examination should include

- Kernig sign: patients cannot straighten knee when hip is flexed
- Brudzinski sign: neck flexion produces knee/hip flexion

Diagnostic Studies

The diagnostic study of choice for CSF analysis is LP (see **Box 6** and **Table 4** for which studies to obtain and typical findings). However, a head CT should be obtained BEFORE the LP to rule out mass effect in those that are of advanced age (greater than 60 years), in immunocompromised patients, in those with AMS, focal neurologic findings, and/or papilledema. MRI with and without contrast is often obtained for those patients with suspected encephalitis and/or brain abscess and should be considered in all immunocompromised patients. Additionally, blood and urine cultures, complete blood count with differential, PT/PTT, electrolytes, and toxicology studies may be indicated.

Box 6
Cerebrospinal fluid tests to obtain for patients with suspected central nervous system infection

Routine tests

White blood cell count with differential

Red blood cell count[a]

Glucose concentration[b]

Protein concentration

Gram stain

Bacterial culture

Selected specific tests based on clinical suspicion

Viral culture[c]

Smears and culture for acid-fast bacilli

Venereal Disease Research Laboratory

India ink preparation

Cryptococcal polysaccharide antigen

Fungal culture

Antibody tests (IgM or IgG, or both)[d]

Nucleic acid amplification tests (eg, polymerase chain reaction)[e]

Cytology[f]

Flow cytometry

[a] Should be checked in the first and last tubes; in patients with a traumatic tap, there should be a decrease in the number of red blood cells with continued flow of CSF.
[b] Compare with serum glucose drawn just before lumbar puncture.
[c] Yield of viral culture may be low.
[d] May be useful for specific causes of meningitis and encephalitis.
[e] Most useful for specific viral causes of encephalitis and causes of chronic meningitis.
[f] In patients with suspected malignancy.
Data from Tunkel AR. Approach to the patient with central nervous system infection. In: Bennett JE, Dolin R, Blaser M, editors. Mandell, Douglas, and Bennett's principles and practice of infectious diseases. 8th edition. Philadelphia: Saunders; 2015. p. 856. Table 90-2.

Treatment

Treatment of meningitis depends on the cause and can range from supportive care with intravenous fluids (IVF), oxygen, antiemetics, and antipyretics to antibiotics,

Table 4
Cerebrospinal fluid findings in patients with selected infectious causes of meningitis

Cause of Meningitis	White Blood Cell Count (cells/mm³)	Primary Cell Type	Glucose (mg/dL)	Protein (mg/dL)
Viral	50–1000	Mononuclear[a]	>45	<200
Bacterial	1000–5000[b]	Neutrophilic[c]	<40[d]	100–500
Tuberculous	50–300	Mononuclear[e]	<45	50–300
Cryptococcal	20–500[f]	Mononuclear	<40	>45

[a] May be neutrophilic early in presentation.
[b] Range from less than 100 to greater than 10,000 cells/mm³.
[c] About 10% of patients have CSF lymphocyte predominance.
[d] Should always be compared with a simultaneous serum glucose; ratio of CSF to serum glucose is 0.4 or less in most cases.
[e] May see a therapeutic paradox, in which a mononuclear predominance becomes neutrophilic during antituberculous therapy.
[f] More than 75% of patients with acquired immunodeficiency syndrome have less than 20 cells/mm³.

Data from Tunkel AR. Approach to the patient with central nervous system infection. In: Bennett JE, Dolin R, Blaser M, editors. Mandell, Douglas, and Bennett's principles and practice of infectious diseases. 8th edition. Philadelphia: Saunders; 2015. p. 856. Table 90–3.

antiviral medications, and consideration to steroids and seizure prophylaxis (both controversial). Table 5 lists the recommended antimicrobial therapy for acute bacterial meningitis.

Table 6 lists empirical therapy for patients with purulent meningitis.

Table 5
Recommended antimicrobial therapy for acute bacterial meningitis

Microorganism, Susceptibility	Standard Therapy	Alternative Therapies
Streptococcus pneumoniae		
Penicillin MIC		
<0.1 µg/mL	Penicillin G or ampicillin	Third-generation cephalosporin,[a] chloramphenicol
0.1–1.0 µg/mL[b]	Third-generation cephalosporin[a]	Cefepime (B-II), meropenem (B-II)
≥2.0 µg/mL	Vancomycin plus a third-generation cephalosporin[a,c]	Fluoroquinolone[d] (B-II)
Cefotaxime or ceftriaxone MIC ≥1.0 µg/mL	Vancomycin plus a third-generation cephalosporin[a,c]	Fluoroquinolone[d] (B-II)
Neisseria meningitidis		
Penicillin MIC		
<0.1 µg/mL	Penicillin G or ampicillin	Third-generation cephalosporin,[a] chloramphenicol

(continued on next page)

Table 5 (*continued*)		
Microorganism, Susceptibility	**Standard Therapy**	**Alternative Therapies**
0.1–1.0 µg/mL	Third-generation cephalosporin[a]	Chloramphenicol, fluoroquinolone, meropenem
Listeria monocytogenes	Ampicillin or penicillin G[e]	Trimethoprim-sulfamethoxazole, meropenem (B-III)
Streptococcus agalactiae	Ampicillin or penicillin G[e]	Third-generation cephalosporin[a] (B-III)
Escherichia coli and other Enterobacteriaceae[g]	Third-generation cephalosporin (A-II)	Aztreonam, fluoroquinolone, meropenem, trimethoprim-sulfamethoxazole, ampicillin
Pseudomonas aeruginosa[g]	Cefepime[e] or ceftazidime[e] (A-II)	Aztreonam,[e] ciprofloxacin,[e] meropenem[e]
Haemophilus influenzae		
β-Lactamase negative	Ampicillin	Third-generation cephalosporin,[a] cefepime, chloramphenicol, fluoroquinolone
β-Lactamase positive	Third-generation cephalosporin (A-I)	Cefepime (A-I), chloramphenicol, fluoroquinolone
Staphylococcus aureus		
Methicillin susceptible	Nafcillin or oxacillin	Vancomycin, meropenem (B-III)
Methicillin resistant	Vancomycin[f]	Trimethoprim-sulfamethoxazole, linezolid (B-III)
Staphylococcus epidermidis	Vancomycin[f]	Linezolid (B-III)
Enterococcus species		
Ampicillin susceptible	Ampicillin plus gentamicin	—
Ampicillin resistant	Vancomycin plus gentamicin	—
Ampicillin and vancomycin resistant	Linezolid (B-III)	—

NOTE: All recommendations are A-III, unless otherwise indicated.

Abbreviation: MIC, minimum inhibitory concentration.

[a] Ceftriaxone or cefotaxime.

[b] Ceftriaxone/cefotaxime-susceptible isolates.

[c] Consider addition of rifampin if the minimum inhibitory concentration of ceftriaxone is greater than 2 µg/mL.

[d] Gatifloxacin or moxifloxacin.

[e] Addition of an aminoglycoside should be considered.

[f] Consider addition of rifampin.

[g] Choice of a specific antimicrobial agent must be guided by in vitro susceptibility test results.

Data from Tunkel AR, Hartman BJ, Kaplan SL, et al. Practice guidelines for the management of bacterial meningitis. Clin Infect Dis 2004;39:1267–84; with permission.

Table 6
Empiric therapy for patients with purulent meningitis

Antimicrobial Agent	Total Daily Dose (Dosing Interval in Hours)			
	Neonates, Age in Days		Infants and Children	Adults
	0–7[a]	8–28[a]		
Amikacin[b]	15–20 mg/kg (12)	30 mg/kg (8)	20–30 mg/kg (8)	15 mg/kg (8)
Ampicillin	150 mg/kg (8)	200 mg/kg (6–8)	300 mg/kg (6)	12 g (4)
Aztreonam	—	—	—	6–8 g (6–8)
Cefepime	—	—	150 mg/kg (8)	6 g (8)
Cefotaxime	100–150 mg/kg (8–12)	150–200 mg/kg (6–8)	225–300 mg/kg (6–8)	8–12 g (4–6)
Ceftazidime	100–150 mg/kg (8–12)	150 mg/kg (8)	150 mg/kg (8)	6 g (8)
Ceftriaxone	—	—	80–100 mg/kg (12–24)	4 g (12–24)
Chloramphenicol	25 mg/kg (24)	50 mg/kg (12–24)	75–100 mg/kg (6)	4–6 g (6)[c]
Ciprofloxacin	—	—	—	800–1200 mg (8–12)
Gatifloxacin	—	—	—	400 mg (24)[d]
Gentamicin[b]	5 mg/kg (12)	7.5 mg/kg (8)	7.5 mg/kg (8)	5 mg/kg (8)
Meropenem	—	—	120 mg/kg (8)	6 g (8)
Moxifloxacin	—	—	—	400 mg (24)[d]
Nafcillin	75 mg/kg (8–12)	100–150 mg/kg (6–8)	200 mg/kg (6)	9–12 g (4)
Oxacillin	75 mg/kg (8–12)	150–200 mg/kg (6–8)	200 mg/kg (6)	9–12 g (4)
Penicillin G	0.15 mU/kg (8–12)	0.2 mU/kg (6–8)	0.3 mU/kg (4–6)	24 mU (4)
Rifampin	—	10–20 mg/kg (12)	10–20 mg/kg (12–24)[e]	600 mg (24)
Tobramycin[b]	5 mg/kg (12)	7.5 mg/kg (8)	7.5 mg/kg (8)	5 mg/kg (8)
TMP-SMZ[f]	—	—	10–20 mg/kg (6–12)	10–20 mg/kg (6–12)
Vancomycin[g]	20–30 mg/kg (8–12)	30–45 mg/kg (6–8)	60 mg/kg (6)	30–45 mg/kg (8–12)

Abbreviation: TMP-SMZ, trimethoprim-sulfamethoxazole.
[a] Smaller doses and longer intervals of administration may be advisable for very-low-birth-weight neonates (<2000 g).
[b] Need to monitor peak and trough serum concentrations.
[c] Higher dose recommended for patients with pneumococcal meningitis.
[d] No data on optimal dosage needed in patients with bacterial meningitis.
[e] Maximum daily dose of 600 mg.
[f] Dosage based on trimethoprim component.
[g] Maintain serum trough concentrations of 15 to 20 µg/mL.
Data from Tunkel AR, Hartman BJ, Kaplan SL, et al. Practice guidelines for the management of bacterial meningitis. Clin Infect Dis 2004;39:1267–84; with permission.

SUMMARY

Reviewing the risk factors associated, clinical presentation, diagnostic workup, and initial management of SAH, CVST/CVT, GCA/temporal arteritis, and meningitis/encephalitis has sought to remind the clinician to be ever vigilant in recognizing and treating each patient with headache with the possibility of a life-threatening cause so as not to miss it when it occurs. Taking a meticulous history and performing a complete and thorough but targeted physical examination are critical components to early recognition and treatment of life-threatening causes for adult headache.

REFERENCES

1. Becske T, Jallo GI. Subarachnoid Hemorrhage 2016. Available at: http://emedicine.medscape.com/article/1164341-overview. Accessed March 18, 2017.
2. McCormack RF, Hutson A. Can computed tomography angiography of the brain replace lumbar puncture in the evaluation of acute-onset headache after a negative noncontrast cranial computed tomography scan? Acad Emerg Med 2010; 17(4):444–51.
3. Perry JJ, Stiell IG, Sivilotti ML, et al. Sensitivity of computed tomography performed within six hours of onset of headache for diagnosis of subarachnoid haemorrhage: prospective cohort study. BMJ 2011;343:d4277.
4. van der Wee N, Rinkel GJ, Hasan D, et al. Detection of subarachnoid haemorrhage on early CT: is lumbar puncture still needed after a negative scan? J Neurol Neurosurg Psychiatry 1995;58:357.
5. Sidman R, Connolly E, Lemke T. Subarachnoid hemorrhage diagnosis: lumbar puncture is still needed when the computed tomography scan is normal. Acad Emerg Med 1996;3:827.
6. Sames TA, Storrow AB, Finkelstein JA, et al. Sensitivity of new-generation computed tomography in subarachnoid hemorrhage. Acad Emerg Med 1996;3:16.
7. Lanska DJ, Kryscio RJ. Risk factors for peripartum and postpartum stroke and intracranial venous thrombosis. Stroke 2000;31:1274.
8. Biousse V, Ameri A, Bousser MG. Isolated intracranial hypertension as the only sign of cerebral venous thrombosis. Neurology 1999;53:1537.
9. Ferro JM, Correia M, Pontes C, et al. Cerebral vein and dural sinus thrombosis in Portgual: 1980-1998. Cerebrovasc Dis 2001;11:177.
10. Bousser MG, Russell RR. Cerebral venous thrombosis. In: Warlow CP, Van Gijn J, editors. Major problems in neurology. London: WB Saunders; 1997. p. 27, 104.
11. Coutinho JM, Stam J. Randomized, placebo-controlled trial of anticoagulant treatment with low-molecular-weight heparin for cerebral sinus thrombosis. Stroke 1999;30:484.
12. Caylor TL, Perkins A. Recognition and management of polymyalgia rheumatic and giant cell arteritis. Am Fam Physician 2013;88(10):676–84.
13. Salvarani C, Cantini F, Hunder GC. Polymyalgia rheumatic and giant-cell arteritis. Lancet 2008;372(9634):234–45.
14. Seetharaman M, Albertini JG. Giant Cell Arteritis (Temporal Arteritis) 2016. Available at: http://emedicine.medscape.com/article/332483-overview. Accessed March 18, 2017.
15. Goodwin JS. Progress in gerontology: polymyalgia rheumatic and temporal arteritis. J Am Geriatr Soc 1992;40(5):515–25.

16. Roche NE, Fulbright JW, Wagner AD, et al. Correlation of interleukin-6 production and disease activity in polymyalgia rheumatic and giant cell arteritis. Arthritis Rheum 1993;36:1286.
17. Weyand CM, Fulbright JW, Hunder GC, et al. Treatment of giant cell arteritis: interleukin-6 as a biologic marker of disease activity. Arthritis Rheum 2000;43: 1041.

Ocular Emergencies

Jeffrey Callard, PA-C, BS, James Kilmark, PA-C, MS*,
Hoodo Mohamed, PA-C, MS*

KEYWORDS

- Ophthalmologic emergencies • Retinal tear • Glaucoma • Ruptured globe
- Acute vision loss • Red eye

KEY POINTS

- Visual acuity should be obtained in all patients with an ocular complaint.
- Central retinal artery occlusion presents with the acute onset of painless monocular vision loss.
- Acute angle closure glaucoma is an ocular emergency and should be considered in the patient with a painful red eye and an intraocular pressure greater than 20 mm Hg.
- The erythrocyte sedimentation rate can be normal in up to 10% of patients with giant cell arteritis.
- Endophthalmitis is an infection emergency of the eye and requires emergent ophthalmology consultation.

INTRODUCTION

Ophthalmologic complaints account for approximately 2 million emergency department (ED) visits per year.[1] These complaints can encompass conditions due to primary ophthalmologic abnormality, infections, or traumatic injuries. Eye injuries account for 3.5% of all occupational injuries in the United States, and about 2000 US workers injure their eyes each day.[2] Eye complaints can be minor to life- or vision-threatening. In this article, the authors cover the common ED presentations for ocular emergencies. Specifically, the article focuses on the historical and physical examination findings that will help readers recognize the red flags in eye and vision complaints.

INITIAL EMERGENCY DEPARTMENT EVALUATION

The history of present illness for ocular complaints should focus on the presence of itching, discharge, pain, blurry vision, light sensitivity, or headache. The location of

Disclosure Statement: The authors have nothing to disclose.
Department of Emergency Medicine, St Joseph Mercy Hospital, 5301 East Huron River Drive, PO Box 995, Ann Arbor, MI 48106-0995, USA
* Corresponding author.
E-mail addresses: jkilmark@epmg.com; hmohamed@epmg.com

Physician Assist Clin 2 (2017) 519–536
http://dx.doi.org/10.1016/j.cpha.2017.02.014
2405-7991/17/© 2017 Elsevier Inc. All rights reserved.

physicianassistant.theclinics.com

pain, how vision is affected, and the onset and duration of symptoms are additional key elements of the history. Monocular versus binocular symptoms can help formulate the differential diagnosis. Additional important historical features include whether the discharge occurs throughout the day or just in the morning, any recent ocular surgery, or antecedent trauma. Identifying whether the patient wears contact lenses is imperative. Contact lenses complicate all eye complaints. The presence of any associated symptoms should also be asked.

The physical examination should be performed in an organized manner. Fig. 1 depicts the pertinent ocular anatomy. Visual acuity is the "vital sign" of the eye. Visual acuity should be checked before instillation of any drops when possible and should be done with vision correction. If glasses are not available for correction, looking through a pin hole can help correct the refraction error and compensate for the missing glasses.[3] The visual acuity should be done using a Snellen chart, and the distance should be recorded. Charts with pictures for children or illiterate patients can be used, if unable to read a chart. Documentation of counting fingers, light perception, or lack thereof should also be documented.

A fluorescein stain of the eye should be performed as part of the evaluation of all patients with eye trauma and concern for infection. It is a quick and easy technique that is crucial for the proper diagnosis and management of common eye emergencies. View the fluorescein-stained cornea and conjunctiva under a cobalt light and ideally in conjunction with magnification.[4] Sodium fluorescein is a water-soluble chemical that fluoresces. Contact lenses should be removed before instillation, because it can stain soft lenses. The Seidel test uses fluorescein to detect perforation of the eye. To

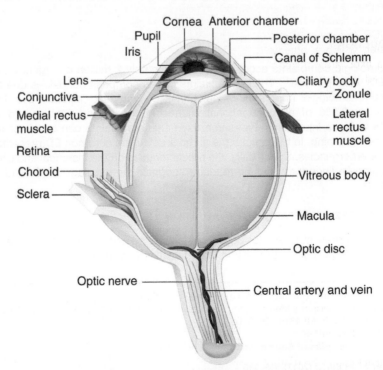

Fig. 1. Essential anatomy of the eye. (*From* Goldman L. Cecil medicine. Mosby's Paramedic Textbook. 23rd edition. Philadelphia: Saunders; 2008.)

perform this test, instill fluorescein onto the eye by wetting the strip. Examine the eye for a small stream of fluid leaking from the globe. This stream will fluoresce blue or green, in contrast to the orange appearance of the rest of the globe flooded with fluorescein.[4] **Fig. 2** illustrates a perforated globe.

The examination of the posterior segment of the eye is performed with either the direct ophthalmoscope or the panoptic ophthalmoscope. The retina should be visualized for tears or abnormalities, along with foreign bodies within the vitreous humor. It is imperative to optimize the ability to visualize the fundus by approaching the examination appropriately. **Box 1** lists the steps to properly perform an examination of the posterior chamber.

The Panoptic ophthalmoscope (Welch-Allyn) may provide better visualization of the fundus compared with traditional ophthalmoscope. In one study, it was found to be superior to both provider and patient in examining and identifying funduscopic abnormalities. The suggested improvement was proposed that the degree of visualization was 25° of field versus only 5° for the direct ophthalmoscope.[5]

Tonometry is the measurement of intraocular pressure (IOP). IOP has been regarded as a core vital sign of the eye, along with visual acuity, the pupillary examination, and an examination of the visual fields.[6] The measurement of IOP in a consistent and reliable manner is fundamental to the diagnosis and management of glaucoma and others disorders. There are several different methods of tonometry. The 2 types of impression tonometry typically used by emergency providers are Schiotz tonometry and a portable handheld battery-operated instrument (pen tonometer) that provides readings that correlate closely with Goldmann tonometry.[7] The electronic indentation tonometry must be calibrated at least once per day for accuracy. As with all tonometers, the pen tonometer is affected by corneal thickness and other corneal parameters and tends to overestimate IOP compared with Goldmann applanation, especially at higher IOP levels.[8,9] The most widely used instrument is the Goldmann applanation tonometer, which is attached to the slit lamp and measures the force required to flatten a fixed area of the cornea.[8,10] New types of tonometers are currently being developed that are aimed not only to be noninvasive but also to decrease the variability of user error, corneal thickness, and rigidity.[10]

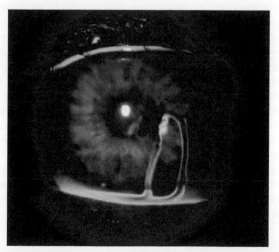

Fig. 2. Siedel's sign with ruptured globe. (*From* Graff J. EyeRounds Online Atlas of Ophthalmology. University of Iowa; 2004. Available at: http://webeye.ophth.uiowa.edu/eyeforum/atlas/pages/corneal-perforation-seidel-posative-.html. Accessed July 22, 2016.)

> **Box 1**
> **Ophthalmoscope examination**
>
> - Darken the room to optimize pupil dilation
> - Use your right hand for the right eye and left hand for the for left eye
> - Set the ophthalmoscope to the small aperture for an undilated eye
> - Ensure that the diopter is at zero
> - Start 15° from lateral about 15 inches away
> - Green light can better optimize blood vessels
> - Adjust diopter once able to visualize vessels of fundus

To perform tonometry, anesthetic solution is instilled into each eye. The patient lies supine and is asked to stare at a spot on the ceiling with both eyes or at a finger held directly in front of the patient overhead. The lids are held open without applying pressure on the globe. The tonometer is then placed on the corneal surface of each eye and the scale reading is taken from the tonometer.[8] Tonometry should be avoided in patients with penetrating eye injuries, patients unable to sit still resulting in rapid eye movements that can potentially lead to corneal injury, and patients with corneal defects.[7] Normal IOP is 12 to 20 mm Hg. If the IOP is 20 mm Hg or more, further investigation is indicated to determine whether glaucoma is present.[9,11]

The slit lamp is the fundamental tool in examination of any emergent condition that may include structures considered to be in the anterior segment of the eye. Using the slit lamp in examining the eye provides significant tiered magnification that is finely focused to provide 3-dimensional views of the structures mentioned. Compared WITH a Woods lamp or ophthalmoscope, it can provide 10 to 25 times the magnification. The focusing of the beam of light (slit) can provide better identification of the anterior eye structures, thus helping better diagnose anterior segment disorders. A good example of the use of the slit lamp can be found at http://www.ophthobook.com/videos/slit-lamp-exam-video.

Bedside ocular ultrasound (US) offers many advantages to the emergency provider. This technique is simple and quick to perform and can diagnose a wide range of medical and traumatic conditions. It is free of ionizing radiation, can show the posterior chamber and retrobulbar structures when hyphema, cataract, or lid edema makes direct visualization impossible, and allows for dynamic evaluation of the eye. Providers trained in bedside ocular US have been found to accurately diagnose many ophthalmic conditions, including intraocular or periorbital foreign bodies, globe rupture, hyphema, lens dislocation, lens subluxation, retinal detachment, retinal hemorrhage, vitreous detachment, vitreous hemorrhage, choroidal detachment, papilledema, increased intracranial pressure, neoplasms, and vascular abnormalities.

Bedside ocular US in the ED is usually performed with the patient supine and the eyelid closed, but not clenched. Place a Tegaderm over the eye and then apply a copious amount of gel over the Tegaderm. Tegaderm and ultrasound gel prevents the need to apply any pressure at all to the globe, which can cause discomfort and/or damage to the eye.

ACUTE MONOCULAR VISION LOSS

When evaluating a patient with a complaint of vision loss, it is important to distinguish whether the vision loss is monocular or binocular. Monocular visual loss indicates disease of the globe or optic nerve, whereas bilateral visual loss, including homonymous hemianopia, indicates a lesion at, or posterior to, the optic chiasm.[2] There are many causes of monocular vision loss, which is why it is imperative to get a full history and a focused physical examination. The history of present illness should include the rate of onset of visual loss, whether it is unilateral or bilateral, painful or painless, and with or without scleral injection. Ophthalmologic examination should emphasize visual acuity and visual field testing. Because most patients have a difficult time distinguishing loss of vision in one eye versus both eyes, it is essential to instruct the patient to alternately cover one eye and then the other to compare. An abrupt onset of visual loss is suggestive of an arterial vascular event, such as central retinal artery occlusion (CRAO), or Amaurosis fugax (AF).[8]

Amaurosis Fugax

AF is a painless, acute transient monocular vision loss lasting seconds to minutes. Although it is not considered a disease, it is a manifestation of systemic diseases that cause a transient interruption of arterial blood flow to the retina. The presentation of AF should be considered an ominous symptom of another serious disease that can lead to permanent vision loss, stroke, or myocardial infarction. In all suspected cases of AF, an embolic source should be considered.

The hallmark symptom of AF is the painless onset of monocular visual disturbance, which could include sudden graying or curtainlike loss of vision occurring to the whole visual field or only a portion, depending on the area of the retina that becomes occluded.[12] Most of the time, the patient will have complete resolution of the symptoms and normal vision at the time of ED presentation.

A facilitated diagnostic workup for an embolic source is a key factor in the patient with AF. If there is ongoing visual loss, emergent ophthalmologic referral is necessary. Diagnostic tests should include an electrocardiogram and echocardiogram. Carotid US should be considered on a more urgent basis, because transient monocular vision loss in a patient with carotid stenosis is associated with an annual stroke rate of 2.2% (95% confidence interval 1.5%–3.0%).[13] Of note, studies have shown that many patients under the age of 40 who present with AF have not gone on to suffer stroke.[14]

Aggressive management of risk factors such as hypertension, diabetes mellitus (DM), smoking cessation, lipid management, and anticoagulation for atrial fibrillation should also be arranged. Pharmacologic treatment to consider until further evaluation can take place should include low-dose aspirin therapy.[15]

Retinal Artery Occlusion

Retinal artery occlusion encompasses both phenomenon of CRAO and branch retinal artery occlusion. CRAO is a sudden painless monocular loss of vision that usually occurs over seconds and often is preceded by episodes of AF. It has an incidence of 1 in 100,000 individuals and 1 in 10,000 ophthalmology visits.[16] The incidence of CRAO is at its highest in the seventh decade of life and appears to affect men more than women.[17] The loss of vision associated with CRAO is profound, and greater than 80% of the time, the loss will be a visual acuity of more than 20/400.[18] Branch retinal artery occlusion also presents with sudden onset visual loss but typically only a partial visual field deficit.[19] Patients presenting to the ED with evidence of CRAO are considered an ophthalmologic emergency.

In CRAO, there will be a distinct loss of visual acuity that varies between only light perception to the ability to see moving fingers. There will often be a Marcus Gunn pupil or relative afferent pupillary defect observed during the swinging-flashlight test. The patient's pupils constrict less, therefore appearing to dilate, when a bright light is swung from the unaffected eye to the affected eye. The funduscopic examination often will be classic for whitening of the retina and the central cherry-red spot.[20] The cherry-red spot is the normal-appearing retina in contrast against the surrounding opacified retina, because the thin retina in this location is nourished by the underlying choroidal circulation and does not become hypoxic or opacified.[21] Fig. 3 illustrates the classic cherry-red spot. Fig. 4 illustrates a patient's right eye showing the classical appearance of a CRAO with diffuse retinal whitening sparing the fovea and the resultant cherry-red spot.

The treatment of CRAO is listed in Box 2.

Optimal return of visual acuity correlates to the time of ischemia to the retina. Hayreh and colleagues[22] showed optimum salvage of retina when blood return was restored before 97 minutes, whereas, beyond 240 minutes, there was massive loss of retinal viability. It is generally accepted that beyond this time the likelihood of appreciable vision return is unlikely. Emergent consultation and evaluation by an ophthalmologist should be obtained as soon as CRAO is suspected.

Central Retinal Vein Occlusion

The prevalence of central retinal vein occlusion (CRVO) increases with age with greater than half of cases affecting patients over the age of 65 years. It is the second most common retinal vascular disorder.[23] The most common risk factors for CRVO include hypertension, hyperlipidemia, arteriosclerosis, DM, and smoking.[24]

Branch retinal vein occlusion (BRVO) can present with peripheral visual blurriness or loss or can be central.[25] Funduscopic examination may reveal venous edema, superficial retinal hemorrhages (dot and blot hemorrhages), vitreous hemorrhage, and "cotton wool spots," which are fluffy white patches on the retina.[25] There will also be dilated tortuous veins with diffuse retinal hemorrhage in all quadrants on funduscopic examination.

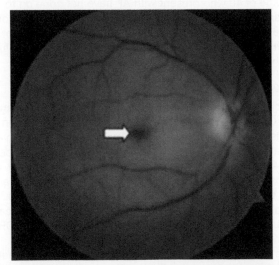

Fig. 3. CRAO of the right eye with retinal edema and the classic "cherry-red spot" in the macula due to the continued presence of the posterior ciliary circulation to the choroid (*arrow*).

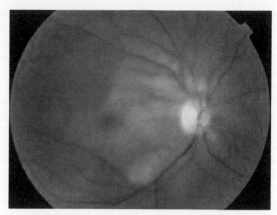

Fig. 4. A color fundus photograph of a patient's right eye showing the classical appearance of a CRAO with diffuse retinal whitening sparing the fovea and the resultant cherry-red spot.

Patients with CRVO will present with sudden painless loss of vision. There may be the presence of a relative afferent pupillary defect. In ischemic CRVO, visual acuity will be 20/400 or worse.[26]

Emergent referral to ophthalmology is imperative when visual loss is present. The ED provider should be aware that the severity of the acute visual loss will correlate to the prognosis of the return of visual acuity. BRVO has a much better prognosis of visual acuity improvement versus CRVO.[27] The extent of visual loss correlates with visual acuity return.[27]

Giant Cell Arteritis

Giant cell arteritis (GCA), previously called temporal arteritis, is one of the most common rheumatologic causes of vision loss. It effects patients starting at the age of 50 and is more prevalent among women, and the peak age is 70 years. Ophthalmic manifestations are commonly seen in patients with GCA. Permanent visual loss is the most-feared complication of GCA. Diagnosis and early treatment are the keys to preventing permanent vision loss.

The primary symptom is the sudden painless loss of vision, usually unilateral initially but can quickly spread bilaterally. Some patients may describe vision changes ranging from blurry, diplopia, to complete vision loss. Patients may also complain of headaches, usually temporal, unilateral, or bilateral. Many will have jaw claudication or pain with chewing.

Box 2 Central retinal artery occlusion treatment	
Treatment	**Purpose**
Digital ocular massage	In an attempt to dislodge any occlusion
Acetazolamide 500 mg IV	By lowering IOP to dislodge emboli
Hypercarbia by rebreathing CO_2	To encourage vasodilation
Hyperbaric oxygenation	Improving potential oxygenation of retina
Intraocular paracentesis	By lowering IOP
Localized intraarterial fibrinolysis	Lysis of emboli

Physical examination is highlighted by temporal and occipital tenderness. The visual field may be reduced. An afferent pupillary defect will be noted on swinging-flashlight test. Visual acuity test will also be reduced. Funduscopic examination may reveal a swollen optic disc with or without pallor. There may also be associated retinal hemorrhages. Patients with vision loss may also have optic atrophy, which is a result of anterior ischemic optic neuropathy.

The diagnostic workup includes an erythrocyte sedimentation rate (ESR), which usually exceeds 50 mm/h and may exceed 100 mm/h. Importantly, ESR may be normal in 7% to 20% of patients with GCA.[28] The gold standard for the diagnosis of GCA is the temporal artery biopsy.

Treatment for GCA should occur promptly. The treatment consists of the use of oral corticosteroids, which should be started as soon as the diagnosis is suspected. Treatment should not be delayed for the temporal artery biopsy, although follow-up should be arranged urgently, but can be done up to 4 weeks later. Prednisone is the first choice for treatment and may be continued for several years following the diagnosis.[29] The usual starting dose of oral prednisone is 40 to 60 mg/d or more (1 mg/kg/d). Intravenous (IV) dose of methylprednisolone in larger doses can be started in a very ill patient.[30]

Retinal Detachment

Retinal detachment can be difficult to diagnose in the ED. Retinal detachment is the separation of the sensory retina from the retinal pigment epithelium. It is a fairly uncommon affliction of the eye, affecting approximately 1 to 2 in 10,000 people per year.[31] The hallmark initial clinical features of retinal detachment is floaters, sometimes also described as lines, strings, dots, flashing, or cobwebs that occur suddenly. The clinical course many times proceeds to peripheral vision loss and then commonly the falling of curtain or veil superior to inferior. Most cases are painless. Funduscopic examination with or without dilation may show the abnormality of the retina. It can have a gray or folded appearance. In some cases, a graying of the vitreous humor pigment can be seen and is called "tobacco dust."

Bedside US reliably detects retinal detachment and is particularly useful when the examiner's view to the retina is obscured by periorbital edema, blood, or other opacities. For the detection of retinal detachment, US performed by an emergency provider has a sensitivity of 97% to 100% and a specificity of 83% to 92%.[32] Fig. 5 illustrates a retinal detachment on US. A retinal detachment is seen as an echogenic undulating membrane in the posterior to lateral globe, protruding into the vitreous humor. Even in complete retinal detachments, the typically folded surface remains bound anteriorly and to the optic nerve head posteriorly. A shallow cuff of subretinal fluid may also be seen along with the detachment.[33]

Retinal detachment treatment goals are to limit or prevent vision loss. Consultation with an ophthalmologist is essential for treatment. If immediate referral is not possible, the patient should be instructed to lie down with the face on the side of the detachment on the pillow (opposite the field defect) to minimize the detachment extending toward the macula. There is no general consensus on how soon patients presenting with a symptomatic posterior vitreous detachment and no other visual symptoms should be referred for a definitive management. Most retinal detachments not involving the macula can be repaired on the same day or the following day.[34]

Optic Neuritis

Optic neuritis is a common cause of unilateral painful vision loss. Most patients describe a retrobulbar nagging or aching pain. It initially causes monocular blurry

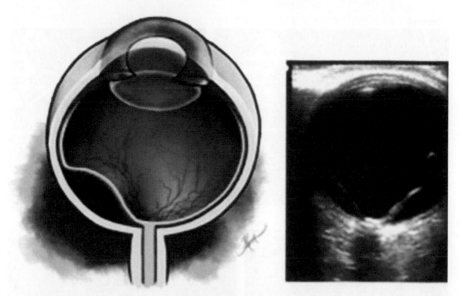

Fig. 5. Retinal detachment illustration and US. (*From* Roque PJ, Hatch N, Barr L, et al. Bedside ocular ultrasound. Crit Care Clin 2014;30(2):227–41; and *Courtesy of* Nicholas Hatch, MD, Denver, CO.)

vision, which then progresses over hours to days. It is an acute demyelinating disease of the optic nerve that is most commonly seen in multiple sclerosis (MS).[35] The inflammatory response against the optic nerve results in edema and breakdown of the myelin sheaths and perivascular cuffing of the retinal vasculature.[36]

Optic neuritis is a clinical diagnosis. Even patients with 20/20 vision at presentation often have defects perceiving color and contrast, often described as blurry or "washed out."[37] Pain is often worse with eye movement. The orbit and fundus are normal in 66% of cases, whereas in 33% of cases, patients present with disc edema, uveitis, or periphlebitis.[38]

Optic neuritis can be confirmed with MRI (**Fig. 6**). MRI can help confirm the diagnosis and risk stratify those likely to develop MS. Optic nerve inflammation can be demonstrated in 95% of patients who have optic neuritis on MRI.[39]

Optic neuritis generally improves over a few weeks even without treatment.[40] Treatment should be considered if the visual loss is severe or if there is an abnormal MRI (higher risk of MS). Treatment is with methylprednisolone 250 mg IV every 6 hours (or 1 g IV daily) for 3 days followed by an oral prednisone taper of 11 days. According to the American Academy of Neurology, although corticosteroids may hasten the return of vision after initial presentation, there is no compelling evidence for long-term benefit for patients who have optic neuritis.[41]

INFECTIOUS CONDITIONS
Endophthalmitis

Endophthalmitis refers to infection within the eye involving the vitreous or aqueous humor. Exogenous endophthalmitis signifies that the infection was introduced into the eye from the outside, by either trauma, eye surgery, or extension of corneal infection (keratitis). It is a true ophthalmic emergency and can result in complete visual loss and

Patient 1

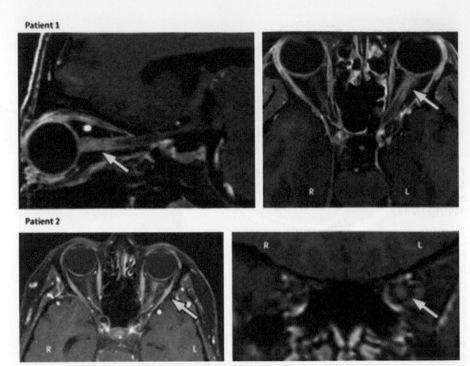

Patient 2

Fig. 6. MRI brain with contrast showing optic neuritis in case of MS. Examples of neuromye-litis optica-optic neuritis in two patients showing left optic nerve enhancement on post-contrast T1-weighted MRI scans. Right optic nerve sheath enhancement (indicated by *arrows*) from a granulomatous optic neuropathy. Patient who presented with an acute right optic neuritis. MRI showed optic nerve sheath enhancement. FDG-PET scan showed hilar/mediastinal avid nodes. Lymph node biopsy showed non-caseating granulomata. *Arrows* indicate FDG-avid hilar/mediastinal lymph nodes in the right-hand figure, and to enhancing optic nerve sheath in the left-hand figure. (*From* Toosy A, Mason DF, Miller DH, et al. Optic neuritis. Lancet Neurol 2014;13(1):89; with permission.)

loss of the eye within 24 to 48 hours. Emergent ophthalmology consultation should be obtained.

Endophthalmitis patients generally present with a red, painful eye, ocular discharge, and progressively worsening visual acuity. They are typically postopera-tive or due to ocular injury. The examination of the anterior chamber frequently shows a hypopyon (a layering of inflammatory cells and exudates in the inferior anterior chamber). The eye and surrounding tissue typically features edema and erythema of the eye lid and conjunctival hyperemia, chemosis, and purulent discharge. A visual acuity helps guide treatment. An IOP less than 5 mm Hg or greater than 25 mm Hg has a poor prognosis. Slit lamp also can show corneal edema and inflammation (Fig. 7).

Treatment may include aspiration of the vitreous or pars plana, vitrectomy, and administration of intravitreal antibiotics and steroids. Systemic antibiotics are also pro-vided. It is important for the ophthalmologist to obtain cultures of the vitreal fluid before starting antibiotics. This culture will help to guide antimicrobial therapy. Admis-sion is required for nearly all cases.

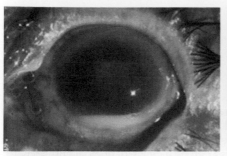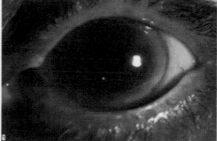

Fig. 7. Endophthalmitis with hypopyon, layering of white cells in anterior chamber. (*From* Major JC Jr, Engelbert M, Flynn HW Jr, et al. Staphylococcus aureus endophthalmitis: antibiotic susceptibilities, methicillin resistance, and clinical outcomes. J Ophthalmol 2010; 149(2):278–83.)

Herpes Simplex Keratitis

Herpes simplex keratitis (HSV) is one of the most common causes of corneal blindness in the world. In the United States, HSV keratitis affects approximately18.2 per 100,000 person-years. The incidence is 1.5 million per year worldwide. Of 1 million new cases of shingles per year in the United States, 25% to 40% develop ophthalmic complications.[42]

HSV keratitis symptoms can include pain, blurred vision, sensitivity to light, red eye, foreign body sensation, or watery discharge. The most common finding on the slit lamp is dendritic ulcers, which consists of a linear, dichotomously branching lesion with terminal bulbs. The central epithelial defect stains with fluorescein[43] (Fig. 8).

The treatment of HSV keratitis especially with lid or dermatologic involvement is oral acyclovir 800 mg 5 times per day, or oral valacyclovir 1000 mg 3 times per day for 7 to 10 days. Therapy is most effective when started in the first 3 days, but may have some efficacy within 5 days of the onset of symptoms.[44] Immune-compromised patients should consider acyclovir 10 mg/kg/8 hours in 1-hour infusions for 7 to 10 days. Topical antivirals have showed improved epithelia healing.[45] For conjunctival involvement, prescribe topical trifluridine (Viroptic), one drop 9 times a day. Idoxuridine (Dendrid), one drop every 1 hour during the first day and every 2 hours at night, can be substituted for those who are allergic.[11] Ophthalmology consultation should be obtained before

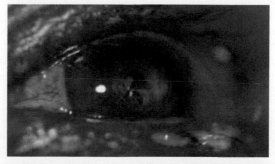

Fig. 8. Fluorescein stained eye under slit lamp showing dendrites in herpes keratitis. (*From* Herpes Zoster Ophthalmicus case report. West J Emerg Med. Available at: http://westjem. com/case-report/herpes-zoster-ophthalmicus.html. Accessed July 22, 2016.)

the initiation of antivirals in order to determine if these agents should be given orally or intravenously. Topical steroids should be reserved for cases of active stromal keratitis and anterior uveitis, under direction of ophthalmology.

CORNEAL INJURIES
Corneal Abrasion

Corneal abrasion is a disruption of the corneal epithelia layer due to trauma. Penetrating or projectile injuries should raise suspicion for a ruptured globe. Patients with a corneal abrasion typically complain of pain, redness of the conjunctiva, sensitivity to light, and excessive tearing. Contact lenses themselves can be a cause of corneal abrasion.

Visual acuity should be done before the administration of any medications. Short-acting anesthetics (eg, proparacaine [Ophthetic], tetracaine [Pontocaine]) can be used for pain control and to improve the eye examination. Fluorescein staining should be done. Areas of corneal damage will fluoresce green, and a foreign body may also be visualized. Also, it is important to examine under the lids for a retained foreign body. When multiple linear corneal abrasions are seen, a foreign body under the lid should be suspected.

Treatment of corneal abrasions is largely based on expert consensus. Primary goals of therapy are pain control, prevention of infection, and rapid healing of the corneal epithelium. In a systematic review of 5 randomized controlled trials, topical nonsteroidal anti-inflammatories, such as ketorolac, diclofenac, and indomethacin, resulted in a modest decrease in pain without a delay in wound healing or an increased risk of infection.[46] A systematic review of cycloplegics showed no clear evidence to support their use in corneal abrasion.[47] Patching of the eye following a corneal abrasion has been shown to be of no benefit in pain relief or rate of healing and is no longer recommended.[48] Patients with contact lens–related abrasions should be instructed to discontinue contact lens use until the defect heals and symptoms resolve. Oral analgesics are typically prescribed for pain control. In cases where oral analgesics are contraindicated, topical nonsteroidal anti-inflammatory drugs may be of benefit. A topical antibiotic ointment, such as erythromycin, is commonly prescribed 4 times per day for 3 to 5 days to prevent infection, although there is no strong evidence to support this practice. Patients with contact lens abrasions should be treated with prophylactic topical antibiotics to cover Pseudomonas, such as gentamycin or ciprofloxacin. There is no convincing evidence in the literature to support tetanus prophylaxis in patients with nonpenetrating corneal abrasions.[49]

Most abrasions heal within 1 to 3 days, although larger defects may require 4 to 5 days to fully heal. Patients with small corneal abrasions will heal quickly and generally require only a single follow-up examination to ensure healing, usually within 24 hours. Patients with contact lens–related corneal abrasions should be reexamined daily to ensure prompt healing and to exclude infection. Referral to an ophthalmologist is indicated for large abrasions, or for patients who develop a corneal infiltrate or ulcer.

Corneal Ulcer

A corneal ulcer is essentially an open sore on the outer surface of the cornea. Corneal ulcers are also referred to as keratitis. Corneal ulcers are a major reason for vision loss throughout the world and require early diagnosis and treatment.[8]

There are many reasons patients develop corneal ulcers. That is why it is essential to take a history that includes recent trauma, contact lens use, and use of steroids or immunosuppressant medications.[11] Patients typically complain of a painful red eye, discharge from the eye, photophobia, and decreased vision.[11,50] Ulcers of the cornea are most often caused by bacteria such as *Staphylococcus*, *Streptococcus*, and *Pseudomonas*.[50] It can also be cause by viral infections, fungal infections, and Acanthamoeba (a protozoan)[50].

Diagnosis is usually made by clinical appearance. To identify the organism, the ophthalmologist normally scrapes the corneal ulcer and cultures the organism.[11] Emergent ophthalmology consult is needed anytime a corneal ulcer is diagnosed. Start the patient on antibiotic drops after obtaining a culture.[11] Current recommendations for antibiotics are to start the patient on a fluoroquinolone, one drop every hour in the affected eye.[8,11] **Box 3** provides a list of organisms and therapy for corneal ulcers. If there is a suspicion that the cause of the corneal ulcer may be a virus or fungus, topical antiviral or antifungal drops should be given[11] in consultation with the ophthalmologist.

ADDITIONAL OCULAR EMERGENCIES
Acute Angle Closure Glaucoma

Acute angle closure glaucoma is an ophthalmic emergency. Glaucoma can cause blindness if left untreated, and that is why it is essential to diagnose and treat promptly. Nearly half of people with glaucoma are not diagnosed, and glaucoma is still one of the leading causes of blindness.[51,52]

As people get older, the lens of the eye becomes less elastic and thicker. These events cause the iris to move forward with greater contact with the lens that can cause pupillary block. Susceptible persons have eyes with shallow anterior chambers, where the angle between the cornea and iris is reduced. Hypermetropic (farsighted) eyes have a shorter anterior to posterior length and a narrower angle, increasing the risk of acute angle-closure glaucoma.[11] Certain medications such as anticholinergic drugs (ie, nebulized ipratropium), adrenergic dugs (ie, systemic ephedrine), and antidepressants can also lead to acute angle closure glaucoma.[53] The underlying mechanism is pupillary dilation subsequently causing pupillary block. Antihistamines can also induce acute angle closure glaucoma due to its anticholinergic affects.[53]

Typical presenting symptoms include the abrupt onset of ocular pain, headache, blurred vision, nausea, and vomiting.[52,53] It is very rare for acute angle glaucoma to present as painless monocular vision loss.[11] Clinical findings on examination are

Box 3	
Corneal ulcer antibiotic guide	
Organisms	**Treatment and Dosing**
No organisms identified; ulcer suggestive of bacterial infection	Moxifloxacin 0.5%, gatifloxacin 0.3%, or tobramycin with cefazolin
Gram-positive cocci = *Streptococcus pneumoniae*	Moxifloxacin 0.5%, or cefazolin Levofloxacin
Gram-negative rods: thin = *Pseudomonas*	Moxifloxacin 0.5%, gatifloxacin 0.3%, ciprofloxacin, tobramycin, or gentamicin; other fluoroquinolones
Yeastlike organism = *Candida* species	Amphotericin B, voriconazole, or posaconazole
Hyphaelike organisms = Fungal ulcer	Natamycin 5%, amphotericin B, or posaconazole
Cyst, trophozoites = Acanthamoeba	Chlorhexidine or neomycin

a significantly elevated IOP above 21 mm Hg, corneal edema, redness, a middilated and fixed pupil, and a shallow anterior chamber.[11,52] When the pupil becomes middilated, the peripheral iris blocks aqueous outflow and the IOP raises abruptly, producing pain, injection, corneal edema, and blurred vision[11,52] (Fig. 9).

IOP that is persistently elevated can cause progressive and irreversible loss of vision.[54] Treatment of acute angle closure glaucoma is aimed at lowering the IOP by blocking the production of aqueous, reducing the volume of aqueous, and facilitating outflow of aqueous. This can be done by treating with acetazolamide (orally or IV), topical beta-blockers, prostaglandin analogues, α2-adrenergic agonists, and pilocarpine to induce miosis.[9,52] Emergent ophthalmology consultation should be done on all patients with suspected acute angle closure glaucoma. If these measures fail, a laser can be used to create a hole in the peripheral iris to relieve pupillary block (laser iridectomy).[50,54]

Globe Rupture

Blunt trauma or penetrating injury to the globe is a major cause of monocular blindness. It has been found that accidental injury followed by violent injury was the leading cause of open globe injuries.[55] Patients presenting to the ED with such injuries may not have obvious signs of actual globe rupture or penetration.

Globe rupture most commonly occurs at the insertion sites of the extraocular muscles or at the limbus where the sclera is thinnest. Accompanying findings may be loss of visual acuity, iridodialysis (teardrop shape to iris), uveal exposure externally, or complete subconjunctival hemorrhage (Fig. 10). An afferent pupillary defect may be present as well as limitation of the extraocular muscle movements. A hyphema may also be present.

Slit-lamp examination should be performed, but extreme care to prevent pressure application to the globe should be of utmost importance, as to prevent expulsion of vitreous contents. When suspicious of penetrating foreign body, slit-lamp examination with fluorescein staining may reveal a positive Seidel's test. Seidel's test will provide evidence of globe leak from rupture or penetration by revealing streaming of fluid that is in contrast to the color of the fluorescein staining the surface of the eye[56] (see Fig. 2).

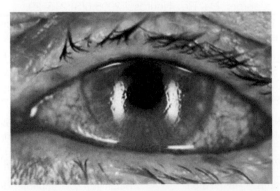

Fig. 9. Acute glaucoma with corneal edema, redness, a fixed and middilated pupil. (*From* Knoop KJ, Stack LB, Storrow AB, editors. The atlas of emergency medicine. 4th edition. McGraw-Hill Education. Available at: http://accessmedicine.mhmedical.com.)

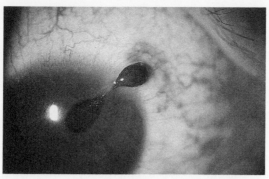

Fig. 10. Ruptured globe. (*From* Howard PK, Steinmann RA, editors. Sheehy's emergency nursing principles and practice. 6th edition. St Louis (MO): Elsevier Mosby; 2010.)

Globe penetration or rupture is an ophthalmologic emergency and requires immediate ophthalmology consultation. Once rupture or penetration is suspected, a protective shield should be placed over the eye, minimizing any manipulation or pressure to the eye itself. Computed tomography (CT) may be helpful in identifying penetrating foreign body but can miss some foreign material. The reported sensitivity of CT for ocular foreign bodies ranges from 65% to 100% in one study.[57] Tetanus should be considered in all corneal traumas.

SUMMARY

Eye complaints are a common reason for patients to present to the ED. Knowing the anatomy and normal physical examination will help to find clues for the abnormality. At stake is the loss of vision either temporarily or permanently. The management of the abnormality depends on the diagnosis. Consultation with ophthalmology is important in most of ophthalmologic complaints.

REFERENCES

1. Nash EA, Margo CE. Patterns of emergency department visits for disorders of the eye and ocular adnexa. Arch Ophthalmol 1998;116(9):1222.
2. Xiang H, Stallones L, Chen G, et al. Work-related eye injuries treated in hospital emergency departments in the US. Am J Ind Med 2005;48(1):57–62.
3. Alteveer J. The red eye, the swollen eye, and acute vision loss: handling non-traumatic eye disorders in the ED. Emerg Med Pract 2002;4(6):1–2.
4. Roberts JR, Hedges JR. Clinical procedures in emergency medicine. 2nd edition. Philadelphia, PA: Massachusetts Medical Society; 1992.
5. Petrushkin H, Barsam A, Mavrakakis M, et al. Optic disc assessment in the emergency department: a comparative study between the PanOptic and direct ophthalmoscopes. Emerg Med J 2012;29(12):1007–8.
6. Okafor KC, Brandt JD. Measuring intraocular pressure. Curr Opin Ophthalmol 2015;26(2):103–9.
7. Babineau MR, Sanchez LD. Ophthalmologic procedures in the emergency department. Emerg Med Clin North Am 2008;26(1):17–34.
8. Biswell R. Cornea. Chapter 6. In: Riordan-Eva P, Cunningham ET, editors. Vaughan & Asbury's general ophthalmology. 18th edition. New York: The

McGraw-Hill Companies; 2011. Available at: http://accessmedicine.mhmedical. com/content.aspx?bookid=387&Sectionid=40229323. Accessed May 28, 2016.

9. Greenberg RD, Daniel KJ. Eye emergencies. Chapter 31. In: Stone CK, Humphries RL, editors. Current diagnosis & treatment emergency medicine. 7th edition. New York: The McGraw-Hill Companies; 2011. Available at: http://accessmedicine.mhmedical.com.proxy1.athensams.net/content.aspx?bookid=385&sectionid=40357247. Accessed June 13, 2017.

10. Arribas-Pardo P, Mendez-Hernandez C, Cuiña-Sardiña R, et al. Measuring intra-ocular pressure after intrastromal corneal ring segment implantation with rebound tonometry and Goldmann applanation tonometry. Cornea 2015;34(5):516–20.

11. Walker RA, Adhikari S. Eye emergencies. In: Tintinalli JE, Stapczynski JS, Ma OJ, et al, editors. Tintinalli's emergency medicine: a comprehensive study guide. 8th edition. New York: McGraw-Hill Education; 2016. Available at: http://accessmedicine.mhmedical.com.proxy1.athensams.net/content.aspx?bookid=1658&sectionid=109444274. Accessed June 13, 2017.

12. Hayreh SS, Zimmerman MB. Amaurosis fugax in ocular vascular occlusive disorders. Retina 2014;34(1):115.

13. Wilterdink JL, Easton JD. Vascular event rates in patients with atherosclerotic cerebrovascular disease. Arch Neurol 1992;49(8):857–63.

14. Poole CJ, Ross Russell RW, Harrison P, et al. Amaurosis fugax under the age of 40 years. J Neurol Neurosurg Psychiatry 1987;50(1):81–4.

15. Antithrombotic Trialists' Collaboration. Collaborative meta-analysis of randomised trials of antiplatelet therapy for prevention of death, myocardial infarction, and stroke in high risk patients. BMJ 2002;324(7329):71–86.

16. Rumelt S, Dorenboim Y, Rehany U. Aggressive systematic treatment for central retinal artery occlusion. Am J Ophthalmol 1999;128:733–8.

17. Kirchhof B. In: Duker JS, Waheed NK, Goldmann DR, editors. Handbook of retinal OCT. Elsevier/Saunders; 2014. ISBN: 978-0-323-18884-5. Graefe's Archive for Clinical and Experimental Ophthalmology 2015;(1):169.

18. Hayreh SS, Zimmerman MB. Central retinal artery occlusion: visual outcome. Am J Ophthalmol 2005;140(3):376–91.

19. Alwitry A, Osbourne A. Central or branch retinal arterial occlusion. Roy and Fraunfelder's current ocular therapy: Elsevier Inc; 2008. p. 616–9.

20. Sadda PSPaSVR. Retinal Artery Obstructions. Retina:1012-1025.

21. Gold D. Retinal arterial occlusion. Transactions. Trans Sect Ophthalmol Am Acad Ophthalmol Otolaryngol 1977;83(3 Pt 1):OP392–408.

22. Hayreh SS, Zimmerman MB, Kimura A, et al. Central retinal artery occlusion.. Retinal survival time. Exp Eye Res 2004;78:723–36.

23. Klein R, Klein BE, Moss SE, et al. The epidemiology of retinal vein occlusion: the Beaver Dam Eye Study. Trans Am Ophthalmol Soc 2000;98:133–41.

24. Ehlers JP, Fekrat S. Major review: retinal vein occlusion: beyond the acute event. Surv Ophthalmol 2011;56:281–99.

25. Rehak J, Rehak M. Branch retinal vein occlusion: pathogenesis, visual prognosis, and treatment modalities. Curr Eye Res 2008;33(2):111–31.

26. Rabinowitz MP. The Wills eye manual: office and emergency room diagnosis and treatment of eye disease. 6th edition. Philadelphia: Lippincott Williams & Wilkins; 2012.

27. Natural history and clinical management of central retinal vein occlusion. The Central Vein Occlusion Study Group. Arch Ophthalmol 1997;115(4):486–91.

28. Hayreh SS, Podhajsky PA, Raman R, et al. Giant cell arteritis: validity and reliability of various diagnostic criteria. Am J Ophthalmol 1997;123(3):285.
29. Aiello PD, Trautmann JC, McPhee TJ, et al. Visual prognosis in giant cell arteritis. Ophthalmology 1993;100(4):550–5.
30. Proven A, Gabriel SE, Orces C, et al. Glucocorticoid therapy in giant cell arteritis: duration and adverse outcomes. Arthritis Rheum 2003;49(5):703.
31. Algvere PV, Jahnberg P, Textorius O. The Swedish retinal detachment register. I. A database for epidemiological and clinical studies. Graefe's Archive Clin Exp Ophthalmol 1999;237(2):137–44.
32. Blaivas M, Theodoro D, Sierzenski PR. A study of bedside ocular ultrasonography in the emergency department. Acad Emerg Med 2002;9(8):791.
33. McNicholas MM, Brophy DP, Power WJ, et al. Ocular sonography. AJR Am J Roentgenol 1994;163(4):921–6.
34. Kang HK, Luff AJ. Management of retinal detachment: a guide for non-ophthalmologists. BMJ 2008;336(7655):1235–40.
35. Balcer LJ. Clinical practice. Optic neuritis. N Engl J Med 2006;354(12): 1273–80.
36. Lessell S. Retinal venous sheathing in optic neuritis: Its significance for the pathogenesis of multiple sclerosis. by S. Lightman, W.I. McDonald, A.C. Bird, et al. Brain 100:405–414, 1987. Surv Ophthalmol 1988;32:437–8.
37. Cole SR, Beck RW, Moke PS, et al. The National Eye Institute Visual Function Questionnaire: experience of the ONTT. Optic neuritis treatment trial. Invest Ophthalmol Vis Sci 2000;41(5):1017–21.
38. Ferri F. Amaurosis Fugax. Ferri's Clinical Advisor. 2017.
39. Rizzo JF 3rd, Andreoli CM, Rabinov JD. Use of magnetic resonance imaging to differentiate optic neuritis and nonarteritic anterior ischemic optic neuropathy. Ophthalmology 2002;109(9):1679–84.
40. Beck RW, Gal RL, Bhatti MT, et al. Visual function more than 10 years after optic neuritis: experience of the optic neuritis treatment trial. Am J Ophthalmol 2004; 137(1):77–83.
41. Kaufman DI, Trobe JD, Eggenberger ER, et al. Abstracts: practice parameter: the role of corticosteroids in the management of acute monosymptomatic optic neuritis. Report of the Quality Standards Subcommittee of the American Academy of Neurology11 Edited by Thomas J. Liesegang, MD. Am J Ophthalmol 2000;130:541.
42. Faroog AV, Shukla D. Herpes simplex epithelial and stromal keratitis: an epidemiologic update. Surv Ophthalmol 2012;57(5):448–62.
43. Yanoff M, Duker J. Ophthalmology. In: Kubal, editor. 1st edition. New York: Elsevier Inc; 2014. p. 700–3.
44. Shaikh S, Ta CN. Evaluation and management of herpes zoster ophthalmicus. Am Fam Physician 2002;66(9):1723–30.
45. Wilhelmus KR. Antiviral treatment and other therapeutic interventions for herpes simplex virus epithelial keratitis. Cochrane Database Syst Rev 2010;(12):CD002898.
46. Weaver CS, Terrell KM. Evidence-based emergency medicine/update: update: do ophthalmic nonsteroidal anti-inflammatory drugs reduce the pain associated with simple corneal abrasion without delaying healing? Ann Emerg Med 2003; 41:134–40.
47. Carley F, Carley S. Towards evidence based emergency medicine: best BETs from the Manchester Royal Infirmary. Mydriatics in corneal abrasion. Emerg Med J 2001;18(4):273.

48. Turner A, Rabiu M. Patching for corneal abrasion. Cochrane Database Syst Rev 2006;(2):CD004764.
49. Mukherjee P, Sivakumar A. Tetanus prophylaxis in superficial corneal abrasions. Emerg Med J 2003;20(1):62–4.
50. Levsky ME, DeFlorio P. Ophthalmologic conditions. Chapter 2. In: Knoop KJ, Stack LB, Storrow AB, et al, editors. The atlas of emergency medicine. 3rd edition. New York: The McGraw-Hill Companies; 2010. Available at: http://accessmedicine. mhmedical.com/content.aspx?bookid=351&Sectionid=39619701. Accessed June 11, 2016.
51. CfDCaP. Available at: http://www.cdc.gov/visionhealth. Accessed June 11, 2016.
52. Horton JC. Disorders of the Eye. In: Kasper D, Fauci A, Hauser S, et al, editors. Harrison's principles of internal medicine. 19th edition. New York: McGraw-Hill Education; 2015. Available at: http://accessmedicine.mhmedical.com/content. aspx?bookid=1130&Sectionid=79725193. Accessed June 11, 2016.
53. Ah-Kee EY, Egong E, Shafi A, et al. A review of drug-induced acute angle closure glaucoma for non-ophthalmologists. Qatar Med J 2015;2015(1):6.
54. Dayan M, Turner B, McGhee C. Acute angle closure glaucoma masquerading as systemic illness. BMJ 1996;313(7054):413–5.
55. Rahman I, Maino A, Devadason D, et al. Open globe injuries: factors predictive of poor outcome. Eye (London, England) 2006;20(12):1336–41.
56. Cain W Jr, Sinskey RM. Detection of anterior chamber leakage with Seidel's test. Arch Ophthalmol 1981;99(11):2013.
57. Mester V, Kuhn F. Intraocular foreign bodies. Ophthalmol Clin North Am 2002; 15(2):235–42.

Low-Risk Chest Pain
What Is the Evidence?

Amanda P. Coté, MHS, PA-C*, Jamie L. Hodes, MSPAS, PA-C, Ryan Voccia, MMS, PA-C

KEYWORDS

- Low-risk chest pain • HEART score • Risk stratification • Diagnostics
- Acute coronary syndrome

KEY POINTS

- The term low-risk chest pain is broadly defined as chest pain with a low short-term risk of a major adverse cardiac event.
- The history, physical examination, risk factors, electrocardiogram, laboratory tests, and sometimes objective cardiac imaging all play a role when determining a patient's risk of acute coronary syndrome.
- The History, Electrocardiogram, Age, Risk Factors, Troponin (HEART) pathway is a scoring system designed specifically for emergency department patients that may be used to determine which patients are at low risk for major adverse cardiac events.

INTRODUCTION

The optimal management of acute chest pain in the emergency department (ED) is a dilemma faced by many clinicians, accounting for more than 8 million annual visits in the United States.[1] Patients present with a spectrum of signs and symptoms reflecting the many potential causes of chest pain, including traumatic and nontraumatic. In order to appropriately narrow the differential, it is useful to evaluate each presentation of chest pain in a stepwise fashion (Fig. 1). The history and physical examination remain the front line of evaluation because they help distinguish among the potential causes of chest pain and lead to appropriate and potentially life-preserving therapy.[2] This, in combination with risk factors and diagnostics, can help disposition patients accordingly. Although most low risk patients do not have a life-threatening condition, clinicians must rapidly identify those who require admission for urgent management and those with a benign cause who can be discharged directly from the ED.[3–5]

This article focuses primarily on nontraumatic, cardiac causes of chest pain with a general overview of acute coronary syndrome (ACS). It also includes discussion of the current, evidence-based recommendations on the evaluation of patients with low-risk chest pain, including the use of novel scoring systems.

Disclosures: The authors have nothing to disclose.
Emergency Medicine, Albany Medical Center, 43 New Scotland Avenue, Albany, NY 12208, USA
* Corresponding author.
E-mail address: amandacote11@gmail.com

Physician Assist Clin 2 (2017) 537–556
http://dx.doi.org/10.1016/j.cpha.2017.02.015
2405-7991/17/© 2017 Elsevier Inc. All rights reserved.

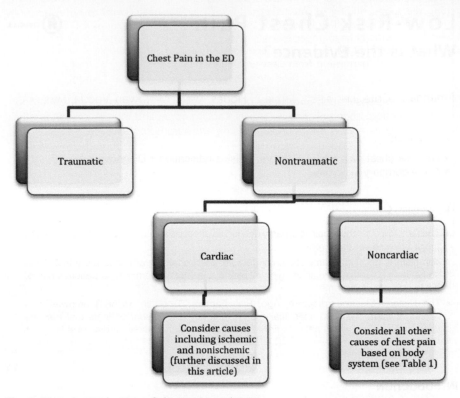

Fig. 1. Stepwise evaluation of chest pain in the ED.

CAUSES OF CHEST PAIN

The differential diagnosis for chest pain is extremely broad; chest pain can be caused by a wide variety of mechanisms, and can originate from almost all body systems (Table 1).[6,7] Cardiac disease accounts for only 8% to 18% of all cases of chest pain, and gastroesophageal reflux disease is the most common cause of noncardiac chest pain.[8,9]

Table 1
Differential diagnosis of chest pain

Cardiac	Noncardiac	
Ischemic	Pulmonary	Psychiatric
• ACS[a]	• Pulmonary embolism[a]	• Anxiety
• Coronary vasospasm[a]	• Tension pneumothorax[a]	• Panic disorder
• Unstable angina[a]	• Pneumonia	• Depression
• Chronic stable angina	• Pleuritis	• Somatoform disorders
• Aortic stenosis		
• Hypertrophic cardiomyopathy		

(continued on next page)

Table 1 *(continued)*		
Cardiac	**Noncardiac**	
Nonischemic	Gastrointestinal/esophageal	Chest wall
• Pericardial tamponade[a]	• Esophageal rupture[a]	• Costochondritis
• Pericarditis	• Esophageal spasm	• Tietze syndrome
• Myocarditis	• Gastroesophageal reflux	• Trauma
• Aortic dissection[a]	disease	• Rib pain
• Mitral valve prolapse	• Biliary colic	• Radicular pain
	• Cholecystitis	• Nonspecific musculoskeletal
	• Peptic ulcer	pain
	• Pancreatitis	
	• Motility disorders	
	Other	Dermatology
	• Acute chest syndrome/sickle	• Herpes zoster
	cell crisis	
	• Diabetic mononeuritis	
	• Tabes dorsalis	

[a] Indicates acute life-threatening pathology.

Data from Papadakis M, McPhee SJ, Rabow MW. CURRENT medical diagnosis and treatment 2013. 52nd edition. McGraw-Hill Professional; 2012; and Lenfant C. Chest pain of cardiac and noncardiac origin. Metabolism 2010;59 Suppl 1:S41–6.

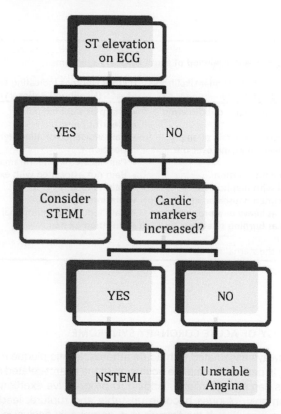

Fig. 2. ACS evaluation. ECG, electrocardiogram; NSTEMI, non–ST segment elevation myocardial infarction; STEMI, ST segment elevation myocardial infarction. (*Data from* Kumar A, Cannon CP. Acute coronary syndromes: diagnosis and management, part I. Mayo Clin Proc 2009;84(10):917–38.)

ACUTE CORONARY SYNDROME

Although the differential diagnosis for chest pain is varied, a type of chest pain that patients and physicians are often most concerned about is ACS. ACS is a spectrum of acute ischemia-related syndromes ranging from unstable angina to myocardial infarction (MI) with or without ST segment elevation (Fig. 2).[10]

- Unstable angina is characterized by myocardial ischemia without infarction; as a result, no increase of cardiac biomarker levels and no pathologic ST segment elevation occur.[10]
- Acute myocardial infarction occurs when myocardial tissue is devoid of oxygen and substrate for a sufficient period of time to cause cardiac myocyte death.[10]
  - Non–ST segment elevation MI (NSTEMI) is characterized by increased levels of cardiac biomarkers without pathologic ST segment elevation.[10]
  - ST segment elevation MI (STEMI) is characterized by ST segment elevation and increased levels of cardiac biomarkers. However, biomarker level increase is not required at onset to make this diagnosis given that the troponin level may take a few hours to become increased after the onset of paint (Table 2).[10]

Table 2 Historical information and likelihood of acute coronary syndrome	
History Findings Indicating Higher Likelihood of ACS (Likelihood Ratios >1)	History Findings Indicating Lower Likelihood of ACS (Likelihood Ratios <1)
• Radiating pain (left, right, or both arms/ shoulders) • Pain similar to prior ischemia or angina • Pain that has been changing over the past 24 h • Pain worsened with exertion • Pain associated with diaphoresis • Pain with associated nausea or vomiting • Pain described as heavy or a pressure • Pain described as burning or aching • Oppressive pain • Pain located in the sternal region	• Sharp or stabbing pain • Pleuritic pain • Pain worsened or alleviated by changes in position • Pain located in the inframammary region • Pain not associated with exertion • Palpitations • Dizziness/syncope • Pain induced by emotional stress • Duration <2 min

Data from Refs.[14–20]

PATHOPHYSIOLOGY OF ACUTE CORONARY SYNDROME

ACS is almost always associated with acute atherosclerotic plaque rupture or plaque erosion resulting in partial or complete occlusion of the infarct-related artery.[11] Atherosclerotic plaques can slowly enlarge, leading to progressive exertional angina. However, more commonly, plaques become unstable and rupture, leading to coronary artery thrombosis (Fig. 3).[12] If the thrombus is completely occlusive, STEMI occurs, but even partial occlusion may result in intermittent angina, rest angina, or NSTEMI. Plaque rupture is unpredictable and commonly occurs in plaques previously shown to be nonocclusive.[11]

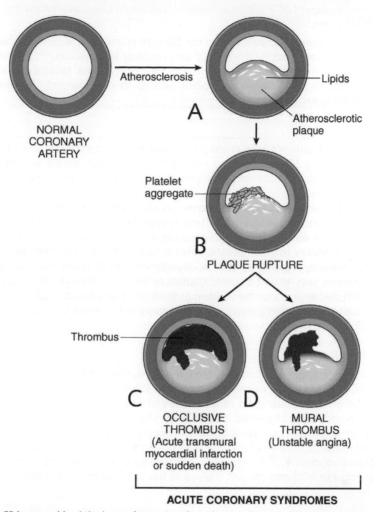

ACUTE CORONARY SYNDROMES

Fig. 3. ACS is caused by (*A*) plaque formation from lipid collection; (*B*) rupture or erosion of the plaque, causing platelet aggregation on the plaque; (*C*) formation of a thrombus that is occlusive, totally blocks the artery, and produces an acute myocardial infarction (heart attack) or sudden cardiac death; or (*D*) formation of a partially occlusive mural thrombus (mural means pertaining to a wall), which causes unstable angina (chest pain at rest or with increasing frequency). (*From* Chabner D-E. The Language of Medicine, Australian Edition, 10th edition. Saunders/Elsevier: Philadelphia; 2013.)

LOW-RISK CHEST PAIN

The term low-risk chest pain is broadly defined as chest pain with a low short-term risk of a major adverse cardiac event (MACE) or death. Patients classified into this group have no objective evidence of acute coronary ischemia or infarction: there are no characteristic electrocardiogram (ECG) changes indicative of ischemia, and cardiac biomarker levels are not increased. These patients also have few to no cardiac risk factors.[13]

EVALUATION

When evaluating patients presenting to the ED with chest pain, a cornerstone in risk stratification is determined by the history and physical examination.[14] By combining information from the history of the event with the patient's risk factors alone, it has been postulated that clinicians can predict with up to 79% certainty the likelihood that the patient is experiencing ACS.[15]

History

Determining which patients have chest pain related to ACS can be challenging, as patients have a variety of presentations ranging from the most classic findings to the most subtle. It is important to retain a high index of suspicion when evaluating these patients for this reason.

Each historical finding individually is only 1 piece of the chest pain evaluation, and ACS should not be excluded based on 1 historical clue.[16,17] For instance, pain that is improved with an antacid or gastrointestinal cocktail does not exclude ACS.[17] Furthermore, contrary to prior beliefs, relief of pain with nitroglycerin does not increase the likelihood that a patient is experiencing ACS given that nitroglycerin may help relieve pain related to other causes as well.[16,17] Women, the elderly, and patients with diabetes are prone to having more atypical signs of ACS so clinicians must remain vigilant in this group.[17–19] A summary of pertinent historical findings is provided in Table 2.

Physical Examination

The physical examination is less useful in the ACS evaluation because patients experiencing ACS often have a normal examination. The physical examination becomes most useful when evaluating for other causes of chest pain or, if severe infarction has occurred, for signs of cardiac insufficiency (Box 1).[19]

Examination findings that may suggest other causes of chest pain include a pulsatile abdominal mass suggestive of aortic aneurysm, and focal reproducible pain suggestive of costochondritis.[17,19,21] However, clinicians must remember that these findings can also occur in ACS and are just 1 piece of the comprehensive evaluation.[14]

Box 1
Physical examination findings suggestive of cardiac insufficiency caused by infarction

- Hypotension (systolic blood pressure <100 mm Hg)
- Lung rales
- Tachypnea
- Tachycardia (>120 beats/min)
- S4, paradoxic splitting of S2, or new mitral regurgitation

Data from Refs.[14–17,19]

Risk Factors

Assessment of the patient's risk factors is paramount in the evaluation of chest pain in the ED. Scores such as the Thrombolysis in Myocardial Infarction (TIMI) score have been developed to aid in risk stratification (Box 2).[17,19,22,23] The TIMI score aids in

---

Box 2
Thrombolysis in Myocardial Infarction (TIMI) risk score for non–ST segment elevation acute coronary syndrome

1 point given for each factor listed. The more points gained, the higher the all-cause mortality.

- Age 65 years or older
- Two or more episodes of angina or equivalent in 24 hours
- Aspirin use in last 7 days
- Three or more coronary artery disease risk factors
- Known coronary artery disease with stenosis greater than 50%
- Increased cardiac biomarker levels
- ECG ST deviation greater than 0.5 mm

Data from Amsterdam EA, Wenger NK, Brindis RG, et al. 2014 AHA/ACC guideline for the management of patients with non-ST-elevation acute coronary syndromes: a report of the American College of Cardiology/American Heart Association Task Force on Practice Guidelines. J Am Coll Cardiol 2014;64(24):e139–228; and Macdonald SP, Nagree Y, Fatovich DM, et al. Modified TIMI risk score cannot be used to identify low-risk chest pain in the emergency department: a multicentre validation study. Emerg Med J 2014;31(4):281–5.

---

determining the patient's 30-day risk for having a MACE, but is less useful as a patient disposition aid in the emergency setting.[23] Therefore, the TIMI score is most useful in the emergency setting when combined with other tools such as the History, Electrocardiogram, Age, Risk Factors, Troponin (HEART) score to improve decision making, and to reduce the rate of missed adverse events.[19,24] The HEART score is discussed in further detail later in this article. Risk factors for ACS are summarized in Box 3.[14–17,19,20]

Box 3
Risk factors for acute coronary syndrome

- History of abnormal stress test
- Peripheral arterial disease
- Dyslipidemia
- Early coronary artery disease in a first-degree relative
- History of cardiovascular disease
- Obesity (body mass index >30)
- Current or recent smoker
- Diabetes
- Hypertension
- History of cerebrovascular accident
- Age (>45 years men, >55 years women)
- Cocaine use

Data from Refs.[14–17,19,20]

DIAGNOSIS

Along with the history, physical examination, and assessment of risk factors, diagnostic tests further aid in the evaluation of patients with chest pain in the ED.

Cardiac Enzymes

There are a variety of laboratory tests that may be ordered during a chest pain evaluation based on the differential diagnosis and clinical impression. When the pain is expected to be cardiac in origin and ACS is considered, one of the most important and recommended tests to order is cardiac troponin.[17] In the past, other cardiac enzymes were included in this panel, including myoglobin, creatinine kinase (CK), and creatinine kinase-MB (CK-MB), although these are no longer recommended given the high sensitivity and specificity of troponin.[17,19] Troponin levels also increase earlier than CK-MB and stay increased for longer than other enzymes (Fig. 4).[19] Troponin levels generally increase 2 to 4 hours after injury and may remain increased for up to 1 to 2 weeks.[17]

Serial troponin testing is a cornerstone of ACS diagnosis because development of ischemia and infarction is a dynamic process, and troponin levels take time to become increased. Although there is much debate on the optimal time spacing for delta troponin levels, the American Heart Association (AHA) suggests obtaining a level on arrival to the ED and 3 to 6 hours after symptom onset in low-risk patients. A troponin level is recommended after 6 hours from symptom onset in patients with higher probabilities of ACS.[17] Current research has discussed the use of high-sensitivity troponin in providing a more rapid disposition for patients with chest pain in the ED; however, this technology is not readily available in the United States at this time.[25]

There are 3 types of troponin: troponin C, troponin T, and troponin I. Troponin T and troponin I are specific to cardiac tissue.[17,21] When there is any damage or infarction to cardiac myocytes, troponin is released.[19] The more extensive the injury, the higher the troponin level. In patients with chronically increased troponin levels, the diagnosis of

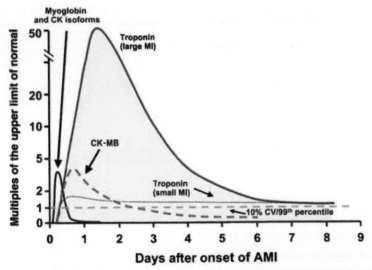

Fig. 4. Cardiac biomarker timescale comparison. CV, coefficient of variation. (*From* Yiadom MY. Acute coronary syndrome clinical presentations and diagnostic approaches in the emergency department. Emerg Med Clin North Am 2011;29(4):693; with permission.)

ACS becomes more challenging. A good rule of thumb is to consider reinfarction if the troponin level is increased more than 20% from baseline.[17]

Although MI is the most severe form of cardiac damage, other types of cardiac stress may also increase troponin levels through different mechanisms.[17,19,21]

Electrocardiography

ECG is the cornerstone screening test for acute MI and ACS. ECGs allow clinicians a quick and simple way to evaluate the electrical conductivity of the heart.[19,21] When ischemia is present, the electrical activity changes in a characteristic fashion.[19] Signs of ischemia on an ECG include:[14,16,17]

- ST segment elevation
- ST segment depression
- T-wave inversion
- Q waves (sign of old infarction)

Note that, in an ED patient with chest pain or with suspicion of ACS, any new ECG changes suggestive of ischemia should raise clinical suspicion.[14,20] MIs are often classified when ischemic changes are present in 2 contiguous leads and therefore suspicion should be raised when ischemic changes are discovered in this pattern.[15,26] ECGs in the setting of chest pain should also be compared with prior ECGs if possible in order to more accurately assess for new changes.[27] The location of ischemia in the myocardium can be determined based on which leads show ischemic changes (**Table 3**).[28,29]

Table 3
Determining location of cardiac damage by examining electrocardiogram changes

Location of MI	ECG Leads Most Likely to Show Changes	Coronary Artery Occluded
Inferior	II, III, avF	Right coronary artery
Posterior	ST depression in V1, V2	Circumflex, right coronary artery
Anteroseptal	V1, V2	Left anterior descending artery
Anterolateral	V3, V4	Left anterior descending artery
Lateral	I, avL, V5, V6	Circumflex artery

Data from Fuchs RM, Achuff SC, Grunwald L, et al. Electrocardiographic localization of coronary artery narrowings: studies during myocardial ischemia and infarction in patients with one-vessel disease. Circulation 1982;66(6):1168–76; and Dubin D. Infarction (includes Hemiblock). Rapid Interpretation of EKG's, An Interactive Course. 6th edition. Fort Myers (FL): Cover Publishing Company; 2000.

Similar to the rest of the evaluation, ECGs should be taken into account with the entire clinical impression. ECGs are a good screening test to rapidly assess life-threatening conditions; however, up 10% of MIs are missed with ECGs, making the test not particularly sensitive.[19] In addition, there are other conditions that can cause changes on an ECG that may mimic ischemia, including pericarditis and coronary vasospasm.[17] Patients with bundle branch block and pacemakers have ECG changes that make detecting ischemia more challenging. Clinicians must be particularly vigilant with this group of patients.[14,17,26] It is important to note that any patient with a new left bundle branch block that is not present on an old ECG has MI until proven otherwise.[17,19]

In clinical practice, any patient presenting to the ED with chest pain should have an ECG performed and read within 10 minutes of presentation.[14,17,19] Given the high morbidity and mortality of ACS, obtaining these tests in a timely fashion is extremely important.[22] In addition, given that the gold standard door-to-balloon time, or time of arrival in the ED to time of cardiac catheterization, is less than 90 minutes, it is critical that these tests are expedited in order to quickly diagnosis STEMI and activate percutaneous coronary intervention as appropriate.[27]

After the initial ECG is performed, continue with the appropriate chest pain evaluation. Note that ECGs are only a moment in time of a dynamic process. Therefore, serial ECGs are important in patients in whom suspicion for ACS remains high, especially in patients who are clinically deteriorating or have uncontrolled and continued pain.[17,19,26] It is recommended that these patients be placed on a continuous cardiac monitor as well.[17,26]

Imaging

Appropriate imaging in patients with low-risk chest pain presenting to the ED is a hot topic of debate in the medical literature. In the immediate evaluation of patients with chest pain in the ED, chest radiograph should be considered as an initial imaging modality. However, chest radiographs are generally not helpful in diagnosing ACS and are not within the guidelines for ruling out ACS, although they may aid in detecting other potential causes of chest pain, such as pneumothorax, pneumonia, aortic aneurysm or dissection. The decision to perform a chest radiograph should be based on the clinician's clinical impression of the patient.[17,30]

Another early imaging modality that may be considered is bedside cardiac ultrasonography, also known as focused cardiac ultrasonography. Bedside ultrasonography can give experienced clinicians expedited information regarding a patient's overall fluid status and cardiac motility, and can detect the presence of pericarditis or cardiac tamponade.[30]

Recommendations for additional objective cardiac testing have been discussed in detail in the literature; however, to date, there is no set guideline for its appropriate use. The clinical challenge is whether the patient requires additional objective cardiac testing and, if so, which modality is optimal. Therefore, clinicians must evaluate each patient individually and determine which, if any, further objective cardiac imaging is required.[14,31–33]

Each imaging modality has advantages and disadvantages that must be considered in the decision-making process. Clinicians must also take into account the availability of each modality at the location of their practice and be cognizant of the protocols in place at their facility.[22] Some of the most common modalities include coronary computed tomographic angiography (CCTA), stress ECG, stress echocardiogram, myocardial perfusion studies (including single-photon emission computed tomography [SPECT]), and coronary artery calcium score (CACS).[14,31,32,34,35] Percutaneous coronary intervention (PCI) is the gold standard intervention for patients with STEMI, but may be used as an elective diagnostic and/or therapeutic measure in the nonacute setting.[32] A summary of some of the most common imaging modalities with sensitivities, specificities, advantages, and disadvantages of each is presented in Table 4.

PATIENT DISPOSITION AND SCORING SYSTEMS

Cardiogenic chest pain is particularly challenging because, despite the significant use of resources, including electrocardiograms, cardiac enzymes, and prolonged observation, missed major cardiac events after discharge from the ED may exceed 2%.[40–43] In contrast, approximately 60% to 70% of patients presenting with chest pain are admitted; however, only 15% to 25% are eventually diagnosed with ACS.[3–5,44] Inadvertent discharge of patients with ACS from the ED is associated with increased mortality and liability, whereas inappropriate admission of patients without serious disease is neither indicated nor cost-effective.[40]

In order to avoid missed events, many scoring systems have been developed over the years, including the Framingham, TIMI, and Global Registry of Acute Coronary

Table 4
Common imaging studies used in patients presenting with chest pain in the emergency department

Imaging Study	Sensitivity (%)	Specificity (%)	Advantages	Disadvantages
CCTA	93–97[14,34]	80–99[14,34]	• Reduced hospital length of stay[17,22,36] • Reduced time to diagnosis[22,32,36] • More direct discharges from ED with fewer hospital admissions[22,36] • Assesses anatomic disease[14,31,34] • Beneficial in assessment of low-risk/intermediate-risk patients with chest pain[14,22,32,37] • May avoid need for further objective cardiac testing[22]	• Some radiation exposure[22,31,34,36,37] • Risk for overdiagnosis potentially leading to unnecessary invasive cardiac testing[17,31] • Only detects anatomic changes without detecting associated physiologic dysfunction[14] • Cannot be used in patients with renal insufficiency, atrial fibrillation, dysrhythmias, or who are pregnant[22,34,37] • Patients with tachycardia may require rate control with β-blockers before testing[22,34,37] • Decreased image quality with patients who cannot hold their breath or who are morbidly obese[14,22,37] • In general, most useful only in the low-risk/intermediate-risk patients with chest pain[14,22,32,37]
Exercise stress ECG	45–68[35,38]	77–85[35,38]	• Low cost[31] • No radiation[31] • Noninvasive	• Less sensitive and specific than other objective tests[31] • May not be useful in patients with other secondary ECG abnormalities, including left ventricular hypertrophy, nonspecific ST-T changes, paced rhythms, or left bundle branch block[14]

(continued on next page)

Table 4
(continued)

Imaging Study	Sensitivity (%)	Specificity (%)	Advantages	Disadvantages
Stress echocardiogram	84[34]	94[34]	• Assesses for inducible angina or inducible wall motion abnormalities suggesting impaired blood flow[32,34] • Noninvasive • No radiation[31,34] • No contrast[34] • Fairly low cost[31,34]	• Operator dependent[32] • Increased risk of false-positive results in patients with prior infarction[32]
SPECT	73–98[34,35]	53–96[34,35]	• Evaluates for defects in perfusion of the myocardium[32,34] • Retains accuracy in patients with arrhythmias[34] • No contraindications to using technetium isotopes[34] • Negative predictive value of nearly 100%[32]	• Expensive[31,37] • Significant radiation exposure[31,32,34,37] • Time intensive; requires prolonged removal from ED[32,34,37]
PCI	Gold standard[14,17,32]	Gold standard[14,17,32,]	• Gold standard for diagnosing coronary artery disease/ACS[14,17,32] • Diagnostic and therapeutic[32]	• Requires contrast[32] • Requires radiation[32] • Invasive[14,32] • Determines only anatomic defects without functional data[14]
CACS	80[14]	40[14]	• Aids in long-term risk stratification[39]	• Minimally helpful in the disposition of ED patients when combined with CCTA[14] • Does not give information regarding acute ACS[39]

Events scores. These scores are beneficial in determining a patient's overall risk in the next 30 days to the next 10 years; however, none are designed to aid in patient disposition in an emergency setting.[45,46]

Given this fact, there has been extensive research in developing and validating such a tool. In 2006, a new scoring system called the HEART score was developed. It remains one of the only scoring systems available to aid in disposition of low-risk patients with chest pain in the ED. The HEART score has gained much traction in recent years and although it is not currently the standard of care, it has gained popularity in clinical practice.[47]

The History, Electrocardiogram, Age, Risk Factors, Troponin Score

The HEART score is a scoring system that has been specifically designed for use as a disposition aid in ED patients. The HEART score is composed of 5 components. These components are:

- History
- ECG
- Age
- Risk factors
- Troponin

Each component is given a score from 0 to 2 and the total score from each component is calculated. The HEART score and its components are summarized in **Tables 5** and **6**.[47]

Table 5 HEART score components	
	Points
History	
Highly suspicious	2
Moderately suspicious	1
Slightly suspicious	0
ECG	
Significant ST depression	2
Nonspecific repolarization disturbance	1
Normal	0
Age	
≥65 y	2
45–65 y	1
≤45 y	0
Risk Factors	
≥3 or history of atherosclerotic disease	2
1 or 2 risk factors	1
No risk factors known	0
Troponin	
≥3× normal limit	2
1–3× normal limit	1
≤normal limit	0

Adapted from Mahler SA, Riley RF, Hiestand BC, et al. The HEART Pathway randomized trial: identifying emergency department patients with acute chest pain for early discharge. Circ Cardiovasc Qual Outcomes 2015;8(2):195–203.

Table 6
HEART pathway assessment form

			Patient ID
			☐ Initial Assessment
			☐ Second Assessment

HEART Score:

History:

High-Risk Features:
- Middle- or left-sided
- Heavy chest pain
- Diaphoresis
- Radiation
- N/V
- Exertional
- Relief of symptoms by sublingual nitrates

Low-Risk Features:
- Well localized
- Sharp pain
- Non-exertional
- No diaphoresis
- No N/V

☐ Highly Suspicious	2 points	Mostly high-risk features
☐ Moderately Suspicious	1 point	Mixture of high-risk and low-risk features
☐ Slightly Suspicious	0 points	Mostly low-risk features

ECG:

☐ New ischemic changes	2 points	• Ischemic ST-segment depression • New ischemic T-wave inversions
☐ Non-specific changes	1 point	• Repolarization abnormalities • Non specific T wave changes • Non-specific ST-segment depression or elevation • Bundle branch blocks • Pacemaker rhythms • LVH • Early repolarization • Digoxin effect
☐ Normal	0 points	• Completely normal

Age:

☐ ≥ 65	2 points
☐ 45-64	1 point
☐ <45	0 points

Risk Factors:
- ☐ Obesity (BMI ≥30)
- ☐ Current or recent (≤90 days) smoker
- ☐ Currently treated diabetes mellitus
- ☐ Family history of CAD (1st degree relative <55 y.o.)
- ☐ Diagnosed and/or treated hypertension
- ☐ Hypercholesterolemia

☐ 3 or more risk factors listed above OR any of the following: ☐ Known CAD=2 points ☐ Prior stroke=2 points ☐ Periphera arterial disease = 2 points	2 points
☐ 1-2 risk factors	1 point
☐ No risk factors	0 points

Troponin (initial)

☐ >0.120 ng/ml	2 points
☐ 0.041-0.120 ng/ml	1 point
☐ 0-0.040 ng/ml	0 points

HEART Score (total points)	_____	Add points from each category above

Serial 3 Hour Troponin Measurement:
- ☐ Normal, 0-0.040 ng/ml
- ☐ Positive, >0.040 ng/ml

HEART Pathway:
- ☐ High Risk = HEART score 4 or more, or any positive troponin.
- ☐ Low Risk = HEART score 0-3 and negative troponin at 0 and 3 hours.

Adapted from Mahler SA, Riley RF, Hiestand BC, et al. The HEART Pathway randomized trial: identifying emergency department patients with acute chest pain for early discharge. Circ Cardiovasc Qual Outcomes 2015;8(2):195–203.

A total HEART score of less than 3 places patients in a low-risk category. In the original HEART score trial, patients in the low-risk category had a 3-month MACE rate of 2.5%.[47] Subsequent studies showed low-risk patients to have a 6 week MACE rate of 0.99% and 1.7%.[48,49] More recent studies have shown low-risk patients with a 0.6% chance of MACE at 30 days.[24] Combining the HEART score with a repeat troponin level at 4 to 6 hours improved the sensitivity of the score from 58.3% to 100% in a study by Mahler and colleagues[24]; however, these statistics require further validation.

The HEART score combined with a 3-hour troponin level is called the HEART pathway. The HEART pathway is designed to aid the clinician in decision making with stable patients and may be used in conjunction with clinical judgment. Unstable patients should be promptly treated according to their presentation. When using the HEART score, a patient with a score of 4 or greater or who has initial positive troponin test is considered high risk and should be admitted to the hospital or observation unit. Patients with a score of 0 to 3 are considered low risk.[28] These patients often provide the greatest challenge for emergency providers.[24,28]

As in all aspects of patient care, shared decision making should be included in determining patient disposition in low-risk patients with chest pain. These patients have 3 options after they have been categorized into the low-risk group using the HEART score. First, they may be discharged for close follow-up within 1 week. Second, they may continue on the HEART pathway and obtain a repeat troponin level at 3 hours. Third, they may remain in the hospital for observation and serial testing (**Fig. 5**).[50] If

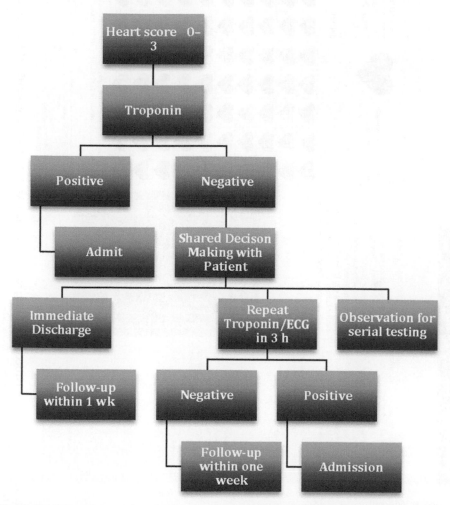

Fig. 5. The HEART score plus shared decision making. (*Data from* Vibhakar N, Mattu A. Beyond HEART: building a better chest pain protocol. Emergency Physicians Monthly. 2015. Available at: http://epmonthly.com/article/beyond-heart-building-a-better-chest-pain-protocol/. Accessed July 26, 2016.)

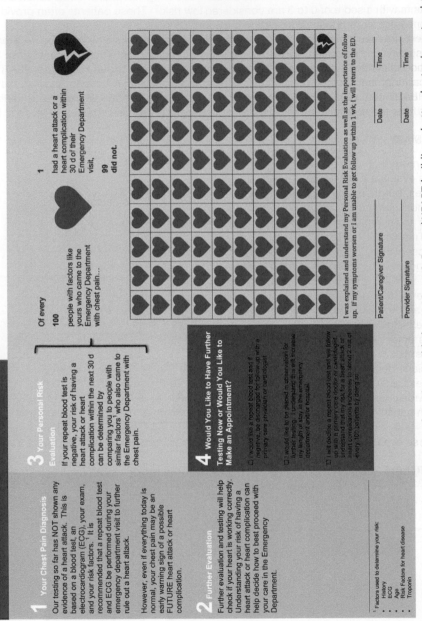

Fig. 6. University of Maryland shared decision-making form. (*From* Vibhakar N, Mattu A. Beyond HEART: building a better chest pain protocol. Emergency Physicians Monthly. 2015. Available at: http://epmonthly.com/article/beyond-heart-building-a-better-chest-pain-protocol/. Accessed July 26, 2016.)

at any point in this pathway the patient has a positive troponin test, ECG changes, changes in clinical impression, or is discovered to be of higher risk, disposition should be reconsidered. The University of Maryland has developed a shared decision-making document to aid clinicians in such discussions with their patients (Fig. 6). Such documents may be used to facilitate discussion regarding the risks and benefits of different options in order to provide the highest quality of care.[50]

There are mounting data that show that the HEART pathway is a useful tool to help risk stratify undifferentiated patients with chest pain concerning for ischemia. As mentioned earlier, this is a tool that can be used to help guide management; however, clinical judgment should continue to be used. Before implementing protocols that use the HEART pathway, it would be beneficial to have a department policy that includes input from the hospital as well as a local cardiologist.

SUMMARY

With more than 8 million annual visits for chest pain in the United States, most clinicians evaluate a patient with chest pain on every shift. Chest pain has many benign causes, but there are also deadly causes that need to be considered. ACS is one of the most common deadly causes of chest pain. Patients who present with concerning signs and symptoms of ACS all have an ECG and laboratory studies performed in the ED. Traditionally, most of these patients are then subsequently admitted or placed in an observation unit for serial testing. Many of these patients are then discharged home with negative work-ups. Admitting all of these patients, only for them to have negative work-ups, is a huge cost to the health care system in both resources and dollars. The challenge for ED providers is to attempt to determine which patients are at low risk for ACS and may safely be discharged home.

The history, physical examination, risk factors, ECG, laboratory results, and sometimes objective cardiac imaging all play a role in helping clinicians determine a patient's risk of ACS. There have been many scoring systems over the years to help clinicians determine which patients are at the highest risk for adverse events. Many of these scoring systems were not developed specifically for ED patients and are not widely used. The HEART score was developed to help ED providers determine which patients are at low risk for MACE. This scoring system has been both prospectively and externally validated. Safely discharging patients deemed low risk for adverse events is likely beneficial for both the patients and hospital systems.

REFERENCES

1. Pitts SR, Niska RW, Xu J, et al. National Hospital Ambulatory Medical Care Survey: 2006 emergency department summary. Natl Health Stat Report 2008;7:1–38.
2. Karnath B, Holden MD, Hussain N. Chest pain: differentiating cardiac from noncardiac causes. Hosp Physician 2004;38:24–7.
3. Koukkunen H, Pyorala K, O Halinen M. Low-risk patients with chest pain and without evidence of myocardial infarction may be safely discharged from emergency department. Eur Heart J 2004;25:329–34.
4. Goldman L, Kirtane AJ. Triage of patients with acute chest pain and possible cardiac ischemia: the elusive search for diagnostic perfection. Ann Intern Med 2003;139:987–95.
5. Boufous S, Kelleher PW, Pain CH, et al. Impact of a chest-pain guideline on clinical decision-making. Med J Aust 2003;178:375–80.
6. Papadakis M, McPhee SJ, Rabow MW. CURRENT medical diagnosis and treatment 2013. 52nd edition. McGraw-Hill Professional; 2012.

7. Lenfant C. Chest pain of cardiac and noncardiac origin. Metabolism 2010; 59(Suppl 1):S41–6.

8. Ruigomez A, Rodriguez LA, Wallander MA, et al. Chest pain in general practice: incidence, comorbidity and mortality. Fam Pract 2006;23:167–74.

9. Flook N, Unge P, Agreus L, et al. Approach to managing undiagnosed chest pain: could gastroesophageal reflux disease be the cause? Can Fam Physician 2007; 53:261–6.

10. Kumar A, Cannon CP. Acute coronary syndromes: diagnosis and management, part I. Mayo Clin Proc 2009;84(10):917–38.

11. Davies MJ, Thomas A. Thrombosis and acute coronary-artery lesions in sudden cardiac ischemic death. N Engl J Med 1984;310:1137–40.

12. Healthwise Staff. How a heart attack happens. WebMD Web site. 2014. Available at: http://www.webmd.com/heart-disease/how-a-heart-attack-happens. Accessed August 1, 2016.

13. Hess EP, Jaffe AS. Evaluation of patients with possible cardiac chest pain: a way out of the jungle. J Am Coll Cardiol 2012;59(23):2099–100.

14. Qaseem A, Fihn SD, Williams S, et al. Diagnosis of stable ischemic heart disease: summary of a clinical practice guideline from the American College of Physicians/ American College of Cardiology Foundation/American Heart Association/American Association for Thoracic Surgery/Preventive Cardiovascular Nurses Association/Society of Thoracic Surgeons. Ann Intern Med 2012;157:729–34.

15. van der Meer MG, Backus BE, van der Graaf Y, et al. The diagnostic value of clinical symptoms in women and men presenting with chest pain at the emergency department, a prospective cohort study. PLoS One 2015;10(1):e0116431.

16. Fanaroff AC, Rymer JA, Goldstein SA, et al. Does this patient with chest pain have acute coronary syndrome?: The Rational Clinical Examination Systematic Review. JAMA 2015;314(18):1955–65.

17. Amsterdam EA, Wenger NK, Brindis RG, et al. 2014 AHA/ACC guideline for the management of patients with non-ST-elevation acute coronary syndromes: a report of the American College of Cardiology/American Heart Association Task Force on Practice Guidelines. J Am Coll Cardiol 2014;64(24):e139–228.

18. Rubini Gimenez M, Reiter M, Twerenbold R, et al. Sex-specific chest pain characteristics in the early diagnosis of acute myocardial infarction. JAMA Intern Med 2014;174(2):241–9.

19. Yiadom MY. Acute coronary syndrome clinical presentations and diagnostic approaches in the emergency department. Emerg Med Clin North Am 2011;29(4): 689–97, v.

20. Mahler SA, Riley RF, Hiestand BC, et al. The HEART Pathway randomized trial: identifying emergency department patients with acute chest pain for early discharge. Circ Cardiovasc Qual Outcomes 2015;8(2):195–203.

21. Mangleson FI, Cullen L, Scott AC. The evolution of chest pain pathways. Crit Pathw Cardiol 2011;10(2):69–75.

22. Raff GL, Chinnaiyan KM, Cury RC, et al. SCCT guidelines on the use of coronary computed tomographic angiography for patients presenting with acute chest pain to the emergency department: a report of the Society of Cardiovascular Computed Tomography Guidelines Committee. J Cardiovasc Comput Tomogr 2014;8(4):254–71.

23. Macdonald SP, Nagree Y, Fatovich DM, et al. Modified TIMI risk score cannot be used to identify low-risk chest pain in the emergency department: a multicentre validation study. Emerg Med J 2014;31(4):281–5.

24. Mahler SA, Hiestand BC, Goff DC, et al. Can the HEART score safely reduce stress testing and cardiac imaging in patients at low risk for major adverse cardiac events? Crit Pathw Cardiol 2011;10(3):128–33.

25. Carlton E, Greenslade J, Cullen L, et al. Evaluation of high-sensitivity cardiac troponin I levels in patients with suspected acute coronary syndrome. JAMA Cardiol 2016;1(4):405–12.

26. Thygesen K, Alpert JS, Jaffe AS, et al. Third universal definition of myocardial infarction. Circulation 2012;126(16):2020–35.

27. O'Gara PT, Kushner FG, Ascheim DD, et al. 2013 ACCF/AHA guideline for the management of ST-elevation myocardial infarction: a report of the American College of Cardiology Foundation/American Heart Association Task Force on Practice Guidelines. J Am Coll Cardiol 2013;61(4):e78–140.

28. Fuchs RM, Achuff SC, Grunwald L, et al. Electrocardiographic localization of coronary artery narrowings: studies during myocardial ischemia and infarction in patients with one-vessel disease. Circulation 1982;66(6):1168–76.

29. Dubin D. Infarction (includes Hemiblock). Rapid interpretation of EKG's, an interactive course. 6th edition. Fort Myers (FL): Cover Publishing Company; 2000.

30. Rybicki FJ, Udelson JE, Peacock WF, et al. 2015 ACR/ACC/AHA/AATS/ACEP/ ASNC/NASCI/SAEM/SCCT/SCMR/SCPC/SNMMI/STR/STS appropriate utilization of cardiovascular imaging in emergency department patients with chest pain: a joint document of the American College of Radiology Appropriateness Criteria Committee and the American College of Cardiology Appropriate Use Criteria Task Force. J Am Coll Cardiol 2016;67(7):853–79.

31. Foy AJ, Liu G, Davidson WR, et al. Comparative effectiveness of diagnostic testing strategies in emergency department patients with chest pain: an analysis of downstream testing, interventions, and outcomes. JAMA Intern Med 2015; 175(3):428–36.

32. Ropp A, Lin CT, White CS. Coronary computed tomography angiography for the assessment of acute chest pain in the emergency department: evidence, guidelines, and tips for implementation. J Thorac Imaging 2015;30(3):169–75.

33. Mahler SA, Burke GL, Goff DC, et al. Avoidable utilization of the chest pain observation unit: evaluation of very-low-risk patients. Crit Pathw Cardiol 2013;12(2): 59–64.

34. Romero J, Husain SA, Holmes AA, et al. Non-invasive assessment of low risk acute chest pain in the emergency department: a comparative meta-analysis of prospective studies. Int J Cardiol 2015;187:565–80.

35. Garber AM, Solomon NA. Cost-effectiveness of alternative test strategies for the diagnosis of coronary artery disease. Ann Intern Med 1999;130:719–28.

36. Hoffmann U, Truong QA, Schoenfeld DA, et al. Coronary CT angiography versus standard evaluation in acute chest pain. N Engl J Med 2012;367(4):299–308.

37. Fernandez-Friera L, Garcia-Alvarez A, Guzman G, et al. Coronary CT and the coronary calcium score, the future of ED risk stratification? Curr Cardiol Rev 2012; 8(2):86–97.

38. Froelicher VF, Lehmann KG, Thomas R, et al. The electrocardiographic exercise test in a population with reduced workup bias: diagnostic performance, computerized interpretation, and multivariable prediction. Veterans Affairs Cooperative Study in Health Services #016 (QUEXTA) Study Group. Quantitative exercise testing and angiography. Ann Intern Med 1998;128(12 Pt 1):965–74.

39. Chang AM, Le J, Matsuura AC, et al. Does coronary artery calcium scoring add to the predictive value of coronary computed tomography angiography for adverse

cardiovascular events in low-risk chest pain patients? Acad Emerg Med 2011; 18(10):1065–71.

40. Amsterdam EA, Kirk JD, Bluemke DA, et al. Testing of low-risk patients presenting to the emergency department with chest pain: a scientific statement from the American Heart Association. Circulation 2010;122(17):1756–76.

41. Pope JH, Aufderheide TP, Ruthazer R, et al. Missed diagnoses of acute cardiac ischemia in the emergency department. N Engl J Med 2000;342(16):1163–70.

42. Schull MJ, Vermeulen MJ, Stukel TA. The risk of missed diagnosis of acute myocardial infarction associated with emergency department volume. Ann Emerg Med 2006;48(6):647–55.

43. McCarthy BD, Beshansky JR, D'Agostino RB, et al. Missed diagnoses of acute myocardial infarction in the emergency department: results from a multicenter study. Ann Emerg Med 1993;22(3):579–82.

44. Graff LG, Dallara J, Ross MA, et al. Impact on the care of the emergency department chest pain patient from the Chest Pain Evaluation Registry (CHEPER) study. Am J Cardiol 1997;80:563–8.

45. D'Agostino RB, Vasan RS, Pencina MJ, et al. Circulation. J Am Heart Assoc. Available at: http://circ.ahajournals.org/content/117/6/743. Accessed August 1, 2016.

46. Amsterdam E, Kirk JD, Bluemke D, et al. Circulation. J Am Heart Assoc. Available at: http://circ.ahajournals.org/content/122/17/1756. Accessed August 1, 2016.

47. Six AJ, Backus BE, Kelder JC. Chest pain in the emergency room: value of the HEART score. Neth Heart J 2008;16(6):191–6.

48. Backus BE, Six AJ, Kelder JC, et al. Chest pain the emergency room. A multicenter validation of the HEART score. Crit Pathw Cardiol 2010;9:164–9.

49. Backus BE, Six AJ, Kelder JC, et al. A prospective validation of the HEART score for chest pain patients at the emergency department. Int J Cardiol 2013;168: 2153–8.

50. Vibhakar N, Mattu A. Beyond HEART: Building a better chest pain protocol. Emergency Physicians Monthly. 2015. Available at: http://epmonthly.com/article/beyond-heart-building-a-better-chest-pain-protocol/. Accessed July 26, 2016.

Printed and bound by CPI Group (UK) Ltd, Croydon, CR0 4YY

03/10/2024

01040391-0002